Voices of Illness: Negotiating Meaning and Identity

At the Interface/Probing the Boundaries

VOLUME 120

The titles published in this series are listed at *brill.com/aipb*

Voices of Illness: Negotiating Meaning and Identity

Edited by

Peter Bray

BRILL
RODOPI

LEIDEN | BOSTON

Cover illustration: *Detail from Kilkenny Castle* (1195), Kilkenny, Ireland. Photographer: Dr. Jytte Holmqvist. Black and white digital photograph. 13 July, 2018.

Library of Congress Cataloging-in-Publication Data

Names: Bray, Peter (Writer on post-traumatic growth), editor.
Title: Voices of illness : negotiating meaning and identity / edited by Peter Bray.
Description: Leiden ; Boston : Brill/Rodopi, [2019] | Series: At the interface/probing the boundaries ; volume 120 | Includes bibliographical references and index.
Identifiers: LCCN 2019002241 (print) | LCCN 2019003900 (ebook) | ISBN 9789004396067 (ebook) | ISBN 9789004390782 (pbk. : alk. paper)
Subjects: | MESH: Narrative Medicine--methods
Classification: LCC R726.5 (ebook) | LCC R726.5 (print) | NLM WB 102 | DDC 610.69/6--dc23
LC record available at https://lccn.loc.gov/2019002241

Typeface for the Latin, Greek, and Cyrillic scripts: "Brill". See and download: brill.com/brill-typeface.

ISSN 1570-7113
ISBN 978-90-04-39078-2 (paperback)
ISBN 978-90-04-39606-7 (e-book)

Contents

Figures

Notes on Contributors

Tineke Abma

is a Full Professor in 'Participation & Diversity' and Vice Chair of the Department of Medical Humanities, and research leader in the Amsterdam Public Health research institute at the Amsterdam UMC. In 2013 she received an ASPASIA laureate from the Netherlands Organisation of Scientific Research (NWO) for excellent female researchers. Her background is in the social sciences, and her work is located at the crossroads of the social sciences, humanities and medical sciences.

Peter Bray

PhD, is Senior Lecturer and Programme Leader for Counsellor Education at the University of Auckland. Peter has recently edited a number of other interdisciplinary collections and articles, which reflect his developing interest in counselling practice and spirituality, and heroic identity and the transformational aspects of grief, loss and trauma.

Verusca Calabria

is a Research Fellow and Lecturer in the Division of Social Work and Health, School of Social Sciences, Nottingham Trent University, Nottingham (UK). Calabria is an interdisciplinary qualitative researcher working across the Social Sciences and Humanities, and an experienced oral history practitioner. Her research interests include the history of asylums and mental health policy in the UK, oral history theory and practice, participatory action research, feminist research methods.

Agnes Elling

PhD, is a Senior Researcher at the Mulier Institute, centre for research on sports in society. Her research interest and expertise include issues of social inequality, such as gender, sexuality, ethnicity, embodiment and belonging throughout elite sporting biographies.

Deborah Freedman

MEd, is a therapeutic storyteller and workshop leader in creating fairy tales. She has authored three books from 'The Quiet Triumph of the Heart' series: *Moments from Portland, Maine*; *Names Project AIDS Memorial Quilt Stories from Maine, The Night Sky is Full of Stars. The Air is Full of Wishes* (a fairy tale).

Alexandra Fidyk
PhD, grew up on a self-sustaining family farm in western Canada, with no running water or indoor plumbing till she was ten. Its way of life shaped who she is and what is of import in her writing, teaching and psychotherapy practice.

Justyna Jajszczok
PhD, is Assistant Professor at the Institute of English, University of Silesia in Katowice, Poland. Her research interests include Victorian science and literature and the language of metaphors of science and medicine in cultural and literary discourse.

Naomi Krüger
PhD, is a Lecturer in Literature and Creative Writing at the University of Central Lancashire. Her research interests include representations of cognitive impairment in fiction and the interface between creative and critical writing. Naomi has recently published her first novel.

Pam Morrison
is an established journalist and writer, a counsellor and supervisor. Her research interests include metaphor, empathy and journaling in the context of illness. She has written for film, radio and magazines and has published academic papers and a book on the impacts of co-journaling following terminal diagnosis.

Miranda Quinney
is a Doctoral student at the University of South Wales and founder of Sharing Stories for Wellbeing. She calls herself a storymaker who works with others, particularly at end of life, to facilitate the sharing and saving of their life stories. Her research looks at how and why creative therapies have a positive effect on mental wellbeing.

Yomna Saber
PhD, is Associate Professor of English Literature at Qatar University. Her research interests include gender studies, ethnic studies and women's literature. She has authored two books, *Brave to Be Involved* (2010), and *Gendered Masks of Liminality and Race* (2017), and published several articles on African American literature.

Elena Sharratt
is a Doctoral candidate at the University of Exeter, UK. Funded by the Economic and Social Research Council (ESRC), she is currently researching the emergence and disappearance of 'transableism' within an online community context. Her research focuses on disability, medical taxonomy and discourses of authenticity.

Victorria Simpson-Gervin
MA, is currently applying to become a Doctoral candidate. Her research interests include narratives of health, illness, and healing.

Hans T. Sternudd
PhD, is Associate Professor at the Department of Music and Art at Linnaeus University, Sweden. He is a member of the Linnaeus University Centre for Intermedial and Multimodal Studies. His research interests include questions about the articulation of gender, corporality and affect.

Mirjam Stuij
MSc, is a medical sociologist at the Department of Medical Humanities of the Amsterdam UMC (University Medical Centres) and the Mulier Institute. Her research interests include meanings people give to sport, physical activity, health and illness, especially those related to discourses and social status positions.

Anja Tramper
has experiential knowledge about living with diabetes and diabetes health care. She was diagnosed with type 1 diabetes and accompanying this experience gained a lot of knowledge about living with diabetes through her engagement with Dutch patient associations.

Alison Ward
is a researcher at the University of Northampton. Her research includes dementia, and creativity and wellbeing. Alison is a Winston Churchill Fellow, currently undertaking a project in Denmark to use photography and storytelling with people with dementia.

Jane Youell
PhD, is a Chartered Psychologist, researcher and Churchill Fellow. Her research focus is that of sexuality, intimacy and dementia. Jane's Fellowship work has researched inclusive aged care services for the LGBTI community, particularly in Australia and the USA.

Introduction: Voices of Illness

Peter Bray

Voice as expressed in the context of illness has rarely been heard with clarity and power. This is undergoing change, thanks to a gradual yet profound shift in the emerging narrative as academics, practitioners and patients challenge the 'old ways' by examining and voicing more of the unmuffled realities intrinsic to illness. Some of those voices are represented in this book, which comprises research findings and insights from individuals in the field of medical humanities.[1] All of the contributors presented at the successful conference Storytelling, Illness and Medicine, held in 2016,[2] and were invited to expand on their use of the concept of 'voice' for a chapter in this book.

The notion of 'voice,' borrowed extensively by medical sociology from narrative studies and also referred to in the field of illness narratives, is used here to interpret the conversational dynamic of interactions that might occur between doctors and other helping professionals with their patients.[3] Similarly, social context is a significant influence on health and wellbeing and institutional experiences of care in illness subsequently serve and shape an individual's perceptions of self and identity.[4] The conference provided an opportunity to share stories of heroic, determined, and sometimes difficult patients, present ideas about what human beings want or need when they are sick and what seems to work for those who find themselves in places of care and caring.

By specifically examining, discussing and applying story making and storytelling practices with those who have to deal directly with illness either as patients or as health practitioners, this book extends that original dialogue and

1 Medical humanities use methods, concepts, and content from humanities disciplines to investigate illness, pain, disability, suffering, healing, therapeutic relationships, and other aspects of medicine and health care practice. Virginia Braun and Victoria Clarke, 'Using Thematic Analysis in Psychology' *Qualitative Research in Psychology* (2006): 77.

2 11th Global Conference of the Health Project: Storytelling, Illness and Medicine, Budapest, Hungary, in March, 2016.

3 Elliot G. Mishler, *The Discourse of Medicine: Dialectics of Medical Interviews* (Norwood, NJ: Ablex Publishing Corporation, 1984). See also: Elliot G. Mishler, *Storylines: Craftartists' Narratives of Identity* (Cambridge, MA: Harvard University Press, 1999).

4 Peter Bray and Ana Borlescu, eds., 'Introduction' *Beyond Present Patient Realities: Collaboration, Care and Identity* (Oxford, England: Inter-Disciplinary Press, 2015), xii.

 | DOI:10.1163/9789004396067_002

advances the ethic of humane caring.[5] Explicitly and critically making a space for the 'non-technical language' and voice of the patient, sometimes described as a 'voice of the lifeworld,'[6] to punctuate and soften the authoritative 'voice of medicine.'[7] The predominant biomedical model of the Western healthcare system is still deeply-rooted but the gradual shift in emphasis from the doctor to the patient is encouraging and confirms the necessity of maintaining personal understanding and relationship in healing. Doctors and professional helpers want to do the best for their patients and the relational fragmentation that both have to endure lies in systemic rather than personal failures. Central to this shift is a growing appreciation that the patient's unique story of illness is a key factor in collaborative enterprise that will effectively assist the patient to move on in their journey despite their suffering and losses.

This collection brings together scholarly work from across the globe that explores the potential of attending to the voices of those who live and work with illness. Illness is broadly characterised here as an opportunity to initiate holistic care through respectful, mutually collaborative relationships between the teller of its story and an audience, between those whose story is of difference and those entrusted to listen. The book is itself a series of stories that respects the empowering and enduring capacity of developing life narratives to provide us with new ways to make sense of a world transformed by illness.

By its nature illness is experienced as a disorder that, to a greater or lesser extent, impairs the normative functions of the body and the mind over a period of time. As Sharon Kaufman[8] observes, serious illness disrupts, highlights and transforms themes in personal narratives to such an extent that they compel individuals to consciously take control of their new biographies. Often expressed in tales of restitution, chaos or quest,[9] illness makes claims upon both its subject and its audience alike. It introduces a voice that not only invites the

5 Elliot G. Mishler, 'Patient Stories, Narratives of Resistance and the Ethics of Humane Care: A la recherche du temps perdu' *Health (London)* 9.4 (2005): 431–451.

6 Mishler, 'Patient Stories, Narratives of Resistance and the Ethics of Humane Care': 437; Christine A. Barry, Fiona A. Stevenson, Nicky Britten, Nick Barber, and Colin P. Bradley, 'Giving voice to the lifeworld. More humane, more effective medical care? A qualitative study of doctor–patient communication in general practice' *Social Science Medicine* 53.4 (2001): 487–505, describing Mishler's everyday 'voice of the lifeworld' they suggest that the individual presents themselves from a 'natural attitude' that depends on their biographical and circumstantial position in the social world.

7 Mishler, *The Discourse of Medicine*, 95.

8 Sharon Kaufman, 'Illness, Biography, and the Interpretation of Self Following a Stroke' *Journal of Aging Studies* 2.3 (1988): 217–227.

9 Arthur W. Frank, *The Wounded Storyteller: Body, Illness, and Ethics* (Chicago: The University of Chicago Press, 1995).

individual to accept and manage change but to take on a new identity, a different lifestyle, a unique set of circumstances, and an unplanned for journey.

Illness stories, although commonly used by anthropologists and medical social scientists to reveal patients' experiences and their relationships with doctors,[10] have more recently been utilised to offset the power-differential, or colonising effect, of handing over one's body to the medical profession for treatment and, by doing so, losing one's voice. By retaining the ability to freely express new life narratives, patients reclaim their bodies, restore their authority and maximise their ability to own and communicate their highly contextualised stories, the symptoms and experiences of their illnesses.

These stand-alone stories of illness, whilst acknowledging the totalising impact of suffering on those engaged in the experience of illness, also communicate truths about what they have and would become and the reality of the changes they have made along the way. There is therefore therapeutic value in their making and telling for both the maker – to be heard and to hear themselves – and the listener who achieves a deeper understanding of the impact of the illness experience. Often witnessed reflectively from positions inside and outside of the self, the stories told and retold in the course of illness can speak for themselves. They are genuinely felt subjective accounts that require little formal analysis or technical interpretation. Thus the stories that we tell about ourselves identify and define us. They touch others with their practical wisdom and inspiration in ways that powerfully initiate relationships with other individuals, groups, families, and communities and reconnect us with the world.

Nevertheless, whilst hearing illness stories can be encouraging, inspiring and powerful they can also be confrontational, unsettling and painful to the listener, or just too distressing to tell about or hear. However, they do provide new ways to view ourselves and illness, and ascribe positive meaning to what can so easily be perceived as a deficit experience in people's lives. In their sharing they signal that we are not alone in our suffering, that there are others to guide and support us and more effective ways to manage painful and disrupted lives. It is increasingly acknowledged that the experience and expression of illness must be a shared project between the patient, loved ones and others within responsive and adapting communities of care.[11] Professional roles, expectations and clinical relationships restricted by bare functionality are no longer enough to enable a collaborative negotiation of the unique pathways

10 Jack A. Clark and Elliot G. Mishler (1992) 'Attending To Patients' Stories: Reframing the Clinical Task' *Sociology of Health & Illness* 14.3: 344–372.

11 Rita Charon, *Narrative Medicine: Honoring the Stories of Illness* (Oxford and New York: Oxford University Press, 2006).

and challenges that will effectively manage individual illness. If it is to be fully understood it is broadly agreed that we must attend to and listen for the diversity and uniqueness of illness's many voices.

All of the contributors to this book in some way interrogate the role that the story and its telling play in the liberation of those voices. Here are examples of the ways in which the different voices and stories of illness emerge and can be heard when individuals and groups personally encounter and share those challenging physical and psychological issues that threaten their ability to thrive. By valuing their potential and providing a space in which stories may be shared, reciprocity and mutual understanding developed and voices honoured in partnership,[12] this interdisciplinary collection demonstrates how people can benefit from engagement with their own and others' illness stories.

The collection is divided into five parts that broadly represent some of our existing understanding of the voices of illness. Using qualitative, phenomenological, autoethnographic and biographic approaches to research and practice, the stories of individuals and groups either working with or experiencing illness are presented in everyday terms. However, in their openness and determination to make meaning and tackle change in their lives and to accept and shape their new identities, these people are in reality exceptional. They generously invite us to fully engage with them in a dialogical understanding of their stories, their lived experience of illness, knowing that their stories will help us to reflect upon our own.[13]

Part 1 of our collection, *The Story, Identity and the Voice,* begins appropriately with a consideration of voice and identity in the context of storytelling and making. In her chapter 'Narrative Medicine and Storytelling,' Victorria Simpson-Gervin addresses the value of using alternative methods of healing in the medical humanities. She specifically examines how the narrative medicine and storytelling methods of Rita Charon, as an aesthetic act, have promoted agency and dignity among patients, specifically those facing death and their family members and caregivers. Her chapter demonstrates that sharing, performing and actively listening to stories in a medical setting with empathy, imagination and caring, provides tools to make sense of the experiences of trauma and pain and can activate a greater understanding between doctors and patients.

We tell stories for many reasons, but often they contribute to the establishment and strengthening of our social identities and to the growth of social

12 See particularly: Arthur W. Frank, *Letting Stories Breathe: A Socio-narratology* (Chicago: The University of Chicago Press, 2010).

13 Dialogical narrative analysis is an analytical approach favoured by Frank, and described in: Frank, *Letting Stories Breathe.*

bonds. In Part 2, *Group Voices and Group Identity*, three authors consider how the processes of creating common narratives and the sharing of personal stories can produce coherent social representations of their illness for the group and 'outsiders' to contemplate and understand. What they create identifies the stand they make over their illness and permits them to use their stories to practice advocacy, build community and personally express their transforming individual identities.

All of the chapters in the second part demonstrate the importance of different creative responses, reminiscence and meaning making in collaborative acts of storytelling at times when individuals are at their most depleted. Through allegory and magical fairy tale Deborah Freedman uses the storyteller's voice in her chapter 'AIDS Awakens Ancient Stories.' Here she responds to the many who, through their experiences of making and contributing individual panels to a memorial quilt to the survivors of AIDS, have remembered the lives of their loved ones who finally succumbed to the fragility of their condition.

In 'Sharing Stories for Wellbeing' a more traditional therapeutic understanding of the voice is presented. Here Miranda Quinney with the research and aid of Alison Ward and Jane Youell set out the origins and applications of a course of facilitated storytelling sessions in palliative care. Through these invaluable workshops, they facilitate life-story discussions in which palliative care patients are encouraged to informally share with a group past memories and present experiences. Highlighting an essential theme from this collection, they suggest that being given the opportunity to be listened to in a community with common interests can produce beneficial outcomes, particularly in self-esteem and feelings of self-worth. Both chapters emphasise that simple pro-social acts free individuals to look beyond their present realities and changed identities to positively reconnect with themselves and take back their autonomy and control.

The final chapter in this section challenges the supremacy of the voice in one-to-one talking therapies. In 'The Collective Production of a Shared Narrative Surrounding Sexual Violence Trauma' Elena Sharratt, by critiquing traditional trauma therapies where survivors specifically recall the experiences that led to their trauma, considers the benefits of collaborative non-vocal participation through meaningful group practices. She demonstrates that in the case of trauma occasioned by sexual violence the survivor's voice and story, pathologised in other therapies, might be potentially less stigmatising to the individual because it does not need to be so overtly voiced in a group who already understand its experience. She convincingly argues that what emerges from practices of 'group narrative telling,' because it transcends speech, is the authentic voice of compassion and political action.

As Part 3, *Irreconcilable Voices: Liminal, Empowered, and Authentic* suggests, disruptive personal stories of illness about difference and loss can compel people to give these experiences a more public voice. Their stories are encouraging reminders of the vulnerability of the human mind and body and the durability of the self; the constancy and reassurance of love and relationship. These stories belong to those that our impatient society regards as Other, those who we disempower and marginalise such as the sick, the grieving, the oppressed and the unfashionably different. These stories, birthed by pain and the desire to manage and control what might otherwise overwhelm us, take many forms but all serve the same purpose. Originating in a cathartic impulse to tell a truth, irrespective of whether the story is crafted to benefit an audience, in the moment of being told they do help others to make meaning, and review, reclaim and restore their lives.

In Part 3 of this book four scholars present work that provocatively illustrates some of the ways that the voice shapes our understanding of all too common real-world experiences. Mental and physical illnesses can be easily identified but not so effectively treated. In her scholarly chapter 'Stories of Journeys Home,' Alexandra Fidyk purposefully documents her personal journey into the dark interior of the psyche, the deep terrain that accommodates the familiar and forgotten, the denied and not yet known stories and voices of the self: all the elements that when recognised, help us balance to our busily conscious lives. It is a heroic story conveyed in an epic style. It is also a deeply uncomfortable and harrowing account of debilitating mental illness that takes its protagonist on a perilous inward journey to the centre of her being. Here, despite her fear at confronting her suffering self, the difficult descent into this transpersonal underworld is also experienced as a return home. What she has feared the most is also the wellspring, the place where she can find the greatest peace.

The second contribution here is Pam Morrison's chapter with her sister, and co-journaler, Annie McGregor. In the tradition of diary and journal keeping, 'Making and Sharing Meaning out of Terminal Illness' demonstrates the positive power of reciprocal writing practices and the endurance of sibling love. Through their shared fascination with language, Pam and Annie's chapter plots their creative project of co-authoring a journal over the last year of Annie's life following her diagnosis of terminal cancer. Exploring their relative experiences of existence through writing together they discovered a way to articulate and ritualise their unique relationship. Co-journaling is a journey of discovery that discloses a shared story and the acceptance and understanding that might accompany the harmony and discord of voices of speaking together to one purpose about the mystery of death and a life well lived. In her analysis of their unfolding narrative, Morrison notes the emergence of themes that call upon metaphors of fabric, sounds, movement and colours to give form to and fluidly shape their familial bond.

A commonly held myth about illness and contagion is that sick people need to be kept away from those who are healthy. Similarly, individuals disabled by birth or culture may learn to accept their stigmatisation by society in ways that reinforce their subservience and marginalised condition in such a way that the oppressed group internalises its own oppression and mutes its own voices.[14] Through the writing of Toni Cade Bambara, and drawing from 20th century African American literature, Yomna Saber traces the voices of disability. In 'Toni Cade Bambara's *The Salt Eaters*: Hearing the Silent Voice of Pain' Saber carefully considers how literature has presented disabled and impaired characters, suggesting that their disabilities signify marks of oppression occasioned by the violence, segregation and exclusion that black people have been subjected to over time. She argues that disability is not only used in a political sense as a metaphor that draws attention to victimisation and othering but is itself identified as an oppressive social construction of the kind associated with gender and race. She claims that like other disadvantaged and voiceless populations who continue to suffer intergenerational cultural abuses and traumas, disabled people are believed to be, and believe themselves to be, insufficient, less than normal, and less capable than others.

In the final chapter in this part of the collection Hans Sternudd examines the growing phenomenon of self-portrayal of mental health problems among teenagers and young adults in Western social media. His provocative portrait of Saraphine Stanier and her You Tube video presentation of depression cautiously reminds us of the dangers of assuming that the patient is ignorant of her illness and has little to contribute to its discussion or amelioration. On the contrary, 'Voices of Depression: An Analysis of a Collective Narrative' highlights social media as a powerful tool to mediate and communicate personal experiences on a worldwide stage in ways that could elicit appropriate care and support. Sternudd suggests that mental health issues like depression have to be communicated with a voice that is culturally recognisable and widely accessible. It is by her courage and the medium of transmission that she is allowed to be fully heard, and by revealing her body and her scars, Saraphine contributes to the discussion on depression and compellingly critiques the established narrative of normative values.

---

14 Bobbie Harro, 'The Cycle of Socialization,' *Readings for Diversity and Social Justice*, eds. Maurianne Adams, Warren. J. Blumenfeld, Carmelita Castañeda, Heather W. Hackman, Madeline L. Peters, and Ximena Zúñiga (New York, NY: Routledge, 2010), 45–51.

When illness stories are co-produced in the context of research, ethical questions regarding the role of all of the participants are likely to arise, as the chapters in Part 4 on *Ethical Stories: Voices in Research* illustrate. Professional rules of conduct commonly restrict the direct use of practitioners' personal stories in their practice with their clients. However, professionals' practices cannot be separated from practitioners' full identities as their personal experiences are reflected in their professional approaches and clinical interactions. The disclosed and unvoiced stories that these relationships together produce remain with them, shaping their identities. In therapy and medicine keeping a professional distance and disclosing only as much of the self as is helpful is encouraged lest we contaminate the interaction or become 'infected' by the other's story and condition. However, even as a listener or witness we are implicated in the stories produced. Thus, when we recall our research participants' stories and consider their origins, whose voice is it that we should use and how does the original story become filtered by the researcher's retelling? In this part of our collection practitioners and researchers consider the ethical implications of their research interactions, planned and incidental, with participants, co-researchers and themselves.

In 'A Shared Story of Professional Practice' counsellor Peter Bray presents the story of his interviews with mental health and addiction therapists who are concerned with their use of spirituality and spiritual interventions in client care. What begins as a discussion group designed to focus on practice with clients quickly becomes a careful exploration of the spiritual needs and experiences of the practitioners themselves. Once disclosed in a group, the similarity between their stories and those disclosed in therapy by their clients soon becomes self-evident. Furthermore, the spiritual dimension was identified as a place of familiar experiences that was understood and valued by therapist and clients alike. A safe place in which to engage with clients and one that may also be used as a positive resource in their work together. However, it is clear that the mutual ground of this story was not shared by the therapists' host organisation – a hospital firmly enmeshed in conventional approaches to patient care and the ethics of disclosure. Consequently therapists, rather than disclose their own quite unique but very similar views on spirituality, find themselves working covertly in a system that has no visible space for spirituality and that they currently believe would have little or no understanding or sympathy with their spirit-centred approaches should they be revealed.

Illness is feared at a fundamental level because it forces unwanted change and can transform and reduce a person's previous identity. Reflecting on the experiences that inspired her writing, novelist and lecturer Naomi Krüger argues that fictional accounts of people suffering with the degenerative disease of dementia can vividly bring symptoms and the experience of illness to life. In 'Dementia Fiction: Giving Voice to an Experience beyond Language' she argues that literature has a role in cutting through the fear that might ordinarily prevent readers from positively engaging with the 'reduced' human being, as well as influencing perception about the way that care and support might subsequently be implemented. The real ethical challenge of managing responses to dementia, she suggests, is for the insider and the outsider to step beyond the confining parameters of disease and the fact and difference of loss, to empathically contact and embrace the richer humanity contained in the patient's bigger story.

In the final chapter in this part, Mirjam Stuij, Agnes Elling, Anja Tramper and Tineke Abma unravel the different voices in the further development of the illness story of Anja, as an incidental result of her participation in a research project. Through 'Developing a Relational Narrative about Diabetes: Towards a Polyphonic Story,' they analyse the interaction between Anja and Mirjam to show how careful reflection and recognition enabled Anja to extend her narrative habitus beyond the restitution narrative, the type of illness narrative most dominant and culturally recognizable.[15] Their detailed analysis, informed by voices from care ethicists, illuminates the importance of interpersonal sensitivity. In spite of advances in medicine and the massive increase in access to medical knowledge over time, it is surprising that the roles of the patient and the professional helper have not changed much in the popular imagination. As the obsession with health becomes a growing Western phenomenon, so tolerance of illness diminishes and ill-health is no longer seen as an inevitable flaw in the human condition. In the formulation of stories, either for ourselves or for an audience, we use cultural definitions of illness and identity which shape both our subjective experience of illness, as well as professional care.

In Part 5 of this collection, *Challenges to the Institutional Illness Discourse*, two final chapters interrogate the following questions: do society's narratives and definitions about illness change over time; do they reflect current theory and practice; or, are they simply responding to the pecuniary and socio-political interests of investors and governments? To conclude, both Verusca Calabria and Justyna Jajszczok demonstrate how the story, its subject, and the voices of the institution are often captured by the work of the contemporary oral historian and disseminated through the language and metaphors of scientific and medical discourse. In a challenge to institutional illness discourse, their chapters illustrate how the institution might influence our own stories and those of more popularised and public narratives.

15 Frank, *The Wounded Storyteller.*

With the closure of mental hospitals in England in the latter part of the 20th century Verusca Calabria's chapter 'Self-Reflexivity in Oral History Based Research' examines perceptions of the total institution of the asylum as a therapeutic environment in which bonds of friendship and networks of relationship were formed and residents were calmed without the use of drugs. Far from the isolated secure units of recent times, these semi-rural hospitals were intentionally located to encourage safety, peace and tranquillity within local communities. Sharing a sympathetic symbiotic relationship, they provided employment as well as positive opportunities for mutual understanding and social interaction. Patients were largely accepted as part of the wider community who shared in their care. By collecting residents' stories of asylum care she discovered that peer-to-peer and peer-to-staff relationships provide fresh insights into the value of inter-personal connections within psychiatric institutions, which were lost in the shift away from asylum care. For some, long-term friendships made in the asylum played a critical role in supporting their recovery. Calabria's work notes what has been lost through the modernisation of mental health services and how relationships between staff and patients have been affected. She challenges us to look beyond normative patient-centred care to offer systems that fully utilise the interpersonal and relational strengths of all those who participate in them.

Depending on who tells the story, modern medical science and Mother Nature are increasingly polarised as they wrestle to be the ultimate arbiter of what it is to be healthy and to be good. However, when health is perceived as normal and illness as temporary, it is perhaps not surprising that poor health is regarded as bad and unnatural, an unfair punishment for a life too long lived. Today, even though illness and disease are clear indicators of the absence of healthy social conditions, they are synonymous with the worst kind of illness, which is difference. In this story the badly transformed host spreads his contagious message of unreason, instability and fear, whilst the heroic doctors of medicine and spin are the only people that stand between human order and inevitable chaos.

Justyna Jajszczok's 'The Voiceless and the Vocal: Infection Literature and *The Sign of the Four*' reviews the impact of 'invasion literature,' specifically the appetites and fears that came to the fore in Britain during her Imperial expansion from 1875 to 1910. In addition she identifies a sub-genre 'infection literature' that simultaneously occurred when the majority of disease-causing agents were discovered in microbiology and similar advances were being simultaneously made in the field of tropical medicine. Significantly, infection literature speaks of a growing belief that, through medicine, man might finally have a way to defeat for all time even the most elusive disease causing micro-organisms. Nevertheless, in the case of tuberculosis, she argues that, even though it was logical to destroy the parasite, it was easier for the authorities to blame the poor lifestyle choices of its infected host. Even today, it is hard to escape the lingering metaphor that infection remains synonymous with the evils of invasion and parasitic colonisation. Reinterpreted through works of literature like Arthur Conan Doyle's *The Sign of the Four*, the detective and the doctor are shown working together with logical deduction and the knowledge of new science, to reach a solution and administer an antidote – endorsing the widely held assumption that any problem in society can be resolved by treating the source of its infection.

In reading this collection you will recognise the many ways that people experience the world. Through their chapters the contributors invite you to give fresh consideration to the rich application of story and voice, to sharpen your sensitivity and enrich your relationships.

The illness story is an exercise in narrative development and narrative autonomy that when shared with others gives a voice to the individual's condition. Heart-felt, pragmatic and often distressing, these stories incorporate details of individual and group engagement with helping professionals, medical procedures and personal losses, the responsibilities that they will take for their health in the future, and ways that they will make their new pathways more tolerable. They are humble manifestos, testaments to hope in the face of hopelessness. Yet the act of making and telling stories does preserve hope, assist in modifying present and future narratives and ultimately maintains closer connection in human relationships and lives.

Working together to create systems of care that are patient-centred, and incorporate the sharing of power and decision making, we are learning that each individual voice has something valuable to contribute to ensure the best outcomes for patients. Taking relationally collaborative positions, accommodating the realities of the differently-abled and seeking mutual understanding, even when there is no cure, might be all that is required. The chapters in this collection provide a simple snapshot of how practitioners and scholars across the globe regard this important goal.

Stories told alone or in communities are empowering to all individuals, and they enrich the lives of everyone. By hearing and telling stories we are able to learn where we stand, which better equips us to act in and upon the world. As we assess our own very unique circumstances in the light of others' experiences it is hard not to resonate with their capacity for optimism and resilience, and their power to adapt.

Bibliography

Barry, Christine A., Fiona A. Stevenson, Nicky Britten, Nick Barber, and Colin P. Bradley. 'Giving voice to the lifeworld. More humane, more effective medical care? A qualitative study of doctor–patient communication in general practice.' *Social Science Medicine* 53.4 (2001): 487–505.

Braun, Virginia and Victoria Clarke. 'Using Thematic Analysis in Psychology.' *Qualitative Research in Psychology*, 2006.

Bray, Peter and Ana Borlescu, eds. 'Introduction.' *Beyond Present Patient Realities: Collaboration, Care and Identity*. Oxford, England: Inter-Disciplinary Press, 2015.

Charon, Rita. *Narrative Medicine: Honoring the Stories of Illness*. Oxford and New York: Oxford University Press, 2006.

Clark, Jack A. and Elliot G. Mishler. 'Attending To Patients' Stories: Reframing the Clinical Task.' *Sociology of Health & Illness* 14.3 (1992): 344–372.

Frank, Arthur W. *The Wounded Storyteller: Body, Illness, and Ethics*. Chicago: The University of Chicago Press, 1995.

Frank, Arthur W. *Letting Stories Breathe: A Socio-narratology*. Chicago: The University of Chicago Press, 2010.

Harro, Bobbie. 'The Cycle of Socialization.' *Readings for Diversity and Social Justice*, edited by Maurianne Adams, Warren. J. Blumenfeld, Carmelita Castañeda, Heather W. Hackman, Madeline L. Peters, and Ximena Zúñiga, 45–51. New York, NY: Routledge, 2010.

Kaufman, Sharon. 'Illness, Biography, and the Interpretation of Self Following a Stroke.' *Journal of Aging Studies* 2.3 (1988): 217–227.

Mishler, Elliot G. *The Discourse of Medicine: Dialectics of Medical Interviews*. Norwood, NJ: Ablex Publishing Corporation, 1984.

Mishler, Elliot G. *Storylines: Craftartists' Narratives of Identity*. Cambridge, MA: Harvard University Press, 1999.

Mishler, Elliot G. 'Patient Stories, Narratives of Resistance and the Ethics of Humane Care: A la recherche du temps perdu.' *Health (London)* 9.4 (2005): 431–451.

PART 1

The Story, Identity and the Voice

CHAPTER 1

Narrative Medicine and Storytelling: An Alternative Method for Healing

Victorria Simpson-Gervin

Abstract

The addition of medical humanities in academia has created a framework for narrative medicine by providing the health care profession with alternative methods for patient care and recovery. This new form of communication allows the patient and physician to build a more meaningful relationship through the embodiment of patient-shared stories. Storytelling as a form of narrative medicine opens up a multitude of possibilities for promoting health and healing. The single act of allowing patients to share their personal stories gives them a certain amount of agency. This study focuses on the benefits of allowing patients to express their fears and concerns through the use of storytelling as a way to come to terms with their illnesses. Additionally, it explores how patients are able to become pro-active in making decisions regarding their personal health care. Lastly, this chapter provides an in-depth discussion through the use of a case study demonstrating how narrative medicine helped an individual process and cope with loss through the use of storytelling.

Key Words

Narrative medicine – medical humanities – deconstruction – reconstruction – stereophonic listening – storytelling – narrative performance – parallel chart – physician/patient relationship – reflective writing – empathy – and caregiver

*****

1 Narrative Medicine

The use of storytelling and narrative language is nothing new. In fact, it is one of the most basic forms of communication, when it expresses matters of the self. Scholars have conducted discourse analysis of storytelling and the

 | DOI:10.1163/9789004396067_003

performance of narrative language for years, researching what effect they have on the human mind and body. However, what *is* new is the integrated use of the less conventional methods employed in medical discourse in conjunction with traditional medicines as an alternative for healing. In their article *Healing through Stories: A Special Issue on Narrative Medicine,* Lynn Harter and Art Bochner acknowledge how limited scientific methods can be in advancing patient care in the areas of performance and healing.

In discussing the work of Barbara Sharf, Kristin Langellier, Bill Rawlins, Richard Zaner, and Terri Thompson, Harter and Bochner suggest that by

> invoking narrative practices, narrative ethics, and narrative theory to enlarge healing practices, these authors offer images of how to live well in the midst of the inescapable suffering, trauma, and disability associated with the lived experience of illness.[1]

In her book *Narrative Medicine,* Rita Charon describes narrative medicine as a performance that encompasses 'the text and bodies, the stories, and selves, which participate in its practice – patients' and physicians' embodied stories as well as the body of medical discourse itself.'[2] The framework of narrative medicine is to undo and redo the way we tell, listen, read, and write these performances. The idea of reading narrative medicine as a performance creates a new form of communication between patient and physician. How might this new way of listening to patients' stories shift the dynamics of the patient/physician relationship? Can we think of storytelling and its healing effect on the soul in the same vein in medical discourse? How and to what extent would the use of narrative medicine impact the patient/physician relationship, the family and the entire health care system? These questions will be analysed as I attempt to explore and respond to the topic of narrative medicine and storytelling.

This chapter examines the holistic effect that the unconventional method of narrative medicine and storytelling has on its patients and how, through the promotion of dignity, patients are allowed to have agency over themselves, even those patients that are facing death. An exploration of the effect storytelling has on family members and patient caregivers will also be presented. How are their lives enriched or impacted by these stories? Furthermore, how

1 Lynn M. Harter and Arthur P. Bochner, 'Healing Through Stories: A Special Issue on Narrative Medicine,' *Journal of Applied Communication Research* 37.2 (2009): 113–17.

2 Rita Charon, *Narrative Medicine: Honoring the Stories of Illness* (New York: Oxford University Press, 2006), 152.

do they create their own stories as a method of healing as they cope with the illness of their love ones?

Charon, a professor of medicine at Columbia University, coined the term 'narrative medicine' to establish another way of enhancing the patient/physician relationship. She created what she refers to as the 'parallel chart,' which functions as a personal journal for her medical students. The purpose of the parallel chart is to serve as a supplement to official hospital charts. Charon writes,

> The goals are to enable them [medical students] to recognize more fully what their patients endure and to examine explicitly their own journeys through medicine. More than a diary, this chart is filled with medical students' reactions to particular patients, enabling them to reflect on their own experiences and be more open and receptive to their patients.[3]

In an article with Sayantani DasGuspta entitled *Personal Illness Narratives: Using Reflective Writing to Teach Empathy* they discuss the difficulty for medical educators to teach students the implications of effective interaction with patients where empathy is the focal point. One method Charon and DasGuspta have found successful is having the students participate in a writing exercise referred to as 'reflective narrative.' They describe the exercise as a

> process of internally examining and exploring an issue of concern, triggered by an experience, which creates and clarifies meaning in terms of self, and which results in a changed conceptual perspective.[4]

Scholars in the field of narrative medicine believe there is a connection between reflection and empathy that affects both the caregiver and the patient. Charon and DasGuspta admit that teaching empathy to medical students remains an 'elusive objective' due, in part, to the lack of concrete definitions of empathy, and the lack of effective pedagogic method in which to teach it. Physicians must be able to feel what their patients are feeling, and place themselves in their patients position in order to experience real empathy for their patients. This process, they explain, is supported through writing reflective narrative, when using the parallel chart. Empathy is built through reflective writing. Reflection is described as 'a process of internally examining and exploring an

---

3 Ibid., 411.

4 Sayantani DasGupta and Rita Charon, 'Personal Illness Narratives: Using Reflective Writing to Teach Empathy,' *Academic Medicine* 79.4 (2004): 351–56.

issue of concern, triggered by an experience, which creates and clarifies meaning in terms of self, and which results in a changed conceptual perspective.'[5] By increasing self-awareness, which focuses on the relationship dynamics of the physician and patient, medical educators such as DasGuspta and Charon believe that this will increase the human side of the health care encounter. Both agree that

> when doctors or medical trainees reflect on their own lives in medicine and when they inspect the memories and associations triggered by their care of the sick, they become all the more available and useful to their patients.[6]

Writing reflective narratives allowed the medical students to examine and articulate their own personal illness and feelings in order to translate their stories, to better understand and shed light on the language of their patients and the meaning of their pain and suffering. It is believed that as we define ourselves through storytelling it allows us to develop bonds with individuals with shared interests. Essentially these activities, in helping us to make sense of the world, also assists us to find meaning within ourselves.

Lori A. Roscoe, a professor at the University of South Florida, believes that the stories shared in medical discourse are often sterile, and can create unsuitable environments between patients and physicians, as well as between physicians in different specialties. In *Healing the Physician's Story: A Case Study in Narrative Medicine and End-of-Life Care*,[7] she explains how storytelling provides the tools of making sense of the pain and trauma suffered by those patients who are in end-of-life care. Roscoe suggests that providing workshops for physicians, which gives them a safe place to share their personal work-related stories and their patient's stories, allows the physicians to enhance their ability to connect with patients. Furthermore, it also allows them to establish trusting relationships with their colleagues. She suggests,

> providing opportunities for physicians to tell stories about their patients' deaths can facilitate the interplay between technical and narrative rationality, and can help physicians to better integrate patients' deaths into the fabric of their clinical practice.[8]

---

5 Ibid., 351.

6 Ibid., 352.

7 Lori A. Roscoe, 'Healing the Physician's Story: A Case Study in Narrative Medicine and End–of–Life Care,' *Narrative Inquiry in Bioethics* 2.1 (2012): 65–72.

8 Ibid., 66.

She believes storytelling fills the gap between technical rationality and narrative rationality. Roscoe describes technical rationality as the information we receive from clinicians, such as classification and lists for illness. Narrative rationality refers to the stories we, physician/patients, family, and care-givers create to describe these illnesses.

Roscoe suggests that, although death is not unexpected for physicians who specialize in oncology and palliative medicine, it never becomes routine. She submits that physicians who practice in specialized fields where patients are in end-of life care, will especially benefit from the use of narrative medicine; they can benefit from practicing such narrative techniques as 'reflective writing that can facilitate relationship building, communication skills, and empathy for patients, colleagues, and oneself.'[9] She advocates for physicians to write and share their stories among colleagues in order to enhance self-awareness, and promote self-care. Like their patients, physicians can find solace in sharing what it's like to specialize in oncology and palliative medicine.

In her chapter, story maker and founder of Sharing Stories for Wellbeing (SS4WB), Miranda Quinney and her colleagues discuss her effective work with the mental wellbeing of end of life patients.[10] With her co-authors, she presents a summary and evaluation of a workshop conducted over five weekly sessions between May and June in 2015. SS4WB provides a supportive and safe space in which patients in palliative care share their stories with others in the programme, 'in a non-linear style and…based on themed topics.'[11] The groups are supported by hospice staff, which include both pastoral and clinical carers. Quinney suggests that 'participation can have positive outcomes fostering choice in the stories shared which then engenders a sense of autonomy and control, reminiscences can also bring feelings of value and self-esteem.'[12] SS4WB uses storytelling as a vehicle for individuals to make meaning of their lives. Through the act of oral storytelling we acquire many important values such as listening, respect, and empathy.

Like Quinney and her colleagues, I believe we must first start with practitioners, making sure that they are adequately trained in the art of storytelling. As Quinney states, 'the process of participating in a life stories workshop will be the first step towards telling and sharing their life stories to others thereby going some way towards dealing with the eulogy situation.'[13] Storytelling is a powerful communication tool for both patients and providers. These shared

9 Ibid., 71.

10 Miranda Quinney, Alison Ward, and Jane Youell, 'Life Story Sharing: A Therapeutic Intervention in Palliative Care,' in this volume.

11 Ibid.

12 Ibid.

13 Ibid.

stories allow practitioners and caregivers to develop a deeper understanding of specific issues and experiences, in an effort to facilitate patient improvement and care. Stories have a transformative power which allows us to see circumstances in a different light. They have a narrative that appeal to the human side of us. I concur with Quinney in acknowledging some of the most effective ways of ensuring patient stories are valued. We must first create the framework which provides a space to accommodate this particular type of narrative. We begin by selecting empathic staff that are trained listeners in storytelling. This allows all staff working with patients to empower them to use storytelling as a way to delve into deeper issues concerning their healthcare. Secondly, and just as important, it's imperative we work with both the bereaved families as well as the children.

2 Medical Humanities

When medical humanities appeared in the 1960s, ethics and the history of medicine were the only topics of interest. The study of medical humanities began to expand as medical faculty with interests in literature, history, and ethics integrated these focuses into their curricula. Gastroenterologist Seamus O'Mahony in his article, *Against Narrative Medicine,* states that while medical faculty members broadened the range of their humanistic and social sciences inquiries, they failed to recognize the change in humanities studies in the late 1960s. Current discourse now includes, 'deconstruction, structuralism, post-structuralism, and relativism, all of which might be placed under the broad umbrella of postmodernism.'[14] Physicians were perplexed by the postmodernist claims that there is no objective truth, and that all written documents, 'even scientific papers were 'narratives."[15] For this revelation, O'Mahony credits Foucault and Derrida, who he refers to as 'postmodernism's high priests.'[16]

O'Mahony suggests that the study of medicine has now become unsure of its capability, particularly regarding the physician/patient relationship. For her part, Charon calls upon healthcare practitioners to be more mindful and attentive to their patients. She calls for more empathy for patients' feelings. O'Mahony believes it is this attitude that has changed the discourse in medical humanities. He argues that, 'discourse in narrative medicine is clouded in

14 Seamus O'Mahony, 'Against Narrative Medicine.' *Perspectives in Biology and Medicine* 56.4 (2013): 611–19.

15 Ibid., 612.

16 Ibid.

impenetrable jargon, strongly influenced by postmodernist literary theory. And much of the language employed has a religious flavor: "witnessing," "professing," "honoring."'[17] O'Mahony further suggests that the medical humanities are regularly filled with phrases such as, 'otherness,' 'postcolonialism,' and 'advocacy,' but the word that has dominated the discourse of medical humanities is *narrative.*[18]

3 Narrative Performance

In *Narrative as Dialogic, Contested, and Aesthetic Performance,*[19] Lynn M. Harter documents the success of one physician that illustrates the impact of narrative medicine and storytelling, as well as the effectiveness of employing a parallel chart to track the progress of one his patients. Pete Anderson, is a clinician and professor at the University of Texas, MD Anderson Cancer Centre. Anna, a teenage patient, was referred to him because of his clinical research and 'expertise in paediatric oncology and multimodality therapies.'[20] Anna was diagnosed with metastatic Ewing's sarcoma, which is a form of bone cancer. Her treatment would include surgery, chemotherapy, and radiation.

Harter, who was given permission by Anna's family and Anderson to write about the case, was not surprised by the treatment Anna received, because her own father's cancer treatment looked very much like Anna's. What did surprise Harter was Anderson's relationship with Anna and her family. Anderson kept a flash drive in which he recorded images of Anna's prom and graduation, her dog, pictures of the family, and a one-page summary. The portable electronic medical record was used in conjunction with the hospital's records. Much like Charon's parallel chart. Harter explains, 'Dr. Pete celebrated these occasions by inserting Anna's prom and graduation photos into his summary of her cancer experience.'[21] Harter suggests that Anderson uses narrative medicine to gather information, to keep records, to build relationships with his patients, and to make therapeutic decisions; thus, it represents '*equipment for* living.'[22]

Six months after her high school graduation, Anna's cancer returned. Anderson asked Anna, 'What other chapters in your life do you want to write?

17 Ibid., 613.
18 Ibid., 614.
19 Lynn M. Harter, 'Narratives as Dialogic, Contested, and Aesthetic Performance' *Journal of Applied Communication Research* 37.2 (2009): 140–50.
20 Ibid., 140.
21 Ibid., 141.
22 Ibid.

How can I help you write those?'[23] Harter writes that she never heard Anderson describe his work as narrative medicine until then; he was consulting Charon's book *Narrative Medicine: Honouring the Stories of Illness.* Anderson agreed that, 'humans reach for storytelling when trying to make sense of expectations gone awry.'[24]

Harter sees Charon's most noteworthy contribution to medical humanities as a way to approach narrative as an aesthetic act. Halter confirms that language still remains 'a chief instrument of self-expression, and a marker of intelligence in western contexts. Yet, sometimes language fails us or may not be the ideal mechanism from which to confer form.'[25] With this in mind, she cites the MD Anderson Cancer Centre, Children's Art Project in which children who may have limited abilities to articulate what they were experiencing in words, used art to allow them to streamline their experiences. By combining imaginative and narrative thought, art provides the children new possibilities of alternative means of self-expression.

In a similar vein, Harter discusses the work of Victoria Marks, a choreographer and professor at UCLA. Marks has employed dance performance in her work with soldiers diagnosed with post-traumatic stress disorder when they return from overseas tours of duty. Her hope is that more researchers will explore the varied forms in which narrative may enlighten us to enhance the patient/physician relationship and to increase quality care for those who are ill, hopeless, and suffering. Quoted in Lynn M. Harter's *Narratives as Dialogic, Contested, and Aesthetic Performances*, Charon suggests that

> [n]arratives invite us to stretch our imagination to grasp events befalling another individual. To exercise our imagination is to affirm our capacity to move beyond the boundaries of own bodies and experiences to appreciate others' storied representations of reality.[26]

By expanding the boundaries of narrative medicine to include aesthetic accomplishments, Charon suggests that 'we enlarge research agendas on the storied nature of health and healing and open possibilities for self-expression.'[27] Her hope is that more researchers will explore the varied forms by which

23 Ibid.
24 Ibid.
25 Ibid., 147.
26 Ibid.
27 Ibid., 148.

narrative may enhance the patient/physician relationship and increase quality care for those who are ill, hopeless, and suffering.

Unlike the example of Dr. Pete Anderson's treatment of Anna, in the case of Arthur W. Frank, he himself was a patient who practiced narrative medicine and storytelling.[28] In his article *Why Doctors' Stories Matter,*[29] he journals his personal experiences with illness. After recovering from what was diagnosed as a virally-induced heart attack, Frank began to have symptoms of what would later be diagnosed as testicular cancer. He chose to write about his experience with illness in the hope that others going through similar ordeals might find companionship in his story.

Frank explains that when he looked for a similar sense of companionship 20 years ago, there was not much available, so he ultimately wrote the book for himself. He further explains how alienated he felt being around physicians as a patient. He wrote *At the Will of the Body* out of his own sense of alienation from medical practitioners. There was a disconnect, or 'gap,' as Charon refers to it. Like Charon, Frank also believes medical knowledge can sometimes create a huge gap between doctor and patient. He states,

> doctors seemed strange to me, and being with doctors made me feel strange to myself. As some part of myself watched me interacting with doctors, I didn't recognize the person who was me; he wasn't expressing what I was feeling.[30]

Frank did not know if his doctors were acting out of choice, or because of how they felt they should act. He suggests that the bedside manners of physicians will continue to leave a gap in the physician/patient relationship until they learn to mourn the deaths of the patients under their care.

Frank stresses the importance of being able to contain sadness and loss within patient narratives. Allowing patients to compartmentalize what they are feeling aids in containing the experiences; patients and caregivers are not then flooded with unpredictable emotions. He further suggests that events do not lose any of their sadness by their containment in a story, but there is a time and a place to be sad. Narrative allows us to revisit feelings when we feel the need to do so.

---

28 Arthur W. Frank, 'Why Doctor's Stories Matter,' *Stories in Family Medicine* (2010): 51–4.

29 Ibid., 51.

30 Ibid.

Annie Parsons and Claire Hooker refer to the use of patient-centred stories as narrative therapy. An essential idea in their article *Dignity and Narrative Medicine* is that

> the narrating of the patient's story is a therapeutically central act, because to find the words to contain the disorder and its attendant worries gives shape to and control over the chaos of illness.[31]

Bradley E. Lewis, in his article *Narrative Medicine and Healthcare Reform,*[32] believes medical science has lost sight of the human side of medicine, and instead has drifted toward:

> overspecialization; technicism; overprofessional; insensitivity to personal and sociocultural values; too narrow a construal of the doctor's role; too much 'curing' rather than 'caring'; not enough emphasis on prevention, patient-participation, and patient education; too much economic incentive; a trade school mentality; overmedicalization of everyday life; inhuman treatment of medical students; overwork by house staff; and deficiencies in verbal and nonverbal communication.[33]

All of which contributes to the separation and struggles patients endure while confronting physicians' bedside manners.

In Nicole Defenbaugh's *A Review of: 'Charon, R. (2006). Narrative Medicine: Honouring Stories of Illness*, she suggests that Charon fills the gap within the current body of narrative medicine literature, outlining an effective way of reading narrative text. She suggests that we must 'understand the reader's act, identify the story's teller, be ready for the story's transformations, and pay attention to source and destination, among others.'[34]

Narrative skills require close reading. In her article *Performing Narrative Medicine*, Kristin M. Langellier understands the interaction of intimacy and power in narrative medicine. Close reading allows the individual both to follow the patient's story and to identify the 'metaphors' and 'images' used in

31 Annie Parsons and Claire Hooker. 'Dignity and Narrative Medicine,' *Journal of Bioethical Inquiry Bioethical Inquiry* 7 (2010): 345–51.

32 Bradley E. Lewis. 'Narrative Medicine and Health Reform.' *Journal of Medical Humanities* (2011): 9–20.

33 Ibid., 12.

34 Nicole L. Defenbaugh, 'A Review of: Charon, R.' (2006). Narrative Medicine: Honoring Stories of Illness,' *Journal of Health Communication* 13.4 (2008): 410.

telling the story. It also allows us to identify the unspoken subtexts. Langellier notes that Charon acknowledges that close reading was coined by the 'New Critics, and it is a practice (she calls it a drill) central to graduate training in literary analysis.'[35]

4 Stereophonic Listening

Another aspect of narrative medicine and storytelling is the act of listening. According to Langellier some of the adjectives Charon uses to describe listeners are, 'dutiful, empathetic, imaginative, and caring.'[36] Charon implies that listening is a skill in itself. She refers to it as 'stereophonic listening,' the ability to 'hear the body and the person who inhabits it.'[37] Practitioners employ this stereophonic listening when engaging with the storyteller's body gestures as well as the silence. The effect of active listening is not only beneficial to the physician/patient relationship, but also for the family member or caregiver caring for the patient. Skilfully listening to these stories provides the listener with a better understanding, and also allows accurate interpretation of the story. Charon suggests that family members and caregiver of the patients should create their own stories as a method of healing and coping with the illness of a loved one by employing these various ways of listening. For those of us that are textual beings, this alternative way of listening to other's stories, allows us to engage in not only the spoken word, but to listen to the body, their gestures, and the silences. It is only then, we can fully understand and create our own stories, beginning with using these performances as an approach to skilful listening.

In his article *Just Listening: Narrative and Deep Illness*, Arthur W. Frank describes patients living in 'deep illness' as individuals who may suffer from illnesses that are critical, chronic, immediately life-threatening, or long-term.[38] Like Charon, he conducts a close examination of narrative medicine, to reveal how those living in deep illness relate their stories, and how clinicians can effectively engage in what Charon refers to as 'stereophonic listening' when listening to the stories of such patients. Frank believes storytelling is based on

35 Kristin M. Langellier. 'Performing Narrative Medicine,' *Journal of Applied Communication Research* 37.2 (2009): 151–58.

36 Ibid., 154.

37 Ibid.

38 Arthur W. Frank. 'Just Listening: Narrative and Deep Illness,' *Families, Systems & Health* 16.3 (1998): 197–212.

the relationships we develop with those living in deep illness – *just listening* to patients' stories is a critical professional role for clinicians.[39]

Frank attributes the clinical importance of stories told by patients living in deep illness to two individuals. The first is psychiatrist and medical anthropologist Arthur Kleinman, who emphasizes 'empathic witnessing … of the patient's and family's stories of the illness, as central to clinical work'[40] and the second, physician Rachel Naomi Remen. Kleinman argues that 'a powerful therapeutic alternative is at hand':

> There is evidence to indicate that through examining the particular significances of a person's illness it is possible to break the vicious cycles that amplify distress. The interpretation of illness meanings can also contribute to the provision of more effective care… This key clinical task may even liberate sufferers and practitioners from the oppressive iron cage imposed by a too intensely morbid preoccupation with painful bodily processes and a too technically narrow and therefore dehumanizing vision of treatment, respectively.[41]

As a professor of medicine, Kleinman stresses to his colleagues and students the importance of allocating time to attend to the stories of their patients, as they attempt to uncover and reveal possible meanings in their suffering. Both Frank and Kleinman cite attending to patient stories as a critical aspect of clinical work with the deeply ill.

Remen, Frank suggests, moves even further in this clinical process, as she steps outside of her role as a physician and places herself squarely in the role of her cancer patients. In doing so, she is able to 'self-consciously place herself as another who is wounded':

> Being here [in the Commonwealth retreat program] opens up opportunities for people to be listened to, and heard, and validated. They're not stuck anymore. If you ask, 'How does that happen?' I have to say I'm not sure – but it does, and I trust that. I think the greatest thing you can give someone else is your attention – not with judgment, but just listening.[42]

39 Ibid., 197.

40 Ibid., 198.

41 Arthur Kleinman, *The Illness Narratives: Suffering, Healing, and the Human Condition,* (New York: Basic Books, 1988), 9, quoted in Arthur W. Frank. 'Just Listening': 198.

42 R N. Remen, *Wounded Healers* (Mill Valley CA: *Wounded Healer Press*, 1994), 345, quoted in Frank, 'Just Listening': 198.

Both Kleinman and Remen emphasize the importance of acknowledging the stories of the deeply ill. Frank suggests that practicing therapy with those living in 'deep illness' is presented as entering relationships based on storytelling.[43] He argues that these stories are not clinical material or charts to be analysed; rather, they are fundamental to entering and developing healing relationships. As noted in the earlier section on narrative medicine, taking time to listen and nurture stories of the deeply ill helps to give meaning to the chaos in patients' lives. The relationships that develop from this alternative method of healing allow care-givers to create their own stories as well.

5 Case Study

In this case study, we will see how an eleven-year old girl employs Charon's concept of 'stereophonic listening' not only as a coping mechanism, but also to create her own story about healing, a story she can revisit and retell as often as need be. From her practice of journaling she hoped to find recovery, wellness, and healing. While she did not know it at the time, writing for transformative change would provide her with her own personal testimony promoting storytelling, activism, and healing.

In 1975, the young girl remembered being told by her older sister why her mother was sobbing uncontrollably, and why the priest was in their home. Her mother had just received the news of her 54-year-old husband's passing. He died of a brain aneurysm while at work. The young girl remembers questioning her older sister as to how her father could have died on the hospital floor where he worked for twenty-five years. How is it possible, not ever being sick or missing a day of work? He went to work one day and collapsed and died instantaneously. She recalls her father leaving for work on that beautiful morning in May, never to return home again. The little girl was not sure how to process all of the events. What would they do now without her dad around? How would her mother survive? How would they survive without their father's love and support? The young girl missed her father terribly; they were extremely close. Her mother kept her father's memories alive by telling her stories of him and how much he loved each and every one of them.

Five years after the passing of her father, this same girl stared death in the face again with the passing of her mother. Her mother passed away two weeks before her sixteenth birthday. Instead of planning a Sweet Sixteen party, she

43 Ibid., 197.

was instead helping her older siblings plan the funeral arrangements for her 54-year-old mother. Her parents died five years apart at the age 54.

She had just begun to cope with the loss of her father, when her mother's unexpected death occurred. She remembers feeling a sense of hopelessness and terrible sadness. She asked herself how would she make sense of this all. Words could not possibly express the deep sadness she experienced from the tragic loss of both of her parents. The pain and emptiness was more than she could bear.

The young girl decided to keep a journal to keep track of what she was feeling, and to try to make sense of the tragedy of her mother's death. She did not know it at the time, but she would journal the loss of three of her siblings before she understood the relevance of the journal. As a further component of this girl's history of loss, she was a triplet, though one triplet did not survive in birth. In 1993, she was informed that her twin brother had stage 3 metastatic lung cancers; this struck her to the core. They were so close, so much so that they would finish each other's sentences. At one point her twin brother lived on the west coast, and she on the east coast, but they could still sense if one was ill or in need of the other.

The sister came home from Israel to help care for her twin brother, a task she thought would certainly send her over the edge. She was racked with grief, yet she still continued to write in her journal. She and her twin brother would sit for hours as she listened to him talk about his life, his past and his present. The more they talked she began to see things through his eyes. She had the ability to see what he could see. Perhaps it was due to their being twins but she was not really sure.

As the brother's health quickly deteriorated, their talks decreased. However, the sister still had her journal to revisit and cherish those memorable moments. Two years after her twin brother's diagnosis, he passed away. The year was 1995. Oh, how she missed him and their talks. How she missed seeing things through the lens of her beloved brother.

In 2008, death came to knock on the family's door again; her older sister was stricken this time. In this case, there was no time for preparation, not that this woman could ever sufficiently prepare herself for the death of another loved one. Her older sister was almost like a mother to her. They were eleven years apart, but it was not the age difference that made her sister a mother figure. After the loss of both parents the older sister had taken the twins in. Figuratively speaking, the older sister was a second mother to the twins. The pain of losing a mother for the second time was almost unbearable for the young woman. She wondered how many more of her family members must succumb to death. The answer to her question came swiftly. In three months, one of her older brothers was also diagnosed with metastatic prostate cancer.

The young woman remembers the day as if it were yesterday, as she sat in the doctor's office with her brother awaiting the test results, only to be told the diagnosis was cancer. She thought this couldn't be so. To both her brother and herself the moment seemed so surreal. Whilst sitting in the doctor's office, she promised her brother that she would be there with him every step of the way. She made good on her promise, as she took over the responsibility of becoming his primary caregiver. All the while she was working, going to school, and caring for her brother. She attended all of his treatments and medical appointments. Her brother gave her Medical Power of Attorney in order to make medical decisions for him, should he become incapacitated.

The brother suffered a long and painful death, with many hospital stays, and near-death experiences. She remembered how it felt to be sitting in class, waiting for her phone to ring, with a nurse on the other end telling her she needed to rush to the hospital right away. She confesses this was the most difficult time of her life. There were many occasions when she just wanted to throw her hands up in the air and give up, but she could not; she remembered the promise she made to her older brother, vowing to be there for him every step of the way. The only thing that kept her sane was journaling her thoughts and conversations with her brother. She now understood the connection between writing for transformative change and healing from traumatic experiences. She believed the two were interconnected.

After fighting the battle against cancer for five years, the brother was no longer able to breathe on his own; at this point, he was placed on a ventilator. After struggling with the decision to do what was best for her brother, she decided to let him die with dignity. She decided to have the ventilator disconnected. It was what he wanted, which is why he trusted her to make the right decision on his behalf. This was the hardest decision she has ever had to make.

The young woman would get a three-year reprieve before receiving word that another brother has been diagnosed with metastatic cancer. Her Sister-in-Law called the remaining siblings to inform them that their brother was recently diagnosed with cancer which had spread to his lungs and his brain. She wanted to know if they could all make a trip to surprise him for his 70th birthday. The Sister-in-Law thought this event would lift the brother's spirits to see all of his siblings together at one time. This was no easy task she admitted, seeing that each of the six siblings lived in different states. Logistics was not the only problem. The siblings seemed to not visit as often after their parents passed away. When their parents were alive, the siblings always made it home for family holidays and major events. Gone were the Thanksgiving and Christmas dinners where they would all be gathered around the table for plenty of food and laughter. Gone now was the frequent visits and most of the laughter. Nevertheless, the Sister-in-Law decided to throw the surprise birthday party anyway. She thought it would do the whole family good to see each other and to catch up. The siblings were unsure how well this would go over considering the circumstances. However, the young woman, who is the youngest of the six siblings was able to capture a rare moment of true celebration in pictures and by journaling the event. She even recorded the event as well. What seemed to be a questionable occasion, turned out to be one she, and the rest of her sibling will always remember and treasure. The event was the dose of medicine they all needed. Pain can sometimes limit our ability to articulate what we feel. This allowed each of her siblings to walk away from the event with their own personal recollection of the event. What she did was help them create their own stories, so that they may be shared with others. She believed this is where healing truly begins. She employed alternative methods for healing, such as those mentioned earlier. In the case of Charon and the parallel chart used as a personal journal for the interns, and Dr. Pete, who recorded images of his patient Anna's prom, and choreographer and professor Victoria Marks who used dance for soldiers suffering from post-traumatic stress disorder. All of these examples give alternatives method for remembering healing and from traumatic experiences.

As an English major studying narrative language and as a caregiver of two brothers whose lives were cut short due to cancer, she was fully aware of the power of narrative medicine. She used her journal to channel all of her emotions and fond memories of her loved ones, and she visits it often. She even sometimes re-visits the not-so fond memories in her journal, the entries that are filled with pain and sorrow. Her journal helps her to compartmentalize the stories, so she can take as much as she need, or as little as she need, depending on the circumstances. Her journal also provides her with a space to navigate through the stories in whatever manner best serves her, and perhaps others with whom she has shared her story. Her hope is that by sharing her story, others may be able to create their own stories in order to make sense of a traumatic experience with which they too may have been unexpectedly confronted.

Now in 2016, although she felt the chain of events in her life would be her demise, she was indeed made stronger. The eleven-year-old girl has grown up into a fifty-eight-year-old woman. I am that girl; this is my story. Journaling has allowed me a safe space to express the many emotions with which I was experiencing during some of the most traumatic times of my life. My journaling and writing became approaches to healing through narrative language. Which opened up a multitude of possibilities for me for promoting health and healing.

Today, I still use my journal for not only reflective writing, but to also revisit those difficult challenges I encountered along the way. By reconstructing the narrative of pain into a positive message of healing, this has allowed me to better understand the person I've become and to recognize my resiliency. I do understand the power of narrative medicine and storytelling, and how it can be used a source of healing, and coping with traumatic experiences; I am a living testament to that.

Bibliography

Charon, Rita. *Narrative Medicine: Honoring the Stories of Illness*. New York, NY: Oxford University Press, 2006.

DasGupta, Sayantani, and Rita Charon. 'Personal Illness Narrative: Using Reflective Writing to Teach Empathy.' *Academic Medicine* 79.4 (2004): 351–356.

Defenbaugh, Nicole L. 'A Review of: Charon, R. (2006). Narrative Medicine: Honoring Stories of Illness.' *Journal of Health Communication* 13.4 (2008): 409–13.

Frank, Arthur W. 'Why Doctor's Stories Matter.' *Stories in Family Medicine* 56.1 (2010): 51–4.

Frank, Arthur W. 'Just Listening: Narrative and Deep Illness.' *Families, Systems & Health* 16.3 (1998): 197–212.

Harter, Lynn M. 'Narratives as Dialogic, Contested, and Aesthetic Performances.' *Journal of Applied Communication Research*: 37 (2009): 140–50.

Harter, Lynn M. and Arthur P. Bochner. 'Healing through Stories: A Special Issue on Narrative Medicine.' *Journal of Applied Communication Research* 37.2 (2009): 113–17.

Langellier, Kristin M. 'Performing Narrative Medicine.' *Journal of Applied Communication Research* 37.2 (2009): 151–58.

Lewis, Bradley E. 'Narrative Medicine and Health Reform.' *Journal of Medical Humanities* 32. (2011): 9–20.

O'Mahony, Seamus. 'Against Narrative Medicine.' *Perspectives in Biology and Medicine* 56.4. (2013): 611–19.

Parsons, Annie, and Claire Hooker. 'Dignity and Narrative Medicine.' *Journal of Bioethical Inquiry Bioethical Inquiry* 7 (2010): 345–51.

Roscoe, Lori A. 'Healing the Physician's Story: A Case Study in Narrative Medicine and End–of–Life Care.' *Narrative Inquiry in Bioethics* 2.1(2012): 65–72.

PART 2

Group Voices and Group Identity

CHAPTER 2

AIDS Awakens Ancient Stories

Deborah Freedman

Abstract

In the beginning…AIDS ravaged humanity all over the globe. People became ill and died quickly. Those who were a part of the gay or haemophiliac communities were going to one funeral after another. Everyone was in the dark and everyone was scared. Those infected cry into the night. Their voices silenced by death.

But there were witnesses. At home there were lovers, friends or parents. Some died alone, the tree outside their bedroom the only witness. It was these people and the earth that knew them who were the witnesses of their stories. Most couldn't speak of it.

One man in San Francisco, Cleve Jones, broke the isolation. He created the 'Names Project AIDS Memorial Quilt.' People were asked to write a name on fabric, a story was too much to ask. The first panels were only a name. Slowly, very slowly, the Quilt grew and grew and grew. Over time images appeared and stories emerged. I was a quilter. I heard the stories from the caregivers at home. The stories shared were not of the illness, but the life of their loved one. Over and over again, tears streaming down their faces, the caregivers' role at home was implanted into my being. Their hearts were exposed. Over and over I listened to narratives until I snapped into fairy tale. The narrative was too small a container for what I was hearing. So, come along with me to my little corner of the world…

Key Words

AIDS – empathy – caregiver – fairy tale – healing – heart – home – legacy – well-being

*****

1 Quilting and Remembrance

Once upon a time a long, long time ago gently, slowly, quietly by witnessing and listening to the stories of others, their voice gives me mine. An unexpected

 | DOI:10.1163/9789004396067_004

format appears. It expresses the depths of love, fear, sorrow and isolation the AIDS epidemic unleashed in those caregivers at home who stayed and chose to love.

Initially I offer what I know. I am a quilter. When a 'Names Project AIDS Memorial Quilt Project'[1] opens in the city where I live, my language is visual, one of an artist expert in her craft with the capacity to hear stories and to transmute this lived tragedy into something beautiful onto a fabric panel 3'×6'. It begins with the name of a loved one. Slowly, mostly women and gay men come to workshops. Quietly they tell their stories and gently we stitch a portrait. Although there is a time when a woman with bright red hair bounds into the room with gusto and states, 'I don't know how to sew and don't want to learn, but I want a panel made for a dear friend.' I smile. 'Tell me the story.' The isolation is broken.

After months pass, I look up. I see on the ellipse in Washington D.C. hundreds of panels, later thousands, gently resting together.[2]

The beauty of each one is a beacon of love. Imagine the courage it takes, especially at the beginning of the epidemic, not only to make a panel, but then to let it go. It is now public.

Quilts were traditionally woman's work at home. Patterns were created from the local landscape and called 'Grandma's Flower Garden,' 'Log Cabin' or 'Church Steps.' Material from worn-out clothing was reused. When the chores of the day were done, women gathered to sew. Between the gentle chatter, something beautiful was created. Quietly a child's bed was covered bringing a sense of comfort and well-being.

What is this sense of comfort and well-being worth? What power does it hold? Value and power are defined one way by the mind and another way by the heart. The mind says money. The heart says love. The mind says authority. The heart says authenticity. The heart's voice, felt just before thought, has been bullied by the mind recently and may need another universal language to release it.

My first heart language appears in visual form as a quilt. The Names Project taps into an ancient memory. A quilt is made in the home, just pick up needle and thread and begin. Old pathways open. Seamlessly I participate in a panel creation. I am guided by the stories. Our hearts beat as one. The result is a co-creation honouring the life of a loved one who has died from AIDS. A new word

1 San Francisco gay rights activist, Cleve Jones conceived of the 'AIDS Memorial Quilt' in November of 1985. In June of 1987, with Mike Smith and others, he went on to formally create the 'NAMES Project Foundation.'

2 History of the Quilt can be found at: www.namesprojectfoundation.org.

is needed now. I invent 'inamore.' The inamore, or inner circle of family, friends and lovers who become caregivers, the people at home between doctors' visits and hospital stays, now have a project on which to focus their grief and love with skills they already have. Feminine power and wisdom is needed now, a steadfast, fierce love.

Ego is put aside. No one knows who has made a panel. A case in point is at one of the first displays in my city of Portland, Maine, there is a display in a large, open, indoor arena. Quilts hang from its walls and on the floor. Eight panels are sewn together to make a 12'×12' quilt. There are over fifty quilts at this display. Schools are busing students over. Students' attitudes are felt… a day off from school to see some quilt. By the time they reach the back of the room the Quilt has worked its magic as silence fills the room. I am at a table sewing on a panel, when a young girl comes over. 'I want to make a panel,' she says. 'Now?' was my question. 'Yes.'

It just so happens I have a bolt of muslin in the trunk of my car, which seems to be normal. I go out and bring the material back into the building. The hug, tears, and emotional release are instantaneous. When the tears stop, the story begins. Her Aunt Shelly had died from AIDS. Her family never even mentions her name. It is as if she had never existed. But the girl remembers. So, we get down on the floor and cut the muslin into the right size for a panel. She takes some magic markers and begins. She draws balloons, hearts and rainbows. Then she writes, 'Aunt Shelly.' At least three times within the ten minutes it takes for her to complete the panel, she looks up. 'Nobody will know who made this panel?' I always reassure her that no one knows who made any panel. 'Are you sure?' 'Yes. I am sure.' When she finishes, I tell her that if it is to join the national Quilt, we need a short biography to accompany the panel. A friend of hers hears me, looks at her and says, 'Hey, we can do that in study hall and bring it back after school.' That is exactly what they do. The panel is now part of the national Quilt. I don't believe she realizes how courageous she was.

After several years of making panels and receiving panels made at home, listening endlessly to stories from inamore whose lives are altered by the experience, I begin sharing these stories before the viewing of the Quilt. My voice deepens the experience. The narrative, combined with the beauty of the panels opens hearts even wider. Little do I know how deep I can go. The very act of sharing brings people to me. Whispered voices speak a name or tell their story. These are people who hadn't the courage to make a panel. The ever after began to stir as I go deeper. As my heart begins to expand to receive all I am hearing I shape-shift not in body, but into an ancient story format.

I am asked to write these stories down. I refuse. I believe nothing is as powerful as the experience. I am wrong. The heart has another language. One night

I put pen to paper and out comes, 'once upon a time and not very long ago…' What is this? I had unexpectedly entered a new realm. Narrative has morphed into a fairy tale, another universal language lying dormant in my bones. It has woken up!

2 The Fairy Tale Emerges

Once upon a time and not very long ago, there lived a queen from the Land of Meld. Queen Eladora had grown up in the palace, although surrounded by many, she was very lonely. Everyone fussed over her, yet her heart did not open. She would often sit at the window seat of her room. An ancient white pine tree grew outside her window. She knew if she were ever to feel love, she needed to leave the castle walls. The safest place for that first step seemed to be into the branches of the white pine. Out she went.

When she sat in the branches of the tree it brought her an aliveness she had never felt before. It was as if they were breathing together. She affectionately called the tree Bolisar. She felt its age, its roots capturing the vibrations of the earth. They came up through its trunk and out through its beautiful long, pine needle fingers to the sky. She spent many hours in the tree learning its language, and she shared her dream of looking for love. The tree was sensitive to the feelings of loss from a new illness in the land of Meld. Its roots picked up the salted moisture from tears. The message flowed through its bark. Sometimes it was so strong it threw Eladora from its branches. The message was clear and she learned to trust it. In place of death grew love.

Eladora sent out a call throughout the land. It was a call spread by eagle by day and owl by night. Any human being who had lost a loved one through this new illness must search their hearts for the words, pictures and patterns that reminded them of the person lost which would be stitched onto fabric. The message was that they had the power to create this new form of love, but in so doing must give it away and share it with the world, so all could feel their love. Not many had the courage at first, but their hearts were so full, just writing a name brought a smile. Each remembered in their own way.

Every day and night Eagle and Owl came by. As everyone looked up to the sky in fear of their work being taken too soon, slowly a strange thing happened. They began to notice the coming of the evening star. It gave them the courage to let go and share their love. Yes, the star lives on, even if you don't see it all the time. Each time the evening star appeared, they remembered their loved one. Now Eladora, touched by love in this new form, began to share the stories with the world, passing on what was good.

One day as Queen Eladora was sitting in Bolisar's branches, a woman walked by and rested by the tree. She sat down, embraced by Bolisar's roots. She was carrying a case from which she took a stringed instrument. She caressed the wooden frame and began playing and singing, unaware of Eladora's presence above:

> *'We were blended on that loving day*
> *Never knowing you weren't to stay.*
> *Your body began wasting away*
> *But I wanted more.*
> *People said you were strange*
> *And I should leave.*
> *The fear in me was strong*
> *To pull me away…I knew it wouldn't be long*
> *But I wanted more.*
> *So, I stayed.*
> *The pain you suffered lasted several years.*
> *Mine was a lifetime of running with my fear.*
> *Who was more ill, I couldn't say.*
> *You made me face life in a different way*
> *And I wanted more.*
> *When your pain was over and I felt*
> *Your spirit soar,*
> *I knew I had more.*
> *More love in my heart,*
> *More strength in my being,*
> *More songs to be sung*
> *And the courage for really living.*
> *I knew I had more.'*

As the woman sang, she kept feeling what she thought were drops of rain on her skin. But it was a beautiful, sunny day. Then one landed on her mouth. It was salty. She looked up and spied Eladora who smiled back and said, "Be at peace." The woman put away her instrument and was gone.

Without a thought this ancient pathway opened to a universal format belonging to every culture.[3] The intensity of the AIDS epidemic has brought forth a new fairy tale into the light of day. Narrative could not contain what I was hearing and feeling. As I go deeper to take in the immensity of the loss, the

3 To view a wonderful history of oral culture, please see Alexandra Fidyk, 'Stories of Journeys Home: Reuniting the Ancestors, Images, and Darkness,' in this volume.

heart speaks its truth as fairy tale. Once leaving the true realm of narrative and entering the truth realm of fairy tale, a life lived is affirmed in a way the heart can hear and love deepens. Nature is the keystone. Our human centred world expands to include all of creation. We belong where we are. We are not alone. Help always comes and we are good enough just the way we are. We are part of the harmony of all creation. All this is revealed through the story. Images move until a story unfolds. The more thought is shut down; the deeper the truth can rise. Fairy tale expands our vision of who we are and our place in the world.

The first time I try telling a fairy tale is in a middle school. The class has just seen the Quilt. As I talk to a class I go back and forth between narrative and fairy tale. Then I hear boys have this exchange, 'What is real?' 'Whatever you believe.'

This keeps me going, for there is much to stop me. In the early nineties' I am at a retreat for social workers on the front line after someone was diagnosed with AIDS. We bring a few panels and I share a fairy tale. The response is immediate. It is one of rage! How dare I trivialize what is happening. They shun me for the rest of the weekend. The one who saves me is a woman living with AIDS. She whispers, 'When I die, will you turn me into a fairy tale?'

I never saw her again, but when the next woman with AIDS entered my life, I create a fairy tale for her. Abandoned by family, it becomes her legacy.

Once upon a time a long, long time ago in a place far, far away lived a daisy named Rose. She was one of many daisies on a rolling field filled with wild flowers. Along with the daisies were Buttercups, Queen Anne's Lace and Black-Eyed Susan. The insects were buzzing around, tickling under the petals of all the flowers. There was much gaiety and singing and giggling. If you were quiet and listened closely, you could hear it. All the rooted plants knew their place. Their roots spread far and wide through the earth. But all of a sudden, the earth shook and nothing was ever the same again.

Our daisy named Rose pulled in her roots and hung onto the earth for dear life. When all became quiet again, she looked around. Most of the field was gone. She checked herself from stem to leaf. She was intact. Then she noticed movement. It didn't seem rooted, yet it was going so slow, it could have been. It took two weeks for a snail to reach our daisy named Rose. 'Who are you?' she asked.

She was soon very sorry she asked. It took twenty-seven minutes for the snail to tell her its name. 'My name is Adolph and I'm looking for the ocean.' Oh, thought our daisy name Rose. I can't talk to him at all. It will take a lifetime. But then he began to sing and as long as he was singing, his tempo was much quicker.

'What a wonder to know
That you grow standing still.

I crawl with my shell
Seeking sounds and smells
Of the ocean.'

Ocean, thought our daisy named Rose. What is that? Then a butterfly came by looking for a place to land and found our daisy named Rose. She landed and spied the snail. Before our daisy named Rose could stop her, she asked. 'Who are you?' There went Adolph for twenty-seven minutes. 'From now on ask him to sing to you,' said Rose. Then Adolph began to sing, 'What a wonder to know that you fly in the sky. I crawl with my shell seeking sounds and smells of the ocean.'

Our daisy named Rose asked the butterfly if she could see the ocean. When she said yes, Rose asked if she could guide Adolph there. Butterfly agreed. Rose watched as they left, listening to Adolph sing, 'What a wonder to know…'

Our daisy named Rose looked around, wiggled a few petals and stood up as straight as she could. She swayed with a gentle wind, testing the security of her roots. Then she felt something nibbling her stem.

It was a family of ants and they were all arguing. 'What's the problem?' Rose asked. Well, their tunnels had collapsed, and no one could agree on where the new one should be built. Rose sighed, 'Aren't you lucky you are here to argue? Shame on you!' They became quiet. Out of the field bounded a bunny. 'Now follow her, said Rose. She will lead you to great tunnelling dirt. Behave and be thankful.' In silent single file they followed the bunny.

Our daisy named Rose was getting weary. It was getting cooler and her stem was getting softer. She knew what this meant. Soon she would be in darkness, just roots. One by one her petals dropped off. They were carried by the wind down Adolph's path to the ocean.

Winnie's family never comes to pick up her ashes. She has a buddy who keeps them and finally comes up with a day to spread Winnie's ashes into the sea. When we all arrive, she says it is Winnie's birthday, so we all sing Happy Birthday to Winnie as her ashes blow over the sea.

Winnie's fairy tale comes to me effortlessly, but I need to know her story. There is no tale without listening to the narrative of another. My offering as storyteller is to shift into the ancient format revealed by the heart… I move from head to heart, from thought to belief and tell a new story…

Only because the AIDS epidemic is so intense, do I go into fairy tale. I realize I am the keeper, as are we all, of a lost language possessed by any culture around the world lying dormant in our bones and being very patient. Not only do we need to believe we are good enough just the way we are, but our world needs to embrace the heart. The heart is home to our authentic self and it does not know how to lie. Your story as fairy tale helps you and those who love you to make the shift into the heart. The storyteller with the narrative meets the storyteller with the fairy tale and together we create a loving gift into the world. I have invented a new word to describe this story. It is a hupa tale.[4]

The voice of the storyteller is not only to chronicle and share the narrative, but to release an old coping mechanism to help us heal. There is an ancient, universal voice of the heart connected to a spiritual truth embedded in all of us and in all of creation. The voice of the heart needs to be heard, not quick or loud or big, but slow and gentle and quiet. It has been silenced for too long. It must pour out one story at a time. When you come home to yourself, then the physical dwelling of home can be a place of comfort, well-being and belonging for all who live there and all who visit.

Welcome to my home, where there is only love, it is noble to cry and no one is alone. It is a place where everyone's inner light shines and any spell blocking it is broken, one hupa tale at a time.

Once this process is awakened, as a storyteller, the focus is on the other. I apply this focus as I branch out away from AIDS after ten years. The last piece of wisdom from the epidemic is spoken to me again by a middle school student. 'There is one thing worse than AIDS. It's Afraids.'

3 An Antidote to Fear

Afraids is everywhere, especially when someone we love becomes ill. Most of the care is for the person diagnosed. But, as caregiver at home or inamore there is something healing we can do without a thought when someone's inner light is blocked by fear we can tell someone their story as a hupa tale. Your ego is put aside as you give the story as a gift. You too are afraid. By giving a gift to another you are given many unexpected gifts as something inside you shifts. I can listen to a narrative thoughtfully. As I create the fairy tale I let go of thought. This is a shift into vision. I can see a landscape from which a story emerges as well as a sense of belonging. You see love is not a thought. The story is then given to you to read or tell to your loved one. It is my creation, but your voice, presence, and love that are transmitted as well. The story becomes a pause, a moment of well-being no matter what the outcome. It is an oasis to be returned to at will and passed on.

---

4 Hupa is derived from the author's imagination. There is no relation to the Hupa tribe in northern California except by sweet accident.

It is my belief, which gives me hope, that there are many like me around the world whom I will never know, living their lives, each in their own way, infused with a fierce, quiet and steadfast love at home.

4 Hupa Tales

The following are three hupa stories. They begin with a short narrative of the person, then the tale. I ask that you try to forget the narrative tale, let it go, before you read the hupa tale. That is what I do when I create the new story. It is my belief that it has already become a part of my subconscious and is invisibly guiding the story. This allows for new images to surface that may have been blocked by the mind. We just need to let go of control. Let us begin without a thought.

Nichole grew up in a large, poor family. She was the only one of the children who broke the cycle.

Once upon a time a long, long time ago in a place far, far away it just kept raining. Cobblestone streets were filled with puddles. Everything was wet and smelled wet. Days were various shades of grey. Rats scurried around, their tails leaving a trail of water behind. Dampness soaked into everything. A family of turtles found their way into the city, hopelessly lost. They had wandered far from home. The puddles were never deep enough. Food was scarce. They were slow. The pace of the city was confusing and they did what they could to survive.

One of the youngest turtles poked her head out from beneath her shell. She smelled the air and tasted the rain. Something was missing. What was it? It was a whisper from the wind. A memory stirred as fleeting as the breeze.

She was a curious one and often went exploring alone. Her pace was a little bit faster than the rest of her family. As she turned a corner, she ran into a frog, who had lived in the neighbourhood for a long time. Turtle asked if there was any water around deeper than a puddle. He said, 'Absolutely!' He slowed his hop down, so she could keep up. They arrived at a small pond. 'I'll race you,' she said. He looked at her shocked! He didn't believe 'race' was even in her vocabulary. Then he chuckled to himself. No one had ever beaten him in the water, let alone the poky turtle. The race was on. They both jumped in. She felt great and soon glided past a disbelieving frog. Once in the water she was powerful, graceful, fast and happy. She began coming to the pond every day, but there was still this gnawing sense that something was missing. Every day she learned something new and everyday was an adventure. Her family refused to turn the corner, but no one could stop her from going.

Time passed. Now she had many friends to encourage her. She became known as the adventuress. Bird came by one day and told her stories that his father had told him which were told to him by his father, which were told to him by his father. They were stories of a place called 'the sea.' It was a place where the sun shone and one could swim and never touch bottom, but also had many dangers. Something stirred inside our turtle and her heart did a flip-flop. Nothing could be more dangerous than staying put. It would be an adventure and she was an adventuress. She left her family, guided solely by a story from a bird.

It was hard and slow going and she hid in her shell often. But one day the ground became warm and soft and sandy. There was a new fragrance in the air. She looked up and there was water as far as the eye could see. She approached cautiously and dove in. She swam until she tired, then sunned herself on nearby rocks. The water felt perfect. It had a taste, the missing something was salt. She played and explored her new home. She was after all an adventuress. As she gained confidence, she went out even further. Zipping by her swam a sleek creature with large brown eyes and an invitation to play. She introduced herself. 'I am seal and I am an adventuress.' Turtle couldn't believe her ears, 'Me too!' They played and explored together, both the happiest they had ever been. One day turtle dove down further than ever before and disappeared. She reached the bottom of the ocean floor and began exploring alone. She went into the netting of a wooden crate and couldn't get out. She was trapped. Seal eventually saw her, but turtle was too far down. She kept herself in sight so turtle wouldn't feel alone, then went back home to see if anyone could figure out what to do. Word was sent to other sea turtles. This was not good. Seal ached for turtle, but she was free to come and go. She made sure she swam as close as she dared, so turtle wouldn't give up.

One day a boat came by and men hauled up the trap. They saw turtle and threw her back into the sea. As she rested with a family of sea turtles, seal approached. They went off together and all the old feelings returned. 'Forgive me for not doing more,' said seal. 'There is nothing to forgive,' said turtle. They swam off to seal's old haunts and settled down. 'Once in a while I just might have to turn a corner,' said turtle. 'We'll do it together,' said seal.

This next story was created for John. He is an avid outdoorsman. His constant companion was a dog named Rapid. When Rapid became ill and died, this was the story given to him as a gift.

Once upon a time a time a long, long time ago in a place far, far away a man sat tending an open fire. He was at the edge of a field, next to a river. He sat crouched down, poking the fire with a stick from time to time. He was alone. The river was high yet calm. Up from its banks walked a turtle. In its mouth was a pebble from the bottom of the river. If you looked closely, in just the right light, you could see a silk thread running through it. It went as high as the stars and as deep as the river. The turtle dropped it at the man's feet. 'Excuse me sir.' It spoke. There was no answer. 'Hum, hum, excuse me,' he spoke a little louder. There was no answer. He just about popped out of her shell. 'Excuse me!' The man looked down. Now our turtle put on her very best voice, 'You are alone and I have brought you this pebble. If you wish I can turn it into a creature with three traits of your choice, but after doing the three courageous acts using these traits, it will turn back into a pebble.' The man agreed. He thought and then spoke, 'I want a creature who is gentle.' The pebble began to spin. I want a creature who is funny.' The pebble began to get larger. 'I want a creature who is loyal.' The pebble then turned into a dog. The man was totally delighted by his new companion. He thanked turtle, who slid back into the river. Off the two went.

They hadn't gone far when night approached. They camped and quickly went to sleep, the man and his gentle, funny, loyal dog. Soon the dog awoke to the sound of a woodpecker in a tree. It was odd for a night sound. She was all ears. The man snored on. Then she heard a snake slithering closer. She jumped up without making a sound. She moved from side to side distracting the snake. When the snake slithered one way, she jumped the other way. Away they went far from the campsite until the snake was plumb worn out. Our dog scampered back to the campsite and fell fast asleep. The man snored on.

Years passed and the two were inseparable. He remembered what the turtle had said, but didn't believe the dog had done any courageous act, so thought they had plenty of time together. Off they would go, the man and his gentle, funny, loyal dog. One night as they lay sleeping inside a cabin the howl of wolves could be heard in the distance. It was a common sound and the man snored on. Soon the sound became closer. The dog awoke. A wolf was sniffing around the cabin. There was a window partially open. Our dog got up on her hind legs just as the wolf peered in, they were nose to nose, scaring them both! The wolf flew back to the hills and the dog flew under the bed. The man, well, he snored on.

Time passed with many adventures and the bond between the two deepened. He was a man with a gentle, funny, loyal dog. One night as they lay sleeping, the man in a bed and the dog curled up on a braided rug next to him, there was a scratching at the door. The man snored on. Out dog went to open it with her paw. Outside was a pack of dogs begging her to come with them and be free. She looked back at the sleeping man, closed the door and curled up onto the braided rug. The man snored on.

The next morning the man awoke and on the braided rug was a pebble. It had a silk thread going through it, up to the stars. He remembered the turtle's words. Grief stricken, he brought the pebble back to the river and dropped it in.

The third story was told to me directly. Ed's life was falling apart and he didn't know where to turn. As he spoke it was revealed that he was a gambler, womanizer and heavy drinker whose second marriage was falling apart. I created this story for him.

Once upon a time a long, long time ago in a place far, far away it was winter. A herd of deer stood at the edge of a meadow ready to flee to the protection of the woods nearby at a moment's notice. They stood there knee deep in snow, soaking in the warmth of the sun. This was a hard winter and they were thin and hungry. This place had been their winter home for many generations. Gathered were old, young, male, female, brother, sisters, aunts, uncles, cousins, etc. There was one stag in this herd with an impressive rack of antlers that had served him well and had withstood many battles both within and outside the herd. His impulse this winter was to leave in search of food for all.

Without looking back on this cold, sunny day, he took off across the meadow. His instincts were keen and he soon saw tracks in the snow. He followed them to a large tree where they disappeared. His body tense, he looked around. A sound came from inside the tree. Surely there was food to be shared there. Without listening any further, he put his head down and butted that tree over and over again, leaving scars on the tree and several broken antlers on the ground. Bear was inside and just chuckled. He had tried to tell the stag the only food around was right inside him. But the stag wasn't listening. The tree withstood all the insults, as exhausted our stag walked away. Night moved in and his keen instincts found another tree under which he bedded for the night. In the silence of the night starlight came down to cover him. When he awoke, mushrooms and fungus were aglow around the tree and he ate heartily.

He looked around trying to get his bearings. (No pun intended.) He heard a rustling sound and saw the flash of a red tail. The chase was on! Panting, fox stopped alongside of a bolder. The stag looked into its eyes. Fox, clever as he was, began talking. 'Stag, I bet there are juicier morsels than me burrowed right under this rock. I bet they have a large stash of food stored for the winter, one for me and two for you.' Fox started to say more, but stag wasn't listening. Without hesitating he butted and heaved at that stone, leaving several more antlers on the ground. Fox shook his head, dug deep and disappeared. Despondent, the stag slowly walked away. He found the bank of a frozen stream and fell asleep. In the silence of the night starlight covered him. When he awoke a small hole appeared through the iced stream. Some small fish popped through. He caught them easily and had a meal.

He looked around and his keen instincts told him to follow the stream for a while. Soon he spied several old apple trees on the other side of the stream. Slowly he made his way across using his antlers to steady him. A few were left on the ice, but he made it across. There were many apples on the ground, a few for a meal and plenty to take home. He began to eat the old fermented ones, became disoriented and lost all track of time. Days passed. When he was finally ready to leave, he put all the apples he could find on old white pine branches. With some roping vine around his neck, he began pulling them home. His keen instincts found the way. He never looked back. If he did he would have noticed that many of the apples had bounced off.

When he reached the herd, no one greeted him. They looked well. Somehow, together, they had figured out how to survive. He looked down at his feet. Green shoots were beginning to appear. Spring was being kind and came early. He had been gone a long time. He looked around. Finally, his oldest son recognized him and then his three other children. 'Dad, where are your antlers?' They were gone. Slowly his mate came forth. He began to show her what was now a meagre offering of apples. Then he stopped. He got down on his knees to meet her eyes. 'How did you do it? I am listening.'

Legend has it, if you lived in that part of the country and saw the profile of a lone stag that winter, you survived. You see the bounced apples fed many.

May inamore know the value of their work.
May hupa stories bring a sense of comfort and well-being.
May you come home to love in your heart and hearth.

Bibliography

Abram, David. *Spell of the Sensuous.* New York: Vintage Books, 1996.

Chinen, Allen. *Waking the World.* New York: Jeremy P. Thatcher/Putnam, 1996.

Erdrich, Louise. *The Master Butcher's Singing Club.* New York: Harper Collins, 2003.

Hoffman, Alice. *The Probable Future.* New York: Doubleday, 2003.

Hogan, Linda. *Power.* New York: WW Norton & Co., 1998.

Larsen, Stephen. *The Mythic Imagination.* Rochester, Vermont: Inner Traditions Intl., 1996.

Luth, Max. *Once Upon a Time on the Nature of Fairy Tales.* Bloomington, Indiana: Indiana Univ. Press, 1970.

Manitonquat (Medicine Story). *Return to Creation.* Spokane, Washington: Bear Tribe Pub., 1991.

Meyer, Rudolph. *The Wisdom of Fairy Tales.* London: Cromwell Press, 1988.

Sawyer, Ruth. *The Way of the Storyteller.* New York: Penguin Books, 1970.

Shlain, Leonard. *The Alphabet versus the Goddess: The Conflict between Word and Image.* New York: Penguin Putnam, 1998.

Smith, Alexander McCall. *Dream Angus.* New York: Canongate Pub., 2006.

Yolen, Jane. *Briar Rose.* New York: Tor/Tom Doherty Associates, 1992.

Zafon, Carlos Ruiz. *The Angel's Game.* New York: Doubleday, 2009.

CHAPTER 3

Life Story Sharing: A Therapeutic Intervention in Palliative Care

Miranda Quinney, Alison Ward and Jane Youell

Abstract

This chapter presents a personal reflection by Sharing Stories for Welbeing (SS4WB) workshop facilitator and programme founder Miranda Quinney with observational input from Alison Ward and Jane Youell of the University of Northampton following the University's evaluation of the programme in May 2015. SS4WB provides facilitated storytelling sessions in palliative care. Workshops foster life-story discussions which participants share with the group, that are delivered in a non-linear style and are based on themed topics. Groups are supported by hospice staff, who provide both pastoral and clinical care. Informal observational feedback suggested that the potential benefits for participants were improved self-esteem, feelings of being valued and of being listened to at a time of personal distress. The running of new SS4WB sessions at Watford's Peace Hospice Care gave the opportunity to conduct a formal evaluation and to understand the potential value of participation. The evaluation was conducted over five weekly sessions between May and June 2015.

Four broad evaluation themes emerged: 'pleasure'; 'what makes you, you'; 'more than just a patient'; and 'benefits beyond the group'.[1] Participants reported enjoyment and felt a sense of autonomy and control in deciding on the stories shared.[2] Sessions provided an opportunity for social engagement, giving a sense of togetherness and were a means to explore the participants' sense of self and feelings of being valued as a person, not a patient. The telling of biographical reminiscences was reported to bring positive reminders of changing times and lived experiences. Workshop engagement also led some participants to experience improved confidence and reduced social isolation, as evidenced through staff and family views and participation in new activities. SS4WB enables people in palliative care to share their life-stories in a supportive and safe environment. Participation can have positive outcomes fostering choice in the

1 Jane Youell and Alison Ward, *Sharing Stories for Wellbeing: An Evaluation.* (Northampton: Institute of Health and Wellbeing, 2015), 9.

2 Pam Morrison and Annie McGregor, 'Making and Sharing Meaning Out of Terminal Illness', in this volume.

 | DOI:10.1163/9789004396067_005

stories shared which then engenders a sense of autonomy and control, reminiscences can also bring feelings of value and self-esteem.

Key Words

Storytelling – palliative care – wellbeing – life story – training

*****

Banksy is often credited with saying: 'They say you die twice. One time when you stop breathing and a second time, a bit later on, when somebody says your name for the last time'.[3] There is confusion about the exact origin of the quote, some say the words were those of Irvin D. Yalom, others David Eagleman, and yet others that the words have been passed down through the ages. Irrespective of its source, it is the sentiment behind it that resonates.

Life Story Sharing is a way of delaying that second death by keeping the story alive. By sharing individual life stories towards the end of a life with friends and family, the teller takes control of the preservation of their part of the family's history for future generations. Whilst the practical results of this process are obvious, it is the unintentional but powerful effect on the wellbeing of the teller that is being embraced by Britain's hospice community. Over the past year over thirty hospices based in England and Wales have asked for training in the techniques developed by SS4WB when running Life Story Sharing workshops. The aim of this chapter is to share some of the learning gathered in the course of developing the workshops and when evaluating the programme. Pseudonyms are used for workshop participants where necessary to maintain confidentiality.

1 How Did the Programme Come About? Miranda's Story

The eldest child of Anglo/Iranian parents, I have grown up with the stories of their youthful globe-trotting adventures. What I hadn't realised was that so many of their friends had also had extraordinary adventures, not until I heard about them as part of a eulogy. The stories were thought-provoking and often led me to reconsider my perception of the protagonist. I wished that

3 'Banksy'. *Wikiquote*, Viewed 21 June 2018, https://en.wikiquote.org/wiki/Banksy.

I had had the opportunity to hear those stories before death, at a time when the teller was still around to talk to and to question.

I soon found that I was not alone – others in the congregation were often also hearing these stories for the first time. I set up a service to record, write and publish personal life stories. I had a lot of willing clients who wanted their parent's stories written, but I came up against a problem, a reluctance or taboo to talk about issues related to death as this made the topic more real.[4] Whilst family and friends were keen to commission me to write the life stories of their parents and grandparents, the parents and grandparents sometimes interpreted the invitation to tell and record their stories as an indication that there was a general consensus that they were about to die. Talking about death and dying is something the British public find difficult to do, so much so that Britain's National Council for Palliative Care has spearheaded Dying Matters Week, a public awareness initiative to encourage people to talk about death and dying. Despite this many remain reluctant to discuss the subject and the practical result, in terms of recording their life story, was that the story was not told, shared or recorded. We were back to the first public sharing taking place as part of a funeral. I struggled with how to overcome this powerful superstition but could not see a way through.

Several years later I was presented with an opportunity. The circumstances were quite unexpected, some might say morbid. A close family friend was diagnosed with cancer and had a short life expectancy. She was admitted to my local hospice. I knew little about hospices or the hospice movement. I had never heard of palliative care. I will openly admit that I was terrified at the prospect of my first visit to see her there. Everything that I had heard about hospices suggested that they were places to be avoided; the final stop before death, the Hotel California of the medical world where you'd check in but never out again.[5] I was taken to the In-Patient Unit. There were nurses and medical equipment, but there was no *ward*. Each patient had a private room, well decorated, comfortable and, most importantly, there was none of the antiseptic smell so often associated with hospitals and care homes.

As I visited my friend Beverley again and again over the next few weeks I was impressed by the level of care she received. When she died a few weeks later, I wanted to do something for the hospice which had cared for her so magnificently. I approached the hospice manager and offered my services as a

4 Marilyn Kirshbaum, Ian Carey, Brigid Purcell and Seamus Nash, 'Talking About Dying and Death: A Focus Group Study to Explore a Local Community Perspective', *Nursing Reports* 1.1 (2011): 29–34.

5 Eagles, 'Hotel California', Hotel California (Asylum, 1977).

biographer. This entailed helping patients to record and share their life stories. As hospice patients, all workshop participants were aware that death could be imminent but at least the psychological impediment of talking about death was removed.

I received a speedy and positive response to my offer and was surprised to be introduced to the Hospice Day Services Manager. My limited experience of the hospice to date was of the In-Patient Unit, which had supported my assumption that all hospice service users were on the point of death. My assumption was wrong. I was shown around the hospice and it was explained to me that the In-Patient Unit constituted a very small part of the services offered. Indeed, at that particular hospice, a far higher proportion of time was spent working out in the community with the patients in their own homes. In addition, they also offered Day Care support for both patients and carers. Furthermore, the range of individuals entitled to benefit from the services offered by the hospice was far broader than I had imagined. Rather than working only with those with a very limited life expectancy, the hospice also had a variety of services that they offered to the patient's family and support networks, including respite care and ultimately bereavement counselling. The next surprise was to discover that it was not just those patients with an extremely short life expectancy who could go to the hospice and ask for support. The day care service's key criteria was that a patient should have a limited life expectancy and in some cases this could be three, four or five years. It was in this later context that the hospice wanted to take up my offer to write life stories; as a service for patients and carers using day care services.

2 The Programme

I was unsure as to the precise form the service would take. One thing however was clear, the service would differ from that offered by narrative therapists where clients are encouraged to organize and give meaning to their experiences through the medium of story with the intention of further shaping their lives and relationships.[6] As a storyteller and biographer, I was not a trained counsellor, nor was I an oral historian recording full length biographies to be archived for future research. I experimented with different ways of encouraging people to tell. Working one to one had the advantage that both I and the participant could really concentrate on the stories being shared but had the

6 Jeffery Kottler, *Stories We've Heard, Stories We've Told: Life-Changing Narratives in Therapy and Everyday Life* (Oxford: Oxford University Press, 2015).

disadvantage that the participant often lapsed into a form of narrative which asked for a therapist's response. Inviting individuals to share anecdotes with me on a one-off basis as part of a large group activity did not give the activity sufficient weight.

What was eventually devised was a workshop programme run over a five-week period for a small closed group of up to six patients. Keeping the group closed preserved the group dynamic and provided a sense of safety for participants when sharing their stories. Whilst holding the workshops in series, rather than as a one-off event meant that participants sometimes missed sessions, the benefit was that they got to know each other well over the weeks. It soon became clear that given the diverse range of backgrounds of participants, following a linear format for life story sharing would be problematic. Participants came from widely differing cultural and socio-economic backgrounds, I could make no assumptions about the experiences of their past. Accordingly, I turned to themes, with a simple theme for each session to which I hoped each participant could relate. Even then I had to consider carefully whether the themes carried with them an obvious element which might result in a participant feeling uncomfortable about the sharing process. For example, on one occasion I suggested the theme of holidays, assuming this would be relevant to all participants. Observing the session, I soon realised it had been a mistake; the lady who followed the story of a grand world cruise with her camping trip looked uncomfortable and apologetic. Next time around, I changed the session that had been about holidays to one entitled celebrations. That worked a lot better. Other themes I used include the senses, nature and colour. At the end of each session, I would set the next week's theme and participants came with a story to tell from any stage in their life. The result was participants chose which stories to share from any period of their life. The experience felt positive and uplifting.

Each workshop was an hour and a half long, run at the same time and at the same place on consecutive weeks giving the programme consistency. Whilst I facilitated the workshops I also received supervision from the hospice's senior social worker. Access to supervision was crucial. As a palliative care specialist she was available to provide emotional support to participants and also to me as a facilitator.

As facilitator I took long-hand notes of the stories told in each session. As I did not record them electronically, they were not verbatim transcripts. My reasons for this approach were simple; firstly, the technology itself can be intimidating and I am not very good at managing it, secondly the time and therefore cost involved to type a verbatim note is significant and could have been enough to scupper the entire process. After each session I typed up my notes into a simple word document, trying to be as faithful as possible to what I had been told. I did not conduct any additional research, fact check, or make any observations or judgements concerning what I had heard.

Following the final session each participant received a simple folder containing type written copies of the stories that they had told. At the start of the workshop series I made it clear that the notes were my best effort at writing down what they had said. I explained that I would not be conducting any additional research or checking their account of events. There was an acknowledgement that I may have misheard certain statements but that any mistakes were unintentional. I included a disclaimer with the final written format. As it turned out, the documents were received with delight, none of the participants asked for changes or corrections to be made.

3 Next Steps: Sharing the Programme

In observing the weekly sessions, the social worker soon took me to one side and asked whether I had any idea what I was doing. A flutter of fear coursed through my body as I worried that perhaps there was some protocol I was unaware of that applied in the palliative care sector about which I knew nothing. After all I had created a programme from grass roots rather than adapting it from an existing activity. I felt instinctively that what I was doing was good. Patients seemed to enjoy it and didn't want to leave at the end of each session. However I was acutely aware that I had no training as a therapist or in any form of counselling, I was very aware that there was no obvious precedent for what I was doing and that as a result there was an element of creating the process as we went along. Quickly responding to the concern in my face, the social worker smiled and said:

> I'm watching the patients both inside and outside of these sessions. I can see that they are responding very well. I can see them becoming more confident, their self-esteem is growing, I'd say that their general wellbeing is improving and I think that these life story sessions are a key factor. We need to share this with others.[7]

My goal from that point was to find a way to make life story sharing sessions available in other hospices. This was not something I could do alone. A solution

7 Extract from Miranda Quinney supervision, 2011. Contemporaneous note following supervision.

was to train a team of practitioners who, in turn, could train their colleagues. The resulting cascade could then make it possible for every hospice patient to have the opportunity to tell and save their story. In 2014 Hospice UK, the national charity for hospice care displayed a poster about the work at their annual conference. They went on to invite me to speak at their 2015 conference, which provided an international audience of individuals responsible for the strategic development and care in 220 or more hospices. Persuading the chief executives of these hospices to adopt a group storytelling programme as part of their in-house services for patients was going to need more than enthusiasm and anecdotal feedback. I needed evidence.

An introduction was made by Hospice UK to Alison Ward of the University of Northampton which provided the solution to that need. Alison agreed to take my evaluation proposal to her team and they in turn approved the funding to conduct an evaluation of the sharing stories for wellbeing programme.

3.1 *Evaluation*

Alison Ward and colleague Jane Youell used a mixed method approach in conducting the Evaluation.[8] Patients (n=5) were asked to complete a paper questionnaire prior to the commencement of the workshop series and a second paper questionnaire was completed after the final workshop had taken place. Two participant observations were undertaken by the evaluation team; one mid-way through the workshop series and one at the end. Finally, participating patients (n=3), hospice staff (n=3) and a patient family member (n=1) attended face to face interviews with the researchers.

Following presentation of the evaluation outcomes at the 2015 Hospice UK conference, I was invited to run a series of one day master classes for clinicians, spiritual advisors, counsellors, palliative care nurses and volunteers interested in offering life story sharing in end of life care. Currently, as I write this, over ten per cent of the UK's hospices now have access to a trained life story group facilitator and the number continues to grow. International interest in the programme is also growing with palliative care professionals from Singapore, Hong Kong and Canada also expressing interest in developing the programme for use in their own practice areas.

8 John W. Creswell, et al., 'Advanced Mixed Methods Research Designs', *Handbook of Mixed Methods in Social and Behavioral Research*, ed. Abbas Tashakkori and Charles Teddlie (Thousand Oaks, CA: Sage, 2003), 209–240.

4 Why Do It?: The Observations of Jane Youell and Alison Ward of Northampton University

Analysis of the results, feedback and observations supported the key themes we had observed in the course of running the life story sharing workshops:

- Participants enjoyed the sessions;
- Sessions provided an opportunity for participants to be truly heard;
- Participants experienced a renewed sense of identity beyond the patient;
- Participants felt that the sessions were one of the few situations where they were fully in control.[9]

4.1 *Enjoyment*

Groups were closed with no more than six members, each of whom joined the group following referral from a hospice clinician. The closed group format, as Mary Anne Boyd suggests, guaranteed no new additions to the group in the course of the workshop series, thereby maintaining the group dynamic, promoting group bonding and cohesion.[10] Referral into the group by palliative care staff helped ensure an appropriate mix of attendees. There were no strict participant criteria applied other than an acknowledgment on a practical level that participants would need to be able to communicate verbally. Attendees of the hospice day care were offered leaflets about the programme and invited to apply to join the next available workshop series. Coordination was carried out by the hospice creative activities coordinator. Limiting the numbers helped create a supportive environment. What we observed was a rapid development of friendship bonds. Participants seemed enthusiastic about catching up with each other from week to week and some arranged to meet each other socially between sessions. The development of social networks, the enjoyment of meeting people and developing friendships was emphasised by the evaluation, where the sessions were reported to be fun and engaging and their friendship bonds increased confidence and rapport with others.[11]

As the weeks passed the participants became more attuned to the needs and interests of their co-participants. At most sessions, participants were able to share two or more stories. Whilst the first tale was usually something prepared in advance of the session, the second and sometimes third stories were often

---

9 Youell and Ward, *Sharing Stories for Wellbeing: An Evaluation*, 7.

10 Mary Ann Boyd, *Psychiatric Nursing: Contemporary Practice* (Philadelphia: Lippincott, Williams and Wilkins, 2005).

11 Youell and Ward, *Sharing Stories for Wellbeing: An Evaluation*, 9.

inspired by the stories shared by co-participants. One example took place in an introductory session where participants were encouraged to introduce themselves to one another by telling a story inspired by something they were either wearing or had with them. Jane introduced herself to the group using her art gallery membership card. Henry followed on pulling a postcard from his wallet of a painting in an exhibition he had been visiting when he met his wife. On another occasion George told his story of celebration describing D-Day in his home village. Alice followed on with her experiences of Liberation in Belgium. George listened with rapt attention; he had never heard a first-hand account of the end of the War from someone from another country.

Participants clearly enjoyed both telling their own stories and listening to those of others in the group. Where some participants in the first session had expressed difficulty in finding a story to tell, by session three they were clearly engaged, allowing the stories to flow, one leading to the next. The role of the facilitator throughout was to ensure all participants were heard and that there was some link to the theme for the week. From time to time the discussion would take an unexpected turn, as in the week when the theme of celebrations led to a family visit to Mexico, a discussion of the Day of the Dead and then a very upbeat discussion of the variety of coffins on offer. This was an occasion when the facilitator turned to the supervisor for emotional support. By the end of the workshop series, trying to draw the sessions to a close had become quite challenging.

4.2 *Therapeutic Activity vs. Therapy*

The key difficulty with running a closed group, particularly in palliative and end of life care is that group numbers can dwindle to just one or two. Participants may be too unwell to attend or may have died in the intervening week. As a facilitator with a small group of one or possibly two, it was important to guard against drifting away from the therapeutic activity into offering narrative therapy. With just one participant working with the facilitator there was a real risk that the self-censorship which existed in the group environment no longer applied. It was harder to stop the story from becoming more self-reflective with the teller potentially turning to the facilitator as a counsellor or therapist. Using a thematic approach to each session helped to avoid this pitfall. Even where just one participant attends, themes such as the senses, colour and nature can all be extended to encourage a series of linked stories and allow the facilitator to redirect the participant away from a timeline.

4.3 *Identity beyond Being the Patient*

Post session feedback suggested that participants noticed the very real interest we as facilitators had in their stories, they felt that they were being seen as individuals rather than as patients. This became an important aspect of their enjoyment of the programme. As a facilitator I had to find a way to avoid focussing on the illness. The solution was quite simple, to not be told the diagnosis or prognosis of any of the workshop participants. Sessions started not with the more usual 'how are you?' as that invites a response reverting to illness, but instead something on the lines of 'how lovely to see you' and a quick sidestep to the theme for the day's session. This way it became easy to see past the illness to the person and an equal. In the process, the patient becomes a storyteller and their identity goes beyond that of the 'patient', finding their connections as mothers, sons, teachers, etc. One memorable session led to sharing recipes where one participant, Jean, found great joy in sharing her best cake recipe and, in a later session, bringing in a cake to share with the group. This not only brought with it a sense of purpose but also a sense of self-identity as a provider and baker, linking to Jean's former notions of self and not just her current identity as a patient.[12]

4.4 *Being Heard*

Many of the participants joining a life story sharing group announce at the start of the first session that they have nothing to say and question why anyone would be interested in their stories. When asked why they have chosen to attend, they might explain that they would like to listen to the stories others have to tell. They simply lack or have lost the confidence to tell their own story, to know that it will be interesting and of value. The key is to encourage them to tell. The story sessions can develop a sense of self-worth and confidence in being given an opportunity to have your story and your voice heard. This has a strong association with the patient vs. person concept already discussed, as the story process encourages people to share aspects of their life story and be more than the person with an illness and instead draw on care which is multi-disciplinary and help to maintain identity.[13] Being heard is not just about sharing your stories but also knowing that these stories will be heard after the person has passed away, giving a sense of legacy or passing on to the next generation. This feeling of sharing experiences before they are lost was expressed by participants in the evaluation who saw value in telling their story, as one storyteller stated, to 'pass them onto future generations of the family.'[14]

---

12 Kathrin Ohnsorge, Heike Gudat and Christoph Rehmann-Sutter, 'What a Wish to Die Can Mean: Reasons, Meanings and Functions of Wishes to Die, Reported from 30 Qualitative Case Studies of Terminally Ill Cancer Patients in Palliative Care', *BMC Palliative Care* 13.38 (2014): 1–4.

13 Peter G. Coleman, 'Adjustment in Later Life', *Ageing in Society*, ed. John Bond and Peter G. Coleman (London: Sage Publications, 1990), 97–132.

14 Youell and Ward, *Sharing Stories for Wellbeing: An Evaluation*, 13.

This not only provides a sense of self-worth through passing on lessons learned but also strengthens self-identity as the person can be seen as more than their family role-identity through the stories.[15] Furthermore, sharing the stories can have a profound effect on the way the clinician or care giver sees the patient. On one occasion, George was wheeled into the session by one of the hospice nurses. She asked if she could stay for the session and all present gave their consent to this. She went on to hear George tell tales of his days as a young competitive cyclist regularly travelling hundreds of miles on a bicycle with solid wheels. The nurse was fascinated and acknowledged that this made her consider George in a new light. She and George went on to spend quite some time together looking through his cycling photos. I often wonder if hospital based geriatric care would change if nurses could be given the opportunity to hear their patients 'stories'?

4.5 *Finding the Time to Listen*

Participants often say that the stories they tell in the group have not been shared for many years, if at all. They explain that they are concerned about encroaching on the busy lives of friends and family. Having now listened to hundreds of stories, my belief that each of us has a story to tell is stronger than ever. Finding the space to tell and listen is key. In one story that stands out Clara told of her time working in a mission led school in Kenya in the 1960s. She described a weekend safari visit when her husband needed to pay a visit to the toilet after dark. She begged him to stay in the hut and use the potty provided for occasions like this, but he refused. When he returned a little later she breathed a sigh of relief. The next morning the camp director ushered her and her husband to see a series of lion paw prints which had appeared overnight, they travelled the length of the camp and circled the toilet block. Clara's husband had been lucky to survive.

After I heard this story, told beautifully with a lot of description and emotion, I asked whether Clara had shared it with her young grandsons. 'Oh no' she answered 'they are all too busy to listen to me'.[16] I hope that my transcript finds its way into their hands at a time when they can ask Granny more questions and that the first time they hear it is not in a eulogy.

4.6 *Listening Properly*

Persuading a participant to tell their story is just one part of the process, listening to it is the other. So often we only half listen, thinking about the question

15 Rebecca Redhouse, 'Life-Story: Meaning Making through Dramatherapy in a Palliative Care Context', *Dramatherapy* 36.2–3 (2014): 72–78.

16 Extract from Sharing Stories for Wellbeing Session, 2015.

we would like to ask, what story we will tell in response, worrying about the text that just came through on the phone or what has to be done next rather than paying full attention to what is being said. Listening properly is a skill many of us have fallen out of the habit of using. Storytelling can be beneficial for both the storyteller and the listener, with both being active in the telling process.[17] The creative techniques employed in Sharing Stories help to develop active listening skills, enabling the teller to be really heard, which is crucial to the story sharing sessions.[18] However, trying to do this in a group can be difficult. To address this I introduce a telling and listening technique into the session often used in drama schools called *mirroring*.[19]

Mirroring involves splitting the group into pairs. In each pair participant X listens closely to the story told by participant Y without interruption. X and Y then reverse roles with Y listening to X's story. Each having heard the other's story, then tells the story that they have heard out loud to the rest of the group. Accordingly X tells Y's story and Y tells X's story. As a result, the level of concentration used when listening is significantly higher than that usually adopted. Most participants want to make a good job of retelling the story that they have heard. They want to honour both the words and the spirit of the story. Accordingly, I usually allow for a short period for clarification between partners before asking the whole group to feed back the stories that they have heard.

Watching the process, I notice that tellers often ask for an acknowledgement from their partner either during or after the retelling that the story they have re-told was largely accurate. The confirmation that usually comes provides a sense of achievement and gives the teller confidence to proceed. Where there are inconsistencies, then this moment provides an opportunity for any corrections. This is important given our predisposition as listeners to personalise the stories we hear, quite often unknowingly. On one occasion Y told X's story about a box of buttons that his grandmother had had. When he finished the retelling, X thanked Y for honouring the story whilst also adding that the original story had in fact been about a bag rather than a box of buttons. Y then realised that he had personalised the story recalling a box of buttons his own grandmother had had.[20]

---

17 Jennifer De Jong and Linda E. Clarke, 'What Is a Good Death? Stories from Palliative Care', *Journal of Palliative Care* 25.1 (2009): 61–67.

18 Youell and Ward, *Sharing Stories for Wellbeing: An Evaluation*, 17.

19 Monica Prendergast and Juliana Saxton, *Applied Drama: A Facilitator's Handbook for Working in Community* (Bristol: Intellect, 2013).

20 Extract Training Session: Sharing Stories for Wellbeing, 2016.

Mistakes of this kind are not uncommon and it is the job of the facilitator to ensure that there is space to rectify any misunderstandings or glaring inaccuracies. Whilst this often happens naturally, on occasion it is important to intervene. This can be done once the teller has finished recounting their partner's story. In one session the teller referred to his partner as Yvette rather than Yvonne throughout the retelling. His partner did not intervene or make any comment. It was my job as facilitator to set the record straight but only at the end of the telling thereby ensuring that the teller did not lose confidence.

It is also sometimes necessary to intervene where X tells Y's story but does so without honouring its spirit. One memorable session involved stories of taste. Marion told her story about the first time she went to the market in South Africa and saw an unusual prehistoric looking fruit. When she opened the fruit, she discovered its creamy white interior and delicious taste. This was her first avocado, a fruit she had never eaten before. Marion described the look and feel of the fruit to her partner Mary in detail going on to express her surprise when she returned home some ten years later and was amazed to find the same fruit on sale in the supermarket of her local town.

When it came to Mary retelling the story she provided a short summary – Marion tried her first avocado in Africa and was then surprised to find them in the supermarket when she returned to England.[21] Factually accurate, the story had lost all its beauty. Did Marion feel heard? Probably not. As facilitator it was my job to capture and air that story in the spirit in which it was told. Having monitored the group as the mirroring between partners was taking place I had been able to overhear elements of each of the stories being shared, including this one. I was therefore able to supplement the telling after its initial delivery honouring the story as best I could. Going forwards, I was careful to ensure that Mary and Marion were not always partnered together. By maintaining a small closed group, it is possible to develop a knowledge of the strengths and weaknesses of its participants making it easier to ensure that each of its members is properly heard.

Indeed, as the sessions progressed, some groups like the discipline of mirroring, others preferred to abandon it and tell their own stories directly out into the group. Both approaches are perfectly fine and the approach the facilitator adopts will depend on the dynamics of the group in question. Where the group reduces down to one participant, then rather than mirror the single story, the storytelling usually develops organically with the facilitator listening carefully allowing the participant to speak before asking more questions with

21 Extract Sharing Stories for Wellbeing Workshop, 2015.

a view to encouraging another story. On these occasions a 90-minute session can be quite exhausting and as facilitator I am usually prepared to share a few of my own stories in order to allow some recovery time for the sole participant.

4.7 *Recording the Stories*

Writing up the stories is the final step in ensuring the stories are heard. I take notes throughout each session; other facilitators record the sessions digitally. Producing the stories as something tangible is a powerful physical reminder that the story has been heard. The methodology for recording the story appears to be less important than the end product. Again I take a practical view. Transcribing audio recordings verbatim is costly and time consuming. Many hospices have limited resources and requiring this approach may be the reason why a life story sharing programme does not get adopted. I find that a simple printed document is all that is needed. Provided the patient is aware of the limitations, they are comfortable that reasonable care has been taken to accurately write up the stories shared each session. The participants are often delighted that someone has gone to the bother of writing up the stories for them. In addition to verbally explaining the process and providing patients with a written outline of the process at the start of each workshop series. We also use a series of disclaimers reminding patients that the story has been written down as it is heard, without interpretation, research or reflection and that any inaccuracies are unintentional. The following is a typical example:

> Notes/disclaimer
> I hope that I have got the details right in this. I have not checked or verified the accuracy of any of the information contained in it – it is purely a representation of your story, as I heard it.[22]

This seems to be sufficient to satisfy most participants. I do not offer to carry out additional research or check the accuracy of the tale I have heard, if a participant wants to present a fabrication, then that is their choice. It is not the intention behind these sessions to produce a factually accurate biography, indeed one person's perception of the story will often be quite different to that over another who was also there. That said, given memories are often unreliable and the stories shared may be factually inaccurate and inaccuracies are not going to be corrected, other members of the participant's family group cannot be assumed to have the right to access them.

22 Extract Miranda Quinney Training Notes, 2015.

4.8 *Control*

All participants in the story sharing groups will be drawn from the hospice's palliative care community. It follows that each has a diagnosis, or in the case of a carer's group, is caring for someone with a diagnosis. In either case, the schedule of their day to day life is often heavily influenced by various practical medical processes running concurrently.

A key theme to emerge from the evaluation data was a resounding recognition that participation provides an opportunity for patients to take back control of at least a part of their life – their story.

Lisa is categorical, 'It was my time to tell my story'.[23] Lisa's nephew was asked to provide some feedback on the effect attendance at the sessions had had on his aunt and he too noted that the sessions appeared to have played a part in helping her to resume her pre-illness identity. This is supported through the programme evaluation, which found the storytelling enabled a sense of feeling valued and having choice in the story you retold. One member of the hospice staff reported that one of the storytellers:

> ... felt she was a bit more individual again, a bit more in control because she was actually telling people about her life story... she felt she was doing something worthwhile. That's what she described it as and she felt humble because other people were interested in it, because other group members were asking her about it.[24]

The accuracy of the content of the story is largely unimportant; the fact that the patient can tell the story without worrying about its accuracy removes a barrier and encourages fluency. In the first of the workshop sessions I run through the ground rules for subsequent sessions:

- The facilitator will write up the stories that are told to the best of their ability without conducting any additional checks or research;
- Full copyright for the stories lies with the teller;
- Confidentiality in relation to the stories told will be maintained by all attendees.

4.9 *Writing Up*

The limits to the writing up service are covered in the preceding paragraphs. Before the mirroring exercise I remind participants of these limitations – namely

23 Extract from Evaluation Interview with Lisa, Patient, 2015.

24 Youell and Ward, *Sharing Stories for Wellbeing: An Evaluation*, 16.

that the story we hear may not be true to the story told and indeed the story told may not be the story the teller intended to tell. This has the effect of easing any concerns participants may have about their personal ability to retell the stories that they hear. I also remind participants that as the facilitator I am there to support the retelling. I also explain that I will be taking notes at the completion of the mirroring exercise as each X tells their partner Y's story aloud to the group.

When it comes to the process of writing up after each session I write each participant's story in the first person. This allows me to integrate any original words or phrases the teller has shared whilst also making it very clear that the story is told from the perspective of the participant. Given each session is relatively short with up to six participants, the resulting transcripts are also quite short. Sarah's transcript is a good example:

> During the War, when the Germans came to my native Belgium we had to capitulate. On 6 June 1945 we heard that the Allies had landed in France. There was a great celebration. Me and my family were in the countryside, staying at my grandparent's home. Brussels had been liberated the week before, we were now waiting for our turn.
>
> The day we were liberated there was an electricity cut. The first we had for the whole war. First there came the Germans into the village on stolen bikes – we knew they were stolen because of their number plates. They came to our home. They wanted food. We fed them as quickly as we could, they lit the table with a light from their bikes. When they left they thanked us and as they went they muttered 'wir werden zuruck kommen' – we will come back. We understood their mutterings as we had had to learn German in school from the time of the Occupation. German language, approved version new atlases and new text books with the approved version of history had all been compulsory.
>
> Next thing we heard was the planes. They were flying overhead, so low we could see the pilots and wave at them, they were American. The hens and the dogs in the village were terrified. They rushed into the stables away from the noise. Next came a deep rumbling sound. It was the tanks. As they got closer we could see that they were American and we asked where they were headed, the answer Berlin.[25]

25 Extract Story Transcript, Sarah, 2013.

The key point here is that the transcript is the story as told by the teller incorporating any inaccuracies and personal opinions. Naturally there is no reason why a facilitator should not go one step further and include relevant supporting images they may find online provided they explain to the participant that they will be doing this and then ask for their approval to insert it into the text. Equally the participant must be given the opportunity to request its removal. For the facilitator with the time and resources, inserting illustrations can add to the end product. On one occasion participants were telling stories relating to the senses. We started to consider the sense of sound and this led naturally to songs at which point Laura led a short chorus of the 'ABC song' which she used to sing along with her friends at the Saturday morning cinema club. She stumbled a little on the words for the verses but remembered every word of the chorus. The facilitator on that occasion went ahead after the session and found the full lyrics. Laura was delighted to see them reprinted in her personal story file.

On another occasion, again looking at the senses, we came to the sense of taste. Jean shared with us her love of baking and how although she can no longer eat the cakes she bakes, she enjoys watching others devour them. Jean provided a recipe for all members of the group and the following week arrived with a cake for us to share, it was delicious. We fondly refer to the cake as Jean's sponge cake.

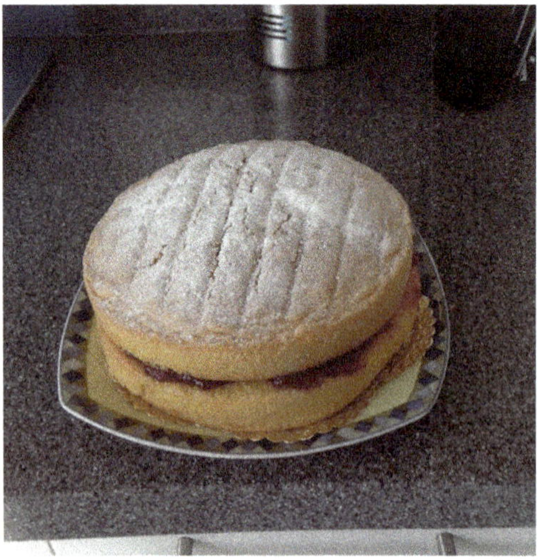

FIGURE 1 Jean's cake
© 2015, SS4WB. COURTESY OF SS4WB

Jean's Victoria Sponge Cake

8oz self-raising flour
+
1 teaspoon baking powder
Sweep these together
8oz butter and marge
+
8oz caster sugar
Beaten well together till light

4 large eggs
Add eggs one at a time and a teaspoon of flour
Add sieved flour
Put into 8" sandwich tin, well-greased, bottom and sides covered with a little flour
Heat oven to 160 degrees
Add to tins and cook for 20 minutes.
Check if ready by feeling the top of the cake. If it is firm and coloured gold, leave in tins for at least 10 minutes then turn out.[26]

Making it clear to participants that they have complete control over the process at a time when many other decisions and actions may be very much out of their personal control goes a long way to encouraging the feelings of wellbeing.[27]

4.10 *Ownership*

Since we are working with individuals with limited life expectancy, there must be an acknowledgement that the workshop participants may die during or shortly after their participation in the life stories workshops. Given also that there is no supporting research or corroboration of the facts contained in the stories it may be possible that the content of the stories is not appropriate for view by others. It is also to be expected that family members may want to see the stories. However it cannot be assumed that the teller wanted them shared. This dilemma can be pre-empted by using a simple consent form at the start of the workshop series. Participants are asked to complete a short form considering who can or cannot have access to the printed stories:

26 Sharing Stories for Wellbeing storytelling session, personal communication, Anon, 2015.
27 Ohnsorge, Gudat and Rehmann-Sutter, 'What a Wish to Die Can Mean', 8.

> You will be presented with a story file containing your stories at the end of the workshop series. Please indicate what you would like done with the electronic copy of the document:

- Delete it immediately;
- Make copies available to my immediate family on their request;
- Automatically make copies available to my immediate family;
- Make copies available to (hospice) staff on their request;
- Automatically make copies available to (hospice) staff.[28]

Addressing this situation at the start of the workshop process also minimises any anxiety the participant may have about the end recipient(s) of the stories. In the early stages of my work, before I had introduced a system to address the point, I was often asked by the patient about the intended recipient of the stories; were they for the vicar or the hospice marketing team? The answer of course was neither. By reassuring the patient that they own the story and control its distribution, this liberates them to tell. However, all of the stories referred to in this chapter and in any training work I undertake have been reproduced with the permission of their owner and pseudonyms have been used to preserve privacy.

5 Storytelling and Trauma

The process of life storytelling naturally triggers a series of memories and emotions. These are generally good and positive. Nora, a participant in the evaluation study acknowledged:

> It was amazing what it brought back, it was absolutely fascinating and so many things came out that you'd completely forgotten…it was good because you remembered people you were fond of and hadn't thought about you know for sixty years and it's good to do that.[29]

5.1 *Support for Participants*

Not all the memories in the course of a storytelling session will be positive. Supporting the group is crucial particularly where the facilitator is not

28 Extract Miranda Quinney Training Notes, 2015.

29 Extract from Feedback Session, 2015.

a trained counsellor. Running the sessions in a group format encourages self-censorship with participants sharing only the stories they wish to be heard. Avoiding a linear storytelling model helps to minimise opportunities for comparison and negative self-reflection. However, there are still times where a participant may find themselves drawn into an uncomfortable space potentially after the session as they reflect upon what was told. The clear provision of access to professional support is imperative. I identify the *go to* individual on my workshop welcome sheet which is distributed in the first session:

> EMOTIONAL SUPPORT
> Our aim is to offer workshops which are uplifting with participation being a positive experience. The group is not arranged as a therapeutic experience. However sometimes during this process stories can evoke strong feelings we had forgotten. If this occurs there is support there for you. It can be helpful to talk this through with an experienced health care professional, please contact (name, title and contact information).[30]

5.2 *Support for the Facilitator*

Support should not be limited to workshop participants. Facilitators also need help. Working with patients at end of life raises the probability that participants may die in the course of the programme or shortly thereafter. Working with them and their stories means a strong bond may be built in a relatively short space of time. Their death, though not unexpected may also be difficult to deal with. Also, the subject matter of some of the stories can become a little morbid!

I have already referred to the session where discussion turned to the subject of coffins and my relief that I had a supervisor to turn to. Not so lucky was the film and audio biographer whom I met recently. She has been visiting hospices recording the stories of patients from their beds. Her work is fantastic but she has no emotional/clinical supervision. I was not surprised when she freely admitted that she often retires to the ladies loo to weep at the end of the day. Access to supervision for both patient and facilitator is something I cannot over emphasise.

30 Extract Miranda Quinney Training Notes, 2015.

6 Variations on the Programme

At the time of writing I have trained over 150 palliative care practitioners in the use of storytelling techniques and have personally recorded over a hundred life stories. I have no way of knowing how many stories have been recorded by those that I have trained. My hope for patients is that the process of participating in a life stories workshop will be the first step towards telling and sharing their life stories with others thereby going some way towards dealing with the eulogy situation. Feedback suggests that this is certainly happening with patients going on to write their own short stories, paint, make films and have refreshed conversations with their nearest and dearest. Jane started painting again having avoided her paintbrushes following her diagnosis a decade earlier. Michael wrote a full autobiography for his grandchildren.

In the same way I expressly encourage the practitioners I train to interpret and use the story sharing skills in the way that works best for them. The variety of ways they have gone on to work with life stories include:

- Establishing off site storytelling groups in the community;
- Offering storytelling for bereaved families;
- Working with children who have been bereaved;
- Producing individual films and sound recordings of patients telling their stories;
- Running groups linking patients and volunteers to share their stories;
- Offering regular drop in story sessions;
- Training for all staff working with patients to empower them to find another way to start a conversation.

One of the most unexpected uses for group storytelling has been as part of in-house staff development programmes. Group facilitators have reported back on the new bonds built and existing ones strengthened by actively encouraging staff to share their life stories together. I suppose that we shouldn't be overly surprised by this, after all, telling stories is part of what makes us human.[31]

---

31 Tineke A. Abma, 'Learning by Telling, Storytelling Workshops as an Organisational Learning Intervention', *Management Learning* 34.4 (2003): 221–240; Arthur Ransom, *A History of Storytelling: Studies in the Development of Narrative* (Classic Reprint) (Hong Kong: Forgotten Books, 2012).

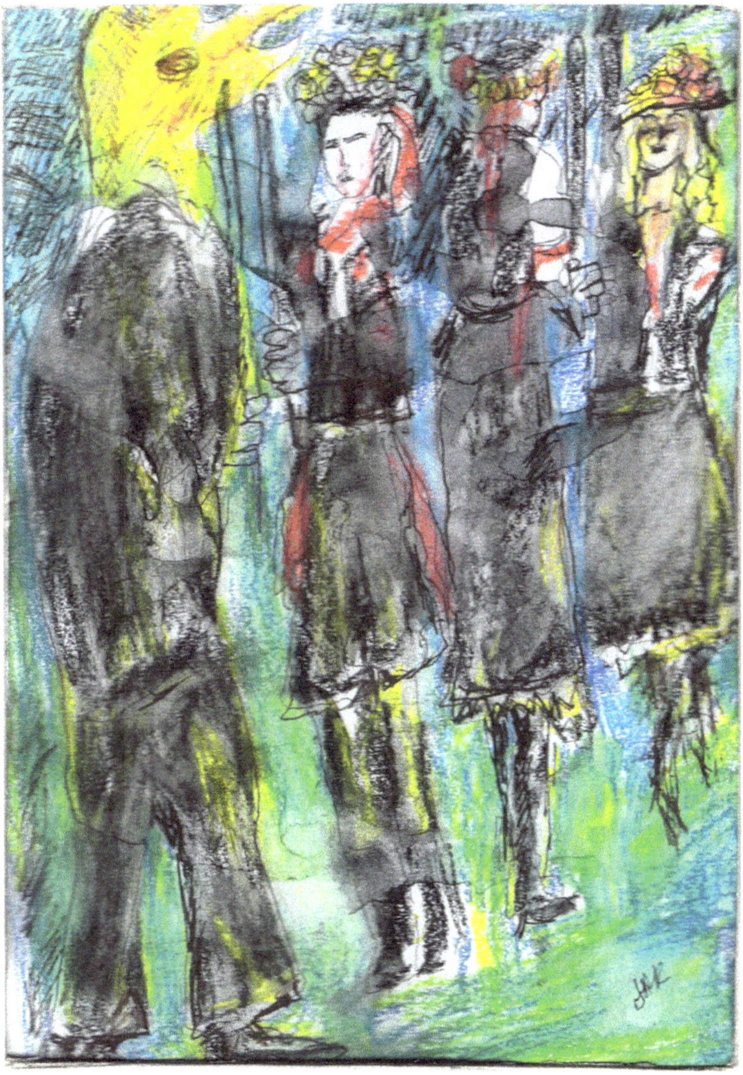

FIGURE 2 Dancing in Cassiobury Park by Jane

Acknowledgements

Thank you to Doreen Pattenson, senior social worker for her continuing support and advice in the development of SS4WB.

Thanks also to Debbie Stewart and Mehri Smyth whose enthusiasm keeps me going when creating and delivering SS4WB is at its most challenging.
Finally, my thanks to Watford's Peace Hospice Care for allowing me to pilot the life stories groups with their patients.

Bibliography

Abma, Tineke A. 'Learning by Telling, Storytelling Workshops as an Organisational Learning Intervention'. *Management Learning* 34.4 (2003): 221–240.

Boyd, Mary Ann. *Psychiatric Nursing: Contemporary Practice*. Philadelphia: Lippincott, Williams & Wilkins, 2005.

Coleman, Peter G. 'Adjustment in Later Life'. *Ageing in Society,* edited by John Bond and Peter G. Coleman, 97–132. London: Sage Publications, 1990.

Creswell, John W., Vicki L. Plano Clark, Michelle L. Gutmann and William. E. Hanson. 'Advanced Mixed Methods Research Designs'. *Handbook of Mixed Methods in Social and Behavioral Research*, edited by Abbas Tashakkori and Charles Teddlie, 209–240. Thousand Oaks, CA: Sage, 2003.

De Jong, Jennifer and Linda E. Clarke. 'What Is a Good Death? Stories from Palliative Care'. *Journal of Palliative Care* 25.1 (2009): 61–67.

Kirshbaum, Marilyn, Ian Carey, Brigid Purcell and Seamus Nash. 'Talking About Dying and Death: A Focus Group Study to Explore a Local Community Perspective'. *Nursing Reports* 1.1 (2011): 29–34.

Kottler, Jeffery. *Stories We've Heard, Stories We've Told: Life-Changing Narratives in Therapy and Everyday Life.* Oxford: Oxford University Press, 2015.

Ohnsorge, Kathrin, Heike Gudat and Christoph Rehmann-Sutter. 'What a Wish to Die Can Mean: Reasons, Meanings and Functions of Wishes to Die, Reported From 30 Qualitative Case Studies of Terminally Ill Cancer Patients in Palliative Care'. *BMC Palliative Care* 13.38 (2014): 1–14.

Ransom, Arthur. *A History of Storytelling: Studies in the Development of Narrative* (Classic Reprint) Hong Kong: Forgotten Books, 2012.

Redhouse, Rebecca. 'Life-Story; Meaning Making through Dramatherapy in a Palliative Care Context'. *Dramatherapy* 36.2–3 (2014): 66–80.

Prendergast, Monica and Juliana Saxton, *Applied Drama: A Facilitator's Handbook for Working in Community*. Bristol: Intellect, 2013.

Youell, Jane and Alison Ward. *Sharing Stories for Wellbeing: An Evaluation*. Northampton: Institute of Health and Wellbeing, 2015.

CHAPTER 4

The Collective Production of a Shared Narrative Surrounding Sexual Violence Trauma

Elena Sharratt

Abstract

This chapter explores the collective production of a shared narrative surrounding sexual violence trauma as found within a support group for female survivors. When I talk of the 'collective production of a shared narrative' I refer to the ways in which collaborative and non-vocal engagement with the support community allowed my participants to present their stories of trauma as common and interconnected. These practices, I argue, can be contrasted to more traditional individual 'talking therapies', which are informed by popular medical and philosophical conceptions of sexual violence trauma and, as a result, often present it as pathological and individually-bound. Alongside outlining a description of these group practices, this chapter seeks to interpret their particular significance and meaningfulness. I suggest that, by implicitly rejecting the more traditional and individualising ways of responding to and treating sexual violence trauma, my participants worked to de-pathologize their experiences and, instead, locate them as pertinent social and structural problems by externalising and reframing them. Ultimately, I argue that, whilst not using their 'voice' in the traditional or vocal sense of the word, the collective voice which emerges from these practices of group narrative telling is one that is both compassionate and powerfully political. Having thus observed the power of this non-vocal message, during the course of my research, I was forced to engage in exploring my own role in translating it into words. As such, this chapter additionally contains a discussion surrounding the ways in which, through the use of feminist-informed critical reflexivity, we, as researchers, might best go about, ethically and meaningfully putting into words that which both evades and transcends speech.

Key Words

Collective narratives – non-vocal narratives – sexual violence – trauma – feminist-informed practice – critical reflexivity

*****

 | DOI:10.1163/9789004396067_006

1 Introduction

This chapter explores the collective production of a shared narrative surrounding sexual violence trauma. My findings are based on evidence gathered from ethnography conducted with an all-female, self-run support group over a five-month period. During my research I observed that, instead of individually narrating their experiences of sexual violence, the women engaged in numerous collaborative, embodied and non-vocal practices. They worked on arts and creative writing projects together and if someone was ever visibly distressed or crying, another group member would offer her tactile gestures of comfort. Here, the unspoken awareness of shared experience, and the genuine empathy that inevitably accompanied this knowledge, was enough to allow the women to effectively connect and support each other, without them feeling the need to speak.

Thus, when I talk of the 'collective production of a shared narrative' I refer to the ways in which this collaborative and non-vocal engagement with the support community, allowed my participants to present their stories of trauma as common and interconnected. These practices can be contrasted to more traditional individual 'talking therapies' which are designed to target symptomatically specific aspects of trauma and, as such, often present it as isolated and pathological.[1]

The point of departure for this discussion is the much critiqued medicalization of trauma within the discipline of medical anthropology in combination with its comparative and, therefore paradoxical, blind spot towards sexual violence. Within the discipline, war, criminal and political traumas have all fallen under scrutiny for their tendency to be over individualized and medicalised. Attention has, instead, turned towards examining the social and structural forces that contribute to these conditions and thus the group narratives and collective practices through which they can be expressed and healed.[2] Contrary to

1 Judith Herman, *Trauma and Recovery: From Domestic Abuse to Political Terror* (London: Pandora, 1994).

2 For critiques of trauma medicalisation see, Arthur Kleinman, *Social Suffering*, eds. Arthur Kleinman, Veena Das and Margaret Lock (Berkeley: University of California Press, 1997); for an examination of the social and structural forces that contribute towards 'suffering' see, Paul Farmer, 'An Anthropology of Structural Violence', *Current Anthropology* 45.3 (2004): 305–325; for local responses to trauma see, Alex Argenti-Pillen, *Masking Terror: How Women Contain Violence in Southern Sri Lanka* (Philadelphia: University of Pennsylvania Press, 2003); Devon Hinton and Laurence Kirmayer, 'Local Responses to Trauma: Symptom, Affect, and Healing', *Transcultural Psychiatry* 50.5 (2013): 607–621; Joop de Jong and Ria Reis, 'Collective Trauma Processing: Dissociation as a Way of Processing Postwar Traumatic Stress in Guinea Bissau',

this, little anthropological effort has been made to similarly problematize the ways in which popular socio-medical conceptions of, and responses to, sexual violence reinforce its effects as pathological and individually-bound rather than shared, common and collective. This is in spite of the fact that culturally normalised and legitimated sexual violence and harassment still routinely affects the lives of women across the world.[3]

In this chapter, I will outline two of these reactions to sexual violence trauma most commonly found within Western influenced, socio-medical cultures. Firstly, I will examine the medical theories which inform trauma related diagnoses in victims of sexual violence and advocate for talking therapy as a way to recover from what are described in the literature as symptoms of these conditions.[4] Secondly, I will outline common philosophical explorations into the impact of sexual violence trauma on 'the self' which describes the narrating of experience as a way to rebuild fractured bonds of 'relationality'.[5] After analysing these models I will then highlight their incongruence with the lived reality of my ethnographic participants' experiences. None of my participants felt that any aspects of their trauma could be outlined as specifically symptomatic, nor did narrating their stories appear to be a way for them to effectively heal a 'relational self'. On the contrary, their trauma appeared to be situated on a continuum alongside commonplace feelings of fear, shame and bodily vulnerability associated with more routine, every day sexual harassments and gender-based micro aggressions, albeit on a much heightened and more debilitating scale. Acknowledging the ways in which these feelings were inextricably intertwined with a particular mode of shared feminine embodied subjectivity, my participants felt that the telling or hearing of individual narratives falsely divided them by causing them to compare experiences and, in doing so, minimise their own distress.[6] As a result, the women in the group implicitly rejected the models which advocated these types of healing and, instead, adopted more collaborative, non-vocal means of support.

Transcultural Psychiatry 50.5 (2013): 644–661; Hanna Kienzler, 'The Social Life of Psychiatric Practice: Trauma in Postwar Kosova', *Medical Anthropology* 31.3 (2012): 266–282.

3 ONS (Office for National Statistics), *Sexual Offences in England and Wales: Year Ending March 2017*, February 2018, viewed on 23 June 2018, https://www.ons.gov.uk/peoplepopulationandcommunity/crimeandjustice/articles/sexualoffencesinenglandandwales/yearendingmarch2017; Rape Crisis England and Wales, *Rape Crisis England and Wales Headline Statistics 2017–2018*, 2018, viewed on 23 June 2018, https://rapecrisis.org.uk/statistics.php.

4 Herman, *Trauma and Recovery*, 34.

5 Susan Brison, *Aftermath: Violence and the Remaking of a Self* (New Jersey: Princeton University Press, 2002), 37.

6 For further discussion of 'shared feminine embodied subjectivity' in relation to sexual violence see, Ann Cahill, *Rethinking Rape* (New York: Cornell University Press, 2001).

As well as being merely a descriptive account of group practices, this chapter seeks to interpret the significance of these collective, non-vocal means of support, specifically as they relate to sexual violence. As Miranda Quinney, Alison Ward and Jane Youell have shown in their work on palliative care, the telling of narrative within a group setting is not always rejected but, within the context these authors describe, it is felt to be extremely positive.[7] This contribution compliments the argument made here. The participants in my study did not reject the telling of individual narrative, *in and of itself*, but rather, the inappropriate use of it for sexual violence trauma specifically. I suggest that by rejecting narrative within this context, my participants were acting to challenge the notion that their responses to sexual violence were individual, pathological 'symptoms' to be treated and overcome. Instead, they implicitly demanded that their reactions be acknowledged as part of the routine, everyday realities of being female, under systems of institutionalised patriarchy. Furthermore, they explicitly highlighted the ways in which narratives of sexual violence trauma frequently produced comparison, minimisation and isolation, in measures incomparable to other types of suffering. By thus doing so, they further drew attention to the danger of narrative telling as a treatment for sexual violence trauma, without an accompanying, much broader, attitudinal shift. I conclude these observations by arguing that, whilst not using their 'voice' in the traditional or vocal sense of the word, the collective voice which emerges from these practices of group narrative telling is one that is both compassionate and powerfully political.

Observing the power of this non-vocal message, I was forced to engage in exploring my own role in translating it. Although how to present rich, complex data is a conundrum that faces all social scientists who do qualitative work, I here felt the challenge all the more strongly given that the information I was interpreting was largely based upon non-vocal practice. In order to overcome these issues and present my findings in as transparent a way as possible, I borrowed from guidelines set by feminist informed methodological practice which highlight critical reflexivity as a core aspect of the research process and, in addition, aim to acknowledge the self as crucially interwoven with both the context and process of data analysis. Through use of these methods I suggest that the researcher can produce narratives that are congruent with the voices of her participants whilst she works to challenge the historically gendered politics of knowledge production.[8] These practices, I argue, can critically

7 Miranda Quinney, Alison Ward and Jane Youell, 'Life Story Sharing: A Therapeutic Intervention in Palliative Care', in this volume.

8 Erica Burman, 'Emotions and Reflexivity in Feminist Education Action Research', *Educational Action Research* 14.3 (2006): 315–332; Natasha Mauthner and Andrea Doucet, 'Reflexive

contribute towards re-inscribing women's voices and realities, which have long been misrepresented and overlooked, into broader conversations.

2 Methodological Background

This chapter is based on an ethnographic study conducted between March and July 2013 in a self-run support group for female survivors of rape, sexual violence and childhood sexual abuse based within Greater London. The group met fortnightly on a weekday morning in the same neutral, public location. The support group formed part of a constituted charity, set-up and run by a woman who was herself a survivor. The charity also worked to raise funds and awareness as well as support a larger community of survivors via its online Facebook forum and charity webpage. These online resources, in addition to books written and published by the community, were also utilised within my research.

During the group sessions, I conducted research in the traditional ethnographic style, engaging in and contributing to activities whilst surveying the dynamics of the group. Alongside this, I conducted short unstructured interviews with members and one unstructured question and answer session with the whole group. I occupied both 'insider' and 'outsider' status in that, as a female research, I was granted access to the female only space, yet I did not identify to the women as a survivor of sexual violence. In keeping with ethical codes, I obtained full informed consent from all the women that attended the group. I made it clear that cooperation with the objectives of my fieldwork were completely voluntary and that, at any point, they could withdraw without having to justify their choice. The women all reported feeling comfortable and pleased to participate. To protect the anonymity of my informants no real names or identifiers are utilised within this chapter.

Whilst it was made clear by the charity that the Facebook forum and webpage were available for use by both female and male survivors of sexual violence, the face-to-face group sessions, from which the majority of this data was collected, were female only spaces. This was a decision made to enhance the safety and wellbeing of the female members. The mixed-gender Facebook forum was also a closed group, a choice which similarly supported this objective. This chapter explores sexual violence trauma in relation to female experience and subjectivity and, whilst this approach certainly does not intend to dismiss

Accounts and Accounts of Reflexivity in Qualitative Data Analysis', *Sociology* 37.3 (2003): 413–431; Gillian Rose, 'Situating Knowledges: Positionality, Reflexivity and Other Tactics', *Progress in Human Geography* 21 (1997): 305–320.

male survivors, it does aim to acknowledge the disproportionately gendered nature of sexual violence and its effects.[9] The use of a female only sample thus reflects both the analytical underpinnings of this research design and the structural reality of sexual violence as a crime.

3 Medical Responses to Sexual Violence Trauma

Nearly a third of victims of sexual violence are diagnosed with post-traumatic stress disorder (PTSD), complex PTSD or rape-trauma syndrome (RTS).[10] In addition, instances of childhood sexual abuse are frequently implicated in diagnoses of borderline personality disorder (BPD) and dissociative identity disorder (DID).[11] Whilst my intention here is certainly not to suggest that these categories be conflated or removed from their context, I do wish to draw attention to the ways in which expressions of traumatic experience are interpreted and treated within a medical context. With these diagnoses, the primary way through which this is done is by defining the feelings, sensations and memories associated with a traumatic event as 'pathological'. They are distinguished from what is considered to be part of the 'healthy' human experience and are thus outlined as indicative symptoms of a condition or disorder. This distinction between what is 'healthy' and 'pathological' can often be made due to the fact that, in the aftermath of a traumatic event, the experiences associated with it are perceived to be more intrusive, overwhelming and somatic, whereas 'regular' events are, comparatively, more cognitive, controllable and coherent. Besides making a distinction between these two 'types' of experiences, these medical models state that, in order to heal from these trauma symptoms, one must work to change these 'pathological' experiences, and, particularly, the intrusive memories associated with them, into healthy memories by talking about them and ordering them into coherent, narrative form.

9 For disproportionate sexual violence statistics by gender see ONS (Office for National Statistics), *Sexual Offences in England and Wales,* Rape Crisis England and Wales, *Rape Crisis England and Wales Headline Statistics 2017–2018.* For the gendered nature of sexual violence see Ann Cahill, *Rethinking Rape* and Rebecca Emerson Dobash and Russell Dobash, eds., *Rethinking Violence Against Women* (London: Sage Publications, 1998).

10 Ann Burgess and Lynda Holmstrom, 'Rape Trauma Syndrome', *American Journal of Psychiatry* 131 (1974): 981–986; Herman, *Trauma and Recovery,* 34.

11 Linda McClean and Ruth Gallop, 'Implications of Childhood Sexual Abuse for Adult Borderline Personality Disorder and Complex Post Traumatic Stress Disorder', *The American Journal of Psychiatry* 160.2 (2003): 369–371; John B. Murray, 'Relationship of Childhood Sexual Abuse to Borderline Personality Disorder, Post Traumatic Stress Disorder and Multiple Personality Disorder', *The Journal of Psychology* 127.6 (1993): 657–676.

As such, individual talking therapy is strongly advocated as a way to transform and regain control over what are outlined as pathological and symptomatic aspects of traumatic experience.[12] My participants' non-narrative responses to trauma, however, suggested that there were other ways to make meaning of these highly activating experiences.

A number of critiques have been directed towards these trauma related diagnoses and models used to describe and treat the effects of a devastating event. These critiques, mostly formulated from within the field of medical anthropology, have been aimed at types of war, criminal and political trauma, in addition to the effects of poverty, malnutrition and illness syndemics.[13] The idea is that, by medicalising these experiences, not only are ethnocentric models applied to contexts wherein Western analytical frameworks may not be relevant or even adaptive but, in addition, the complex structural conditions which contribute towards these 'social', rather than pathological, 'sufferings' are ignored.[14] These broad criteria also ignore and negate diverse individual human responses.

Unfortunately, this timely and much needed critique is yet to extend towards the field of sexual violence trauma. Undoubtedly, there are numerous reasons why this may be the case. Sexual violence, by its very nature, is often a crime that is committed intimately and in private. In addition, victims are frequently shamed and blamed for their own attacks, thus leading them to keep their experiences hidden from public view and underreported to services.[15] This may lead to the belief that, contrary to survivors of other types of more

12 Herman, *Trauma and Recovery*, 34.

13 For critiques of trauma medicalisation see Argenti-Pillen, *Masking Terror*; and, Kleinman, *Social Suffering*; for the social and structural conditions that contribute towards poverty, malnutrition and illness syndemics see, Farmer, 'An Anthropology of Structural Violence'.

14 For local response to trauma see, Argenti-Pillen, *Masking Terror*; Hinton and Kirmayer, 'Local Responses to Trauma'; de Jong and Reis, 'Collective Trauma Processing'; and, Kienzler, 'The Social Life of Psychiatric Practice'; see especially for the irrelevance of Western analytical frameworks, Argenti-Pillen, *Masking Terror*.

15 For estimated underreporting of sexual violence see ONS (Office for National Statistics), *Sexual Offences in England and Wales*, Rape Crisis England and Wales, *Rape Crisis England and Wales Headline Statistics 2017–2018*; Liz Kelly, Jo Lovett and Linda Regan, 'A Gap or a Chasm?: Attrition in Reported Rape Case', *Home Office Research Study* 293 (London: Home Office, 2005); For attribution of shame and blame see, Ronnie Janoff-Bulman, 'Characterological versus Behavioural Self-Blame: Inquiries into Depression and Rape', *Journal of Personality and Social Psychology* 37 (1979): 1798–1809; Collen Ward, *Attitudes Towards Rape: Feminist and Social Psychological Perspectives*, (London: Sage, 1995); Gail Wyatt, Cindy Notgrass and Michael Newcomb, 'Internal and External Mediators of Women's Rape Experiences', *Psychology of Women Quarterly* 14 (1990): 153–176.

'public' trauma, survivors of sexual violence are rare and isolated and, as such, the traumatic expressions that follow it warrant medicalised diagnoses rather than public or social critique. Despite the relatively plausible nature of these assumptions, there are numerous issues associated with them. To begin with, even with gross instances of underreporting, official sexual violence prevalence statistics indicate that these are not rare instances but are, in fact, crimes that affect women[16] with worrying regularity.[17] In addition, the very frequency with which rape survivors who do report receive trauma related diagnoses, appears to indicate that, rather than these responses being pathological or out of the ordinary, they are extremely natural and socially patterned reactions.[18] Whilst these recognitions are, as of yet, rarely brought into public or academic critique, they, nevertheless, appeared to strongly inform the structure of the support group wherein I conducted my research.

4 Group Rejection of the Medical Model

This research draws on ethnographic fieldwork conducted within a support group for women who had experienced rape, sexual violence or abuse. The group had been set up by a woman who was herself a survivor. In comparison to the type of individual and clinical treatment models most frequently offered to sexual violence survivors, as described above, the members of this group described their model as relatively rare. When I first spoke to the leader and founding member, she described the isolation she had felt in the aftermath of her abuse. A great deal of this isolation, she stated, was experienced during one-on-one clinical therapy sessions within which she would often feel a sense of distance and lack of connection between her and her therapist. She stated that her primary goal for establishing the group was to break this sense of solitary suffering and create a space of sociality where survivors could unite in their experiences. In addition to this, she was heavily critical of the ways in which survivors received various mental health diagnoses following rape or sexual abuse. She often, and with great dislike, described these diagnoses as 'labels' and indicated that such 'labels' were rarely felt to be meaningful or

16 The use of the female pronoun does not negate instances of sexual violence that are reported by male survivors. Violence against males does not, however, reflect my expertise or my analytical underpinnings, as I further discuss in my methodology.

17 ONS, *Sexual Offences in England and Wales*, Rape Crisis England and Wales, *Rape Crisis England and Wales Headline Statistics 2017–2018*.

18 For frequency of trauma related diagnoses in victims of sexual violence, see: Burgess and Holmstrom, 'Rape Trauma Syndrome', 981; Herman, *Trauma and Recovery*, 34; Murray, 'Relationship of Childhood Sexual Abuse', 657.

even useful within the group. At this stage, it is important to note that not all talking therapies exclusively operate around individual diagnosis. Importantly, however, this had been the experience of my participants and, as such, their group model could be seen as a direct response to this.

What I saw as particularly significant about the structure and ethos of this group were the ways in which it appeared to explicitly critique the premise that directly underlay the medical model of trauma. It rejected the separation and individuation of survivors, inherent within the model, and was wary of the damage done through the partitioning and 'labelling' of symptoms and effects. Perhaps even more striking, not only was a critique of 'isolation' and 'labels' directly articulated within the group but, in addition, the very practices which occurred there appeared to fundamentally reject the medical model by diverting from the healing pathway it delineated: namely, narrative style talking therapy. Within the group there was absolutely no individual discussion of sexual violence, its impacts or its aftermath. Instead, members would collaborate on painting, drawing and creative writing projects, share food and drink together and display non-verbal expressions of emotion through crying and providing each other tactile offerings of comfort.

Before I had begun my research, I had already been familiar with the medical model of trauma as described above. I was aware of its cultural salience and, particularly, of the ways in which it so strongly advocated talking therapy as key to recovery from sexual violence. As a result, within the support-group, I definitely expected that something akin to this would take place. Whilst I understood it was not a clinical environment and therefore knew that one-on-one therapies would not occur, I assumed that the women would narrate their individual experiences to each other. As such, when I found this not to be the case, and, in fact, witnessed the contrary, I was extremely surprised.

To add to this sense of surprise, I soon discovered that, not only was individual sexual violence narrative absent from group discussions but, furthermore, members would actually actively engage in suppressing it. This appeared to me as particularly ethnographically significant and, as such, warranted further enquiry. Within the group, the most common way by which this was done was through frequent reference to the notion of 'trigger warnings'. These warnings were employed on the group's webpage, on their introductory information sheet and were even, on occasion, used to directly interrupt new group members who seemingly, had anticipated an environment of full disclosure within the group and had attempted to talk about their experiences during their first sessions.

Over the past decade 'trigger warnings' have become increasingly popular within internet forums, media outlets and public spaces such as universities. These warnings are applied in relation to the idea that speaking about traumatic events can potentially induce, or 'trigger', distressing memories and even vivid, sensory flashbacks in those who have previously survived such traumas.[19] As such, within the group, the idea was that any talk of sexual violence could be potentially 'triggering' to members and thus 'trigger warnings' surrounding its content were utilised to supress individual narrative practice. However, during the course of my research, there were a number of times wherein I witnessed the 'trigger warning' mechanism being utilised in ways which could be seen as departing from this more widely understood application.

Firstly, within the group, not only was speech that directly concerned rape or sexual violence recognised to be 'triggering', but particular events and situations were as well. During the course of my research, a newspaper article was published in a popular broadsheet featuring an interview with a well-known celebrity in which he engaged in victim blaming survivors of sexual abuse.[20] The group leader responded to this by writing an angry letter to the newspaper, outlining the ways in which their institutionalised misogynistic attitudes and the actor's irresponsible abuse of power and influence had led many of the group members to re-live feelings of shame and self-blame. On another occasion a group member arrived at a session having been winked at by a strange man on her bus journey. This instigated a conversation surrounding street harassment in general, which was largely acknowledged to illicit feelings of fear, anger and bodily vulnerability. Both of these instances, whilst not directly referencing rape or sexual violence, had aroused emotions so similar and connected to those experiences that they were, understandably, seen to activate its memory and were acknowledged as triggering events. These triggering events, and others like them, were acknowledged and critiqued, without the members seeing need to discuss in specific detail, the more painful memories of sexual violence that they were connected to.

In addition to how, alongside speech, a number of situations were recognised as 'triggering', within the group there was a concern about *who* could potentially be triggered. Here, not only were inner group members who were known to be survivors themselves acknowledged as being vulnerable in relation to events such as those described above but, rather, all women were, including me as the researcher. This was clearly demonstrated through the ways in which both of these incidents were outlined as being profoundly harmful

---

19 Lindsay Holmes, *A Quick Lesson on what Trigger Warnings Actually Do*, 26 August 2016, viewed on 15 July 2018, http://www.huffingtonpost.com/entry/university-of-chicago-trigger-warning_us_57bf16d9e4b085c1ff28176d.

20 Hayley Dixon, *Sex Abuse Victims Bring it Upon Themselves Bill Roache Claims*, 19 March 2013, viewed on 15 July 2018, https://www.telegraph.co.uk/news/celebritynews/9939558/Sex-abuse-victims-bring-it-upon-themselves-Bill-Roache-claims.html.

in routine ways, to all women. Street harassment was described as being almost *designed* to initiate the types of anger and fear responses that the group member had experienced and the newspaper article – and others like it – was expressly critiqued, not only for how it had 'triggered' the current survivors of abuse but for the ways in which it contributed towards a victim blaming culture wherein women, who may be attacked in the future, would find it much more difficult to report or seek help. The salience of these particular observations was made even more apparent to me as I, whilst being an 'outsider' in relation to the group, was invited to contribute towards these conversations and was able to do so easily, empathically connecting with the all too commonplace feelings they incited.

The above practices extended the 'trigger warning' mechanism so that it encompassed not only speech and direct trauma survivors but, in addition, events and those more broadly associated with them. I interpret these as extremely significant in relation to the collective production of shared narrative surrounding sexual violence trauma, as found within my field work. Firstly, by recognising the 'triggering' potential of both talk of sexual violence and more every day gender-based micro-aggressions, these practices noted the ways in which all of these incidents were inextricably interconnected. By doing so, they implicitly acknowledged the structures of patriarchal power through which they were all mediated and legitimated. Also, being aware that all of these incidents held the potential to invoke the self-same feelings of fear, anger, shame and bodily vulnerability, not only within women who had survived the more extreme forms of this structurally legitimated violence, but in all women, confirmed that this structure is an oppression both omnipresent in its operation and routine in its affects.[21]

Whilst the medical model labels expressions of traumatic experience as 'pathological' symptoms, distinguished from 'healthy' human states, it was evident that the narrative surrounding sexual violence trauma which emerged from these group practices stood in sharp contradiction to these descriptions. Here, instead of understanding the experiences associated with a traumatic event as out of the ordinary or particularly symptomatic, the women instead situated them upon a continuum alongside the recognisable and routinized effects of gendered structural violence. By reframing their experiences in this way, they were able to reject the medical model of healing, which advocates individual talking therapy as a way to 'recover' from 'pathological' symptoms.

21 When I write 'the more extreme forms of this structurally legitimated violence' this is not intended as a way in which to rank the severity or impact of these types of violences, rather it is a comment upon the ways in which they are socially and legally perceived.

Instead, they adopted a group model based upon 'trigger warnings'. By utilising these mechanisms, the group not only honoured and respected responses to trauma as extremely commonplace, natural and socially patterned but, furthermore, they created a powerful, collective statement which spoke to the pertinent structural and political issues underlying their practices.

5 Philosophical Interpretations of Sexual Violence Trauma

In addition to the medical model of trauma, there have been numerous philosophical mediations upon this topic which seek to explore the nature and meaning of its impact. These are most commonly found in accounts written by survivors of war and Holocaust trauma. However, they have been specifically applied to the field of sexual violence by the philosopher Susan Brison.[22] Brison, who was herself violently attacked, raped and nearly murdered by a stranger, wrote a text following this incident in order to document and make sense of its devastating aftermath.[23]

In taking a philosophical approach towards the study of her own personal experiences and attempting to understand the particular impact of sexual violence, Brison concludes that, in order to fully interpret the effects of a trauma inflicted by another human being, we must first outline a definition of 'the self'.[24] For Brison 'the self' is fundamentally relational. The way we establish our sense of subjectivity is through our chosen interactions with others. As such, she states that when we experience a human inflicted trauma, the belief that we can freely exist in relation to others becomes destroyed and we are robbed of the very means by which we define our subjectivity. The impact of this is such that the survivor often experiences a 'death of the self'.[25] In order to recover from this sense of self-annihilation, Brison states that, through narrating one's experiences and having those experiences listened to, new bonds of relationality can be formed and thus 'the self' can be re-established.[26]

---

22 For interpretations into war and Holocaust trauma see Jonathan Shay, *Achilles in Vietnam: Combat Trauma and the Undoing of Character* (New York: Atheneum, 1994).
Charlotte Delbo, *Auschwitz and After*, trans. Rosette Lamont (New Haven: Yale University Press, 1995).

23 Brison, *Aftermath.*

24 Ibid., 37.

25 Ibid., 38.

26 For additional discussions concerning existential re-orientations to the world following trauma and loss see also, Thomas Attig, *How We Grieve: Relearning the World* (Oxford: Oxford University Press, 1996); And, Ronnie Janoff-Bulman, *Shattered Assumptions: Towards a New Psychology of Trauma* (New York: The Free Press, 1992).

Whilst this text is, undoubtedly, to be praised for introducing much needed critical examination into the realm of sexual violence, which, as I have highlighted, is profoundly under-theorized outside of the medical sphere, unfortunately, it cannot be said to entirely depart from medicalized conceptions of trauma and healing. As highlighted previously, the medical model distinguishes between 'pathological' and 'healthy' types of memory and dictates the ways in which, through talking therapy, the former can be converted to the latter.[27] Throughout Brison's text, this is a framework that she explicitly endorses and utilises to compliment her notion of the way in which the 'relational self' can be reconstructed through narrative. As a result, she similarly advocates these individual-style models of talking therapy as a way to heal from sexual violence trauma.[28] What Brison overlooks are the many other non-vocal ways through which the 'self' can be seen as relational and thus the non-narrative means through which it can be relationally reconstructed following a traumatic event.

Whilst individually narrating one's trauma in this way is highlighted by Brison as extremely relevant in relation to recovery and, indeed, is revealed to have been beneficial within the process of her own healing, nevertheless, within the support group, this was not a mechanism that was utilised or even deemed to be appropriate. None of my participants welcomed the idea that their traumatic experiences were pathological states that needed to be or, even, could be, healed, a notion implicit within the imperative to narrate. As a result, they rejected these models in favour of group practices which acknowledged and respected their experiences as natural and commonplace, both within the group and, indeed, for women more broadly. As such, it appeared that in addition to the popular medical model, this philosophical model as proposed by Brison was incompatible with the lived reality of sexual violence trauma as experienced by my participants.

6 Group Re-interpretation of the Philosophical Model of Sexual Violence Trauma

Despite this obvious incongruence between the practices within the support-group and the healing pathway outlined by Brison, there was *one* element of her philosophical theory that struck me as significant, most notably for the ways in which, contrary to the rest of the model, it did appear to be relevant to the lives of my participants. This particular element was her notion of the self as 'relational'. Within the group, whilst none of my participants related to each

27 Herman, *Trauma and Recovery*, 34.

28 Brison, *Aftermath*, 62.

other by sharing their individual stories, they would frequently describe to me the extremely strong bonds that connected them and, furthermore, would outline these bonds as a crucial source of comfort and support in the aftermath of their experiences of sexual violence. As a result, as part of my research, I wanted to explore this apparent paradox between the ways in which my participants insisted upon the vital importance of themselves as relational, yet continued to reject the exchange of narrative which, within the philosophical discipline, was highlighted as primarily constituting this relationality. In order to do this, I examined the non-vocal practices that occurred within the group.

When I first began conducting my research, I had observed numerous collaborative, embodied and non-vocal practices occurring within the group. The members would work on arts and creative writing projects together which allowed them to work towards a common goal in a relaxed and non-directional way, organically engaging and integrating them into a solid unit. Also, if someone was ever visibly distressed or crying, another group member would offer her tactile gestures of comfort. Here, the unspoken awareness of shared experience, and the genuine empathy that inevitably accompanied this knowledge, was enough to allow the women to effectively support each other, without them feeling the need to speak. All of these practices appeared to me to demonstrate the ways in which relationality could be constructed in non-narrative ways, a fact completely overlooked within Brison's interpretations. This observation was one that I interpreted as significant enough in and of itself. However, when during the course of my research, I witnessed an occasion which directly concerned the hearing of a narrative, it began to appear as even more relevant.

During this particular incident a member arrived at a session describing how awful she was feeling. She said she had been on the internet all morning reading accounts written by other survivors of sexual violence that had caused her to compare her own experiences and feel as if what she went through 'wasn't that bad'. As a result, she began to think her trauma was unwarranted, which left her feeling guilty and undeserving of the inclusion and support that being a member of the group offered her. Almost immediately, the other members empathised with what she was describing. The group leader even went so far as to state that 'that's always what happens when you read those stories, you end up feeling alone'. After saying this, she then went on to add 'I know we're taught to, but we shouldn't compare each other, abuse is abuse is abuse'.

What was particularly interesting about all of these instances, taken together, was that, whilst group members were able to form and maintain strong and nurturing bonds of relationality in numerous embodied, non-narrative ways, the hearing of individual narrative appeared to threaten these connections.

Not only was the 'triggering' potential of narrative here acknowledged, as was previously described in relation to the medical model, but it was also recognised as something that could fundamentally sever bonds within the group by reactivating the individual members' vulnerable selves and returning them to hypervigilance. Given that my participants appeared to feel so strongly connected and, furthermore, described their shared emotions and experiences as particularly powerful, this at first appeared to me as somewhat contradictory. Upon paying closer attention to the particular language that the group leader used in response to this specific situation, however, it began to make sense.

Here, by stating that 'that's always what happens when you read those stories', the leader not only empathised with the group member's responses, but she also highlighted their very commonality. By doing so she acknowledged comparison, minimisation and guilt to be, seemingly, inevitable effects, directly related to the hearing of other narratives surrounding sexual violence. Even more importantly, by drawing attention to the ways in which women are 'taught to'[29] have these responses, she effectively re-framed them as a constitutive part of the very structures through which violence against women is perpetrated and legitimated.

By advocating the telling of narrative, Brison inadvertently places exclusive focus upon how this practice can re-construct the relational self, following a traumatic event, at the exclusion of all other, non-narrative practices. However, by failing to acknowledge the cultural context within which narratives surrounding sexual violence are located, she crucially overlooks the potentially damaging consequences which may arise as a result of engaging in this type of speech. Contrary to this, the group leader was able to recognise the cultural mechanisms which encourage comparison between women and, in addition, the ways in which these dangerously intersect with narratives surrounding sexual violence trauma to produce feelings of minimisation and self-blame within survivors. Having done so, she could then critically challenge the individual narrative telling model and engage in practices which affirmed and maintained connections. By engaging in these non-narrative relationality practices, not only were individual members able to truly benefit from the supportive bonds they formed with each other, but also the group enacted a powerful critique of patriarchal culture which further contributed towards

29 For the socialisation of comparison and minimisation in relation to sexual violence see Heather Hlavka, 'Normalizing Sexual Violence: Young Women Account for Harassment and Abuse', *Gender and Society* 28.3 (2014): 337–358 and Liz Kelly and Jill Radford, "Nothing Really Happened': The Invalidation of Women's Experiences of Sexual Violence', *Critical Social Policy* 10.30 (1990): 39–53.

their emerging counter-narrative surrounding sexual violence trauma. Significantly, this research was undertaken in 2013, almost four and a half years prior to the #metoo movement. My participants did not appear to envisage the ways in which this movement has enabled many survivors to share their stories without oppression and judgement.

7 The Politics of Narrative Practice

Thus far within this chapter, I have described the practices that occurred during the aftermath of trauma, as found within a support group for survivors of sexual violence. I have argued that these practices can be interpreted as contributing towards the collective production of a shared narrative surrounding sexual violence trauma. This narrative can be described as fundamentally counter to those more commonly portrayed in that it rejects the individual pathologization of sexual violence trauma and, instead, emphasises its shared, collective elements. By doing so, it forces us to examine the broader mechanisms which contribute towards sexual violence trauma as an effect. As I have frequently drawn attention to within this chapter, unlike investigations into other types of trauma, sexual violence trauma is comparatively and grossly undertheorized within academia. Whilst disciplines such as medical anthropology have been able to present types of war, criminal and political trauma as socially patterned and naturalised responses to systemic structural issues, this is yet to be the case for sexual violence trauma.[30] Here I suggest that it is, in large part, due to this critical oversight that the narrative that emerges from my field site is still perceived as 'counter'.

Whilst this observation may, at first, appear to be entirely pessimistic, I do not feel that this has to be the case. This paper, whilst certainly intending to critique the under-theorization of sexual violence trauma, has also, quite evidently, attempted to initiate further exploration into this arena. This has been a task that I have felt to be both important and immensely necessary. However, it has also been one that has required much thought, sensitivity and critical reflection. Almost paradoxically, I have here attempted to 'narrate' the ways in which, through various embodied, emotional and intuitive ways, my participants 'voiced' a message that was, not only in many ways unspeakable, but, in addition, a fundamental critique of narrative practice. As a result of this, both during the course of my research and in the interpretive process that followed

30 Kleinman, *Social Suffering.*

it, I was inevitably faced with the question of how I was to meaningfully put into words that which both evaded and transcended speech.

This question was, and still is, one that I see as both methodological and political. Firstly, the question of methodology relates to how I, as a researcher, when faced with data so rich, complex and nuanced, could effectively interpret and portray it in a way that remained congruent towards those I was representing. Whilst this is, of course, a conundrum that faces all social scientists who work with highly qualitative data, I here felt the challenge all the more strongly given that the information I was interpreting was largely based upon non-vocal practice. In order to overcome these issues and present my findings in as transparent a way as possible, I borrowed from guidelines set by and now common within, all feminist informed methodological practice. These guidelines highlight reflection and criticality as core aspects of the research process and, in addition, aim to acknowledge the self as crucially interwoven with both the research context and the process of data analysis.[31] As such, following these suggestions, rather than obscuring or erasing my 'voice' within this chapter, I aimed to bring it precisely into view. By transparently documenting my own evolving thoughts and interpretations in this way, I hoped to present the conclusions that I reached in relation to my data, not as absolute or definitive statements but, rather, as reflections which the reader is invited to enter into conversation with.

Alongside these methodological responsibilities that I saw myself as being accountable towards, I additionally recognised the pertinence of particular political and academic issues associated with my project. These issues largely relate to historically established notions within academia which have insisted upon the empirically unsound, 'irrational' or even 'corrosive' nature of particular types of data, namely those associated with subjectivity, embodiment and emotions.[32] In more recent years, however, the masculinist biases behind these types of assumptions have been highlighted as theorists have drawn critical attention to the ways in which the disregarding of these experiences has long been legitimated through their typical association with the 'feminine'.[33]

In response to this obviously gendered politics of knowledge production, feminist informed theorists have begun to advocate that, rather than avoiding investigation into emotion, subjectivity and embodiment, researchers should

---

31 Burman, 'Emotions and Reflexivity'; Mauthner and Doucet, 'Reflexive Accounts'.

32 James Davies and Dimitrina Spencer, eds., *Emotions in the Field: The Psychology and Anthropology of Fieldwork Experience* (Stanford, California: Stanford University Press, 2010), 2.

33 Kay Anderson and Susan Smith, 'Editorial, Emotional Geographies' *Transactions of the Institute of British Geographers* 26 (2001): 7–10; Rose, 'Situating Knowledges'.

centre these types of experiences within their enquiries as a way to resist the institutional and patriarchal norms within the academic canon.[34] This project, by foregrounding the 'non-vocal' aspects of my participants' practices, is thus an attempt to carry out this politically motivated task and, by doing so, re-inscribe previously overlooked realities into broader conversations. As such, in this chapter, by asking the reader to 'tune in' to my participants' collective narrative, which is both counter to popular discourse and 'vocalised' in a non-traditional way, I have aimed not only to promote a message that might otherwise have been disregarded but, in addition, I hope to have challenged the reader to pay critical attention to the types of knowledges she might typically receive and the mechanisms through which she receives them.

8 Conclusion

In this chapter I have explored the various collaborative and non-vocal group practices found within a support group for female survivors of sexual violence. I outlined the ways in which these group practices could be seen as greatly diverging from popular medical and philosophical models surrounding sexual violence trauma, both of which advocate individual talking therapy as a way to either heal from pathological 'symptoms' or re-establish bonds of relationality.[35] Contrary to these understandings and, as I have highlighted, within the group, traumatic experience was interpreted not as pathological but, instead, as inextricably intertwined with a particular mode of shared feminine embodied subjectivity. As a result, the telling of individual narrative was felt to compromise this sense of connection by provoking comparison and minimisation.

By drawing attention to the actual practices that the group engaged in, I additionally highlighted the ways in which they implicitly contributed towards the collective production of a shared narrative surrounding sexual violence trauma. Here I argued that this shared narrative was one that was fundamentally counter to those that are, more typically, presented in relation to sexual violence. I suggested that, by de-pathologizing traumatic 'symptoms' this narrative worked to re-frame reactions to *all* types of gender-based violence, not as medical concerns, but as pertinent structural issues. Alongside this, by explicitly highlighting the ways in which narratives of sexual violence trauma frequently produce comparison and minimisation, I argued that this collective

34 Paige Averett and Danielle Soper, 'Sometimes I am Afraid: An Autoethnography of Resistance and Compliance', *The Qualitative Report* 16.2 (2001): 358–376.

35 Herman, *Trauma and Recovery,* 34; Brison, *Aftermath,* 38.

response problematized these effects as natural and, instead, acknowledged them to be a constitutive part of the undermining and oppressive system through which violence against women is perpetrated and legitimated. Ultimately, I here concluded that, whilst my participants might not be described as having a 'voice' in the traditional or vocal sense of the word, the collective voice that emerged from the group was one that was both profoundly political and deeply compassionate.

By highlighting the meaningfulness of this group narrative I have also engaged in exploring my own role in translating it. Having presented myself with the task of documenting a message that was not only outside of language but was a fundamental critique of narrative practice, I was, inevitably, forced to reflect upon the ways in which I might best present my research findings. I have suggested that, through the use of feminist informed critical reflexivity, both in relation to one's own methodological practice and as applied to the discipline within which one is situated, the researcher is able to produce congruent narratives whilst, simultaneously, challenging the historically gendered politics of knowledge production.[36] Frequently, this chapter has highlighted the issues surrounding the gross under-theorization of sexual violence trauma compared with other aspects of structural suffering.[37] Through the use of these critical reflexivity practices, I suggest that we can begin to remedy this ill by crucially re-inscribing women's voices and realities into broader conversations.

Bibliography

Anderson, Kay and Susan Smith. 'Editorial, Emotional Geographies'. *Transactions of the Institute of British Geographers* 26 (2001): 7–10.

Argenti-Pillen, Alex. *Masking Terror: How Women Contain Violence in Southern Sri Lanka.* Philadelphia: University of Pennsylvania Press, 2003.

Attig, Thomas. *How We Grieve: Relearning the World.* Oxford: Oxford University Press, 1996.

Averett, Paige and Danielle Soper. 'Sometimes I am Afraid: An Autoethnography of Resistance and Compliance'. *The Qualitative Report* 16.2 (2001): 358–376.

Brison, Susan. *Aftermath: Violence and the Remaking of a Self.* New Jersey: Princeton University Press, 2002.

36 Burman, 'Emotions and Reflexivity'; Mauthner and Doucet, 'Reflexive Accounts'; Rose, 'Situating Knowledges'.

37 Kleinman, *Social Suffering.*

Burgess, Ann and Lynda Holmstrom. 'Rape Trauma Syndrome'. *American Journal of Psychiatry* 131 (1974): 981–986.

Burman, Erica. 'Emotions and Reflexivity in Feminist Education Action Research'. *Educational Action Research* 14.3 (2006): 315–332.

Cahill, Ann. *Rethinking Rape.* New York: Cornell University Press, 2001.

Davies, James and Spencer Dimitrina, eds. *Emotions in the Field: The Psychology and Anthropology of Fieldwork Experience.* Stanford, California: Stanford University Press, 2010.

Delbo, Charlotte. *Auschwitz and After.* Translated by Rosette Lamont. New Haven: Yale University Press, 1995.

Dixon, Hayley. *Sex Abuse Victims Bring it Upon Themselves Bill Roache Claims.* 19 March 2013. Viewed on 15 July 2018. https://www.telegraph.co.uk/news/celebritynews/9939558/Sex-abuse-victims-bring-it-upon-themselves-Bill-Roache-claims.html.

Emerson Dobash, Rebecca and Dobash Russell, eds. *Rethinking Violence Against Women.* London: Sage Publications, 1998.

Farmer, Paul. 'An Anthropology of Structural Violence'. *Current Anthropology* 45.3 (2004): 305–325.

Herman, Judith. *Trauma and Recovery: From Domestic Abuse to Political Terror.* London: Pandora, 1994.

Hinton, Devon and Laurence Kirmayer. 'Local Responses to Trauma: Symptom, Affect, and Healing'. *Transcultural Psychiatry* 50.5 (2013): 607–621.

Hlavka, Heather. 'Normalizing Sexual Violence: Young Women Account for Harassment and Abuse'. *Gender and Society* 28.3 (2014): 337–358.

Holmes, Lindsay. *A Quick Lesson on what Trigger Warnings Actually Do.* 26 August 2016. Viewed on 15 July 2018. http://www.huffingtonpost.com/entry/university-of-chicago-trigger-warning_us_57bf16d9e4b085c1ff28176d.

Janoff-Bulman, Ronnie. *Shattered Assumptions: Towards a New Psychology of Trauma.* New York: The Free Press, 1992.

Janoff-Bulman, Ronnie, 'Characterological versus Behavioural Self-Blame: Inquiries into Depression and Rape'. *Journal of Personality and Social Psychology* 37 (1979): 1798–1809.

de Jong, Joop and Ria Reis. 'Collective Trauma Processing: Dissociation as a Way of Processing Postwar Traumatic Stress in Guinea Bissau'. *Transcultural Psychiatry* 50.5 (2013): 644–661.

Kelly, Liz and Jill Radford. "Nothing Really Happened': The Invalidation of Women's Experiences of Sexual Violence'. *Critical Social Policy* 10.30 (1990): 39-53.

Kelly, Liz, Jo Lovett and Linda Regan, 'A Gap or a Chasm?: Attrition in Reported Rape Case', *Home Office Research Study* 293 London: Home Office, 2005.

Kienzler, Hanna. 'The Social Life of Psychiatric Practice: Trauma in Postwar Kosova'. *Medical Anthropology* 31.3 (2012): 266–282.

Kleinman, Arthur. *Social Suffering.* Edited by Arthur Kleinman, Veena Das and Margaret Lock. Berkeley: University of California Press, 1997.

Mauthner, Natasha and Andrea Doucet. 'Reflexive Accounts and Accounts of Reflexivity in Qualitative Data Analysis'. *Sociology* 37.3 (2003): 413–431.

McClean, Linda and Ruth Gallop. 'Implications of Childhood Sexual Abuse for Adult Borderline Personality Disorder and Complex Post Traumatic Stress Disorder'. *The American Journal of Psychiatry* 160.2 (1993): 369–371.

Murray, John B. 'Relationship of Childhood Sexual Abuse to Borderline Personality Disorder, Post Traumatic Stress Disorder and Multiple Personality Disorder'. *The Journal of Psychology* 127.6 (1993): 657–676.

ONS (Office for National Statistics), *Sexual Offences in England and Wales: Year Ending March 2017*, February 2018. Viewed on 23 June 2018, https://www.ons.gov.uk/peoplepopulationandcommunity/crimeandjustice/articles/sexualoffencesinenglandandwales/yearendingmarch2017.

Rape Crisis England and Wales, *Rape Crisis England and Wales Headline Statistics 2017–2018*, 2018. Viewed on 23 June 2018, https://rapecrisis.org.uk/statistics.php.

Rose, Gillian. 'Situating Knowledges: Positionality, Reflexivity and Other Tactics'. *Progress in Human Geography* 21 (1997): 305–320.

Shay, Jonathon. *Achilles in Vietnam: Combat Trauma and the Undoing of Character.* New York: Atheneum, 1994.

Ward, Coleen. *Attitudes Towards Rape: Feminist and Social Psychological Perspectives.* London: Sage, 1995.

Wyatt, Gail, Cindy Notgrass and Michael Newcomb. 'Internal and External Mediators of Women's Rape Experiences'. *Psychology of Women Quarterly* 14 (1990): 153–176.

PART 3

Irreconcilable Voices: Liminal, Empowered, and Authentic

CHAPTER 5

Stories of Journeys Home: Reuniting Ancestors, Images, and the Underworld

Alexandra Fidyk

Abstract

Beginning with a brief historical overview of the oral tale, this chapter discusses its evolution to the literary tale and their differentiation. It then considers language and its relationship with the animate world as well as to magic and its power to enact wondrous transformation within the protagonist. The dominant structure of the oral tale is outlined along with a call for counter structures and themes. In support of the art of storytelling and its importance to the endeavour that maintains our humanity, this chapter frames suffering as a journey of necessity. This journey is highlighted as it unfolds through the particulars of the dominant plot, the heroic quest, and its counter plotline, a descent, or *katabasis*, to the underworld. Counter narratives about illness are less common today because they require different ways of doing and being, rather than the heroic those that seek to strengthen the ego. Through mythological and alchemical amplification, descent and its companion, *nigredo*, are viewed as the most negative, difficult, and dangerous of life's unfolding movements. Read in its characteristic blackening, time spent in the icy underworld is described as a way toward transformation. Descent is also framed as a journey to the home of the dead, to the ancestors, and to the darkness of humanity – a depth that requires one to relinquish ego's centrality in life, to sacrifice rational day-world expectations and preconceptions and to abandon hope. While less popular, this plot carries value, despite the hardships, because it teaches the primacy of the psyche, images, and the ancestors. It also reflects a fate that may have roots in transgenerational trauma. Here, the chapter makes a case for embracing the ways of the underworld, which has its own integrity and wisdom. In this journeying, suffering is seen as a way of knowing and a way of ethics.

Key Words

Oral tale – literary tale – wonder tale – descent – alchemy – katabasis – nekyia – death – empathy – suffering – surrender – ancestors – storytelling – trangenerational patterns

 | DOI:10. 1163/9789004396067_007

*****

1 Storytelling as Ancient Practice

Storytelling is an ancient practice. Passed down through generations, carried across land and sea, stories preserve the journeys of humanity and in their sharing, keep us human. Storytelling contributes to constructing a sense of self[1] as well as creating a sense of community. In its oral form, it has been used as a social and cultural activity to share knowledge, instil morals, entertain, educate, and preserve beliefs and practices. In its earliest form, stories were alive, shape shifting to reflect the context and intended purpose, and they were created between teller and audience – thereby leaving their indelible effect. Combined with gestures, dance, improvisation, theatrics, music, and embellishment, stories stitched us into a web of relations. They wed us to the animals, textures, and terrain of a particular place and time. Stories reflected human consciousness and contributed to its changing nature, especially its increasing separation from wilderness wherein language has become increasingly abstract and ungrounded in the sensorial and sensate.

Early cave art paintings might be read as rock stories created when humans existed in a more symbiotic relationship with nature. The images of beautiful eland, hartebeest, and lines of dancing humans visible on the walls of Cederberg caves and rock shelters in South Africa being one example. These illustrated stories, likely at least 1500 years old, and in many cases twice or three times that in age, depict the deeply held values that needed to be told by one generation to the next.[2] The San people, similar to other hunting and gathering groups, were a society without written records, without the option of committing knowledge and structure to portable means. Likewise, the rock art of the Northwest Pacific coastal tribes of Canada, reveals life lived in tandem with seasons, weather, hunts, and spirits. With the former typically considered pictographs and the latter petroglyphs, although there are also pictographs in the northwest Pacific region as well, both reveal symbolic meaning best understood in contemporary terms as religious. That is, the images were related in part to shamanic activities as well as to rites of passage, vision quests, and

1 This "sense of self" may be as a collective or community of people or as an individual, wherein the former is more common among traditional peoples and the latter to societies arising out of the Enlightenment and its continuing legacy.

2 John Parkington, *Cederberg Rock Paintings* (Cape Town, SA: Creda Communications, 2008), 25.

records of important events. In these examples, we see a kindred relationship between story, art, and life.

2 Voice in an Oral Culture

Remembering that language is rooted in the sounds, movements, and images of nature suggests that human language is not primary. Rather, it is the sensuous, felt, and perceptual life-world whose wild, participatory logic elaborates itself into language. David Abram argues that in Indigenous and oral cultures, 'nature itself is articulate; it *speaks*'.[3] The human voice in an oral culture, he suggests,

> is always to some extent participant with the voices of wolves, wind, and waves – participant, that is, with the encompassing discourse of an animate earth. There is no element of the landscape that is definitively void of expressive resonance and power: any movement may be a gesture, any sound may be a voice, a meaningful utterance.[4]

Abram continues that whenever members of a literate culture seek to engage and understand discourses of predominantly oral cultures, they find it difficult to detach from the habitual impulse to visualize language as a static structure that can be diagrammed and coded structurally. Without a formal writing system, the language of an oral culture cannot be objectified as a separate entity by those who speak it. This lack of objectification influences not only the way in which oral cultures experience the field of discursive meanings, but also the very character and structure of that field – its inhabitants, sounds, and matrix of colour. In the absence of a written analogue to speech, the breathing, textured, porous world remains the primary enactment of spoken utterance – the visible accompaniment of all spoken meaning. Consciousness remains more deeply embedded in the landscape. Just as the intellect objectifies experience, splitting it into an *in here* and *out there*, the alphabet as an abstracted tool for writing has over time done the same thing. It separates landscape and meaning, place and soul, self and other. Besides this splitting capacity, the alphabet has a creative capacity as well, especially powerful when used intentionally. Playfully, even poetically, we invent words. We too manipulate

3 David Abram, *The Spell of the Sensuous: Perception and Language in a More-than-Human World* (New York, NY: Vintage Books, 1996), 116.

4 Ibid., 117.

syntax for effect. More important is the symbolic aspect of language rather than the literal and technical – words that have been flattened because there is no breath to become anything other than the predetermined, predefined. Thus, there are those who have maintained an attentive, artful, and hermetic way with language, who understand words to be a kind of membrane or fibre, stitching us with a place, and comprehend that the aliveness, beauty, and power of verse are contingent upon the very world itself, and so by honouring that beingness, even locatedness, preserve their magic.

It is this magic that is central to storytelling. The distinction between oral and literary traditions is an important one although there exists a tendency among readers/listeners in the West to resist such analysis for fear of disturbing its sacred element. What is it that endows tales with enchantment? Why do some stories hold such a grip on us? Why do we seem to need them?

3 Development and Structure of Oral Tales

As tales were collected and recorded across Europe, distinctions between the oral folk tale and the literary fairy tale grew evident. According to German scholar Jens Tismar, the literary fairy tale as genre is '*written* by a single identifiable author' and is 'synthetic, artificial, and elaborate in comparison to the indigenous formation of the folk tale that emanates from communities and tends to be simple and anonymous'.[5] The differences between the two kinds of tales do not imply that one genre is better than the other; in fact,

> the literary fairy tale is not an independent genre but can only be understood and defined by its relationship to the oral tales as well as to the legend, novella, novel, and other literary fairy tales that it uses, adapts, and remodels during the narrative conception of the author.[6]

There are other important distinctions that help clarify the socio-historical rise of the fairy tale in Europe and North America. An array of writers, artists, filmmakers, musicians, and movements have contributed to the changing nature of the fairy tale as genre, and to its expansion into opera, theatre, photography, film, visual art, and other related cultural forms.

5 Tismar cited in Jack Zipes, 'Introduction', *The Oxford Companion to Fairy Tales*, ed. Jack Zipes (Oxford, UK: Oxford University Press, 2015), xv.

6 Ibid., xvi.

During its progressive development, the literary fairy tale continued to differentiate itself as genre by 'appropriating' many symbols, motifs, and drawings from folklore, embellishing and mixing them with elements from other literary genres. In this way, a certain kind of oral storytelling called the 'wonder tale' was gradually adapted to standards of literacy and made acceptable for diffusion in the public sphere. The fairy tale is only one type of literary appropriation of a particular oral story telling tradition related to the oral wonder tale that existed throughout Europe in many forms during the medieval period.[7] As more wonder tales were collected and recorded during the 14th through 17th centuries, they constituted the genre of the literary fairy tale which began to establish its own conventions, motifs, characters, and plots based on those created in the oral tradition, but revised to suit a reading public of middle class, aristocracy, and clergy. Although peasants were marginalized and excluded in its formation, it was their voices, habits, and beliefs that shaped this new literary tradition.[8]

Recalling the magic of language and its symbiotic relationship with place and people, villages and communities across Europe and North America developed various modes of storytelling in innumerable dialects and diverse forms of tales, reflecting their customs, laws, morals, and beliefs. While the oral wonder tale cannot be readily or simply defined, 'fundamental and constant' elements can be identified.[9] Most plots follow a basic pattern beginning with the protagonist who is confronted by a prohibition that she or he violates in some way. This contravention leads to the banishment of the protagonist or to the assignment of a task related to the prohibition. His or her character is then marked by the task that becomes his or her assigned identity or destiny. As many will remember from their childhood tales, the protagonist will have encounters with all sorts of characters, including animals, birds, and the supernatural. Gifts are usually involved and these are often magical agents. The protagonist is tested and, generally, there is a temporary setback. A wonder or miracle is needed to reverse the wheel of fortune. The protagonist eventually makes use of the endowed gifts to achieve his or her goal. The inimical forces are vanquished and the success of the protagonist usually leads to marriage and wealth. While the structural analysis of a wonder tale is useful, there are innumerable variations in theme and plot line. However, in contemporary renditions, the 'happily ever after' theme or the heroic tale has become

7 Ibid.
8 Ibid.
9 Propp cited in Zipes, *The Oxford Companion to Fairy Tales*, xvii.

all too common, especially in relation to illness narratives, thereby reducing the breadth of material for our own storied lives.

The wonder tale, in reality, is a hybrid formation. It evolved out of the chronicle, anecdote, myth, legend, and other oral forms and constantly changed, depending on the circumstances of the teller. If there is one constant in the structure and theme of the wonder tale that was also passed on to the literary fairy tale, it is transformation – 'miraculous transformation'.[10] 'Everybody and everything can be transformed in a wonder tale'![11] In particular, the social status of the protagonist changes. 'For the peasants who constituted the majority of the population in the Middle Ages, the hope for change was embedded in this kind of narrative, and this hope had nothing to do with a systemic and institutionalized belief system'.[12] That is, the fortuitous changes and happenings that befell the tales cannot be predetermined or guaranteed. Because the tales told by peasants were secular, the fortuitous change implies a kind of agency imbued in the world itself, out of the hands of humans.

Most wonder tales within the oral tradition have happy endings. In fact, they might be understood as wish fulfilment. Nevertheless, they are threaded to initiation rites that usher listeners into the 'appropriate' way to become a member of a given community. Stories are powerful socializing, even educational methods. The particulars of a narrative arise from life experiences and form a paradigm that supports recall for tellers and listeners – a kind of unconscious patterning that binds its kin – be it conservative, subversive, or other. The paradigmatic structure enables tellers and listeners to recognize, store, remember, and recreate the stories and to alter them to fit experiences and desires as needed via easily identifiable characters that are associated with particular assignments and settings. Indeed, this structure is abstract because it is generalized; so the protagonist and setting can be readily identified by listeners because the tale rose directly from common experiences and beliefs. 'Once upon a time in a far off land' offers a context that can be readily personalized. It is this archetypal structure that draws from the deep roots and common inheritance of humanity where magic arises. After all, the characters, settings, and motifs are combined in such a way as to induce wonder. This aura kindles astonishment and thus gives rise to admiration, fear, awe, and reverence. Listeners then and now, in this telling, are made to ponder the workings of the universe where anything can happen at any time, as the tales seek to awaken our regard for the 'marvellous *changing* condition of life and to evoke

10 Ibid.
11 Ibid.
12 Ibid.

in a religious sense profound feelings of awe and respect for life as a miraculous process that can be changed' by other forces, such as, nature, extraordinary encounters, and the creative principle.[13]

4 Storying Our Lives as Survival Technique

In the play of re-tellings, re-figurings and re-visions, not only do we continuously invent our lives, but also we keep ourselves in relation to the ancestry of humanity by drawing upon collectively shared images and emplotments. Thereby, 'the stories we tell produce and find us in the past, and enable us to live through the present's uncertainties by projecting us into the future'.[14] Folklorist W. F. H. Nicolaisen suggests that 'storying' serves as an 'essential component of our intellectual survival kit'.[15] We encounter stories 'not only as narration from knowledge and wisdom but also as a narrative given shape through ideas and relevance through vision'.[16] In this way, stories are interwoven with history and, subsequently, knowledge, values, and visions. As such, s/he who holds mastery of such narrative threads produces power as both privilege and empowerment. That is, traditions may be upheld or overturned, desire scripted or suppressed, and thus the specificities can be configured via the gender, narrativity, and subjectivity that it performs. Although we may not think of them as folkloric, 'preliminary censorship', tradition and consensus go together,

> and it is their dynamic interaction with an 'innovative' or subversive impulse that constitutes folk narratives. As folk and fairy tale, the tale of magic produces wonder precisely through its seductively concealed exploitation of the conflict between its normative function, which capitalizes on the comforts of consensus, and its subversive wonder, which magnifies the powers of transformation.[17]

This tensionality, along with the symbolic nature of language, enables us as listeners to repeatedly open to life and its potentialities, or to close down to it. Constructed as mythic constellations, the universality of their themes is part of their appeal. It is through these ancient tethers to our collective human

13 Ibid., xix.
14 Cristina Bacchilega, *Postmodern Fairy Tales: Gender and Narrative Strategies* (Philadelphia: University of Pennsylvania Press, 1997), 24.
15 Nicolaisen cited in Bacchilega, *Postmodern Fairy Tales*, 24.
16 Ibid.
17 Ibid., 7.

ancestry that something stirs and calls from what has passed and reaches toward what might be. In this way, the numinous artfully appears as natural – and we are caught in its spell.

Even though oral and literary tales often echo the plot line of the traditional oral tale, we see that, despite the persistence of themes across time, place, and language, their breadth has collapsed within contemporary European and American – North, South, Central – culture. Recalling that consensus and censorship aid to preserve cultures and their distinctive qualities, it is no surprise that the theme that holds privilege among illness and medical narratives is the hero's tale. Within this genre, stories about illness typically aim to conquer, overcome, even kill the invading Other, for example, campaigns to fight cancer – a plot line that echoes a similar fate for a dragon or a wicked stepmother. How might we welcome, host, or befriend Other so to offer different lines of flight within both lives?

5 Dominant and Counter Narratives

In response to this call for storytelling, I cobble a tale, a collective composition, which reflects the dramatic structure outlined earlier. In its ancient theme, it hearkens to my Northern European and Eastern European ancestors – indeed, for this telling to be possible, both heroic acts and fortuitous events must have occurred within my generational lineage. If one listens carefully, other versions of the tale, known commonly as a night sea journey or a dark night of the soul can be heard. Within it, however, I weave a counter narrative of descent, one that penetrates below that initial darkness, heat and fire, of the dominant narrative to the numbing chill of the land of the dead. Indeed, this land is not about, or for, heroic conquests. Rather, the aim of this narrative may well be about 'simple survival and acquisition of important knowledge based on experience'.[18] Such tales, if told at all, usually happen before darkness – that is, danger, despair, and depression – sets in and again well after light has returned. In both locations, the listeners are safe, free from the perils of the underworld. Writing during descent is also less common. We do not often write of the hell and agony, destruction and loss that are experienced during difficult times. Similarly, we do not often find pleasure in reading them either. Indeed, such tales have been forgotten, even forbidden, within mainstream education, counselling, and medicine.

18 Zipes, *The Oxford Companion to Fairy Tales*, xvii.

In what follows, elements of the counter tale are amplified with depth psychological insight in an effort to give new meaning to illness journeys – meaning made richer through an increased understanding of storytelling.[19] Stitched to these pieces are personal shards of another narrative – a story partially penned during a time of debilitating illness, and later fleshed out through various writings in an effort to gain insight by making the experience conscious and meaningful, despite the illness's crippling effects. In writing *from* and *of* the hell of the underworld, the aim is not to draw attention to the 'I' but to invite empathy for the human condition, to better understand the complexities involved in soul making, and to mark the difference between being simply overwhelmed and bearing witness to the extremity. Such attention acknowledges our shared human ancestry as well as our capacity for transformation, especially during critical times. As Annie Dillard advises, even in dark times, we must:

> Push it. Examine all things intensely and relentlessly… . Do not leave it, do not course over it, as if it were understood, but instead follow it down until you see it in the mystery of its own specificity and strength.[20]

The alchemists likewise assure us that there is a shining even in the blackest of black and this is where light and rebirth may be found.[21]

6 Mythological and Alchemical Amplification of Descent

Within depth psychology, with its mythological and alchemical roots, descent to the land of the dead is known as *nigredo* because it is characterized by blackening and known experientially through darkness, despair, and depression. It is known throughout history and across cultures because it refers to an 'innate, necessary psychic movement which must take place sooner or later when the conscious ego has exhausted the resources and energies of a given

19 As the event upon which this chapter derives spanned seven years of my life and was at play both before and after that particular period, my understanding and expression of it continues to evolve. Versions of this paper were given at the 5th *International Symposium of Poetic Inquiry* (October 2015) at the University of British Columbia and at the *Art & Psyche Conference* (September 2015) in Sicily, Italy.

20 Annie Dillard, *The Writing Life* (New York, NY: Harper & Row, 1989), 78.

21 Alexandra Fidyk, 'An Ethics of Humility', *A Heart of Wisdom: Life Writing as Empathetic Inquiry,* eds. Cynthia M. Chambers, Erika Hasebe-Ludt, Carl Leggo, and Anita Sinner (New York, NY: Peter Lang, 2012), 306–315.

life attitude'.[22] At one time or another, most people arrive here due to a prolonged period of loss, sadness, illness, overwhelm, or failure – whether they will enter or retreat remains to be seen. The experience is feared and cultural practices, institutions, and belief systems that promote avoidance or denigration of this journey are dangerous. To deny its call is to miss the depth, wisdom, and mystery that beckon.

Viewed as a symbolic art, alchemy has been used to illustrate that lifelong process of becoming an 'in-dividual, that is, a separate [yet interconnected] indivisible unity or whole', woven into all that has ever been or will be.[23] Alchemy locates the death experience at the heart of the alchemical process. The root of the term alchemy, *khem*, refers to Egypt as the 'land of black soil' or 'black land', and its *techne* can be traced through the 'black art' of Egyptian embalming, jewellery making, and dyeing cloth.[24] While there are four variations of unification in alchemy – *nigredo*, *albedo*, *citrinitas*, and *rubedo* – *nigredo* is the initial process. Like illness, it is a world of its own, 'another plane of reality', with 'its own geography "beneath deeps of darkness", [and] its own gravity at the farthest bottom of life'.[25] *Nigredo* marks a descent into the unconscious, *and* it signals an accomplishment for beginning to separate out from the collective. Historically, to preserve a given culture, only a few are chosen and so called on such a journey – one deemed beneficial to the collective – like a healer, teacher, artist, or visionary. To return the world, individual and collective, to order and balance, their bodies bear the untold lessons and scars of history. As these protagonists suffer their 'wounds in the extremities of illness, they become the offerings, [the] means of realizing and remembering' what is necessary to bring their lives and their world back into balance.[26] 'Consciously lived suffering', wrote Jungian analyst Marie-Louise von Franz, 'has a redeeming effect upon the past and future of [hu]mankind, an effect which is exerted invisibly from the Beyond', from the collective unconscious.[27]

Of the alchemical process, *nigredo* is 'the most negative and difficult operation', and it is also one of the most numinous.[28] Such a journey requires a

22 Edward Edinger, *Melville's Moby Dick: A Jungian Commentary: An American Nekyia* (New York, NY: New Directions, 1975), 21.

23 Carl Gustav Jung, *The Archetypes and the Collective Unconscious, The Collected Works of C.G. Jung* Volume 9i. Bollingen Series, trans. R.F.C. Hull (Princeton, NJ: Princeton University Press, 1959/1969), par. 490.

24 James Hillman, 'The Seduction of Black', *Fire in the Stone: The Alchemy of Desire*, ed. Stanton Marlan (Wilmette, IL: Chiron, 1997), 45.

25 Kat Duff, *The Alchemy of Illness* (New York, NY: Bell Tower, 1993), 4.

26 Ibid., 123–124.

27 Marie-Louise von Franz, *On Dreams & Death* (Boston, MA: Shambhala, 1987), 109.

28 Stanton Marlan, *The Black Sun* (College Station, TX: Texas A&M University Press, 2005), 11.

transmutation, a transformation, from one state of being to another, as in the dissolution of a solid to a liquid. It requires a willingness to be acted upon even though 'it comes as violation'.[29] And it requires 'a sacrifice of the upper-world aspects of the Self', of the surface of things such as status, relationships, even preferred ways of knowing and doing, 'to and for the sake of the dark, different, or altered-state [of consciousness] aspects'.[30] Like a sacred contract, there can be no breach, no forfeiture. Here in the process of psychic unfolding, in adherence to 'the rhythmic order of nature', the destructive-transformative side of cosmic will, death occurs – death as a psychological event not as a corporeal one, although there are exceptions, especially in regards to illness.[31] As John Donne wrote, 'health is a long and regular work; but sickness summons us, seizes us, possesses us and destroys us in an instant'.[32]

This journey is not analogous to the night-sea journey although many narratives use the terms synonymously, and the former may contribute to the latter. The heroine returns in better shape for the tasks of life. She has endured, battled 'past her personal and local historical limitations'[33] and so she returns enlightened and fortified for what follows. On the rough seas, she conquers the 'villain' often with the aid of magical talismans or helpful forest animals, in this case treatment – medical professionals, family members, other 'survivors' or those to whom she was kind. That is, her ego has strengthened instead of its unthinkable dissolution. At the end of the journey, of the wonder tale, she is rewarded – happiness, marriage, or wealth – and in the case of illness, renewed health by 'beating cancer', for example, indeed, a kind of wish fulfilment.

7 Descending to the Land of the Dead

In the ancient world, *katabasis*, the Greek word for 'descending', referred to the journey to the underworld, to the land of the dead. *Nekyia*, in Greek, was a ritual by which ghosts were called up and questioned about the future; it was not an actual descent. C. G. Jung used the concept of *nekyia* as an integral part of analytical psychology: the 'introversion of the conscious mind into the deeper

29 Hillman cited in Marlan, *The Black Sun*, 77.

30 Silvia Brinton Perera, *Descent to the Goddess: A Way of Initiation for Women* (Toronto: Inner City Books, 1981), 14.

31 Ibid., 13.

32 John Donne, 'Devotions', *Complete Poetry and Selected Prose of John Donne and Complete Poetry of William Blake* (New York, NY: Random House, 1941), 309.

33 Joseph Campbell, *The Hero with a Thousand Faces* (Princeton, NJ: Princeton University Press, 1949/1968), 19.

layers of the unconscious psyche'. However, he often used it interchangeably with a night sea journey.[34] For Jung, the *nekyia*, is 'no aimless or destructive fall into the abyss, but a meaningful *katabasis* into the cave of initiation and secret knowledge ... its object [is] the restoration of the whole [person]'.[35] James Hillman however made clear distinctions between the two terms – a distinction considered vital to the stories that give shape and meaning to our lives. Here in their telling and amplification, the night sea journey requires heroes and heroines to take up the call to adventure; to leave the ordinary world; and to traverse the threshold to the unknown. While demanding and difficult, it ends with successful results. In the descent, that which supported the hero offers no aid. While it unfolds incomprehensibly and chaotically, a *katabasis* is by aim and design. Those who, in actuality, are destined, journey through the psychic history of humanity, to the ancestors, to the dead; 'This is no mere metaphor'.[36] It is a leave-taking from the upper world, its light, and its knowing, to the land of 'blacker than black'.[37] All brightness becomes veiled by the mists of Hades, 'infecting it with deadly decay, and finally, like an earthquake, dissolving it into fragments, fractures, discarded remnants, debris, shreds',[38] where she is swallowed into the cold, dark depths, devouring her soul into 'a depth for its own sake' – a movement necessary for psychological maturation – and specific contribution to society.[39] Here, like Odysseus, Odin, or Gilgamesh, she sinks 'below that pressurized containment [common to the night-sea journey], that tempering of the fires of passion, to a zone of utter coldness', 'to a realm of ice – deep, deep down'.[40] The heroic modes of doing, acting, and conquering no longer have power. Said otherwise, the descent is a psychological and physiological process that is real for the protagonist, intentionally initiated – a sealed fate. In Hillman's reading of the mythologem of Hades, 'descent to the underworld is to frozen depths' and 'archetypal crystallizations' for it takes one to a place beyond the human imaginary of flame,

34 Carl Gustav Jung, *Analytical Psychology* (London: Routledge, 1976), 41.

35 Carl Gustav Jung, *The Spirit in Man, Art, and Literature. The Collected Works of C.G. Jung*, trans. by R.F.C. Hull (Princeton, NJ: Princeton University Press, 1966/1978), 15: par. 213, emphasis in original.

36 Shamdasani in James Hillman and Sonu Shamdasani, *Lament of the Dead. Psychology after Jung's* Red Book (New York, NY: W.W. Norton and Company, 2013), 2.

37 Hillman cited in Marlan, *The Black Sun*, 51.

38 Jung, *The Spirit in Man, Art, and Literature*, par. 210.

39 James Hillman, *The Dream and the Underworld* (New York, NY: Avon, 1979), 168.

40 Ibid.

heat, and fire.[41] 'Cold is misery'[42]: it immobilizes, paralyzes, and it is necessary. Cold 'preserves, holds, protects, isolates, suspends'.[43] 'For those destined to it', like Inanna in the Sumerian tale with Ereshkigal, the Dark Goddess, 'it forces us to go deep to reclaim modes of consciousness which are different from the intellectual', and

> it forces us to the affect-laden ... [realm] and archaic depths that are embodied, ecstatic, and transformative: these depths are preverbal, often pre-image, capable of taking us over and shaking us to the core.[44]

From this journey, there is no return.

For this protagonist, death is twofold: first, as she descends, she is stripped. All traces of outer world adornment, and all inner world constructs which were meant to insulate and protect her, must go. When she reaches the ends of the earth, like Inanna, she is hung on a meat hook and left to rot. This is the elongated time when her ego reconfigures; it must accept a secondary position to life's unfolding. Unlike the hero who prevails over adversity, this character undergoes failed attempts to overcome misfortune, suffering, and death. She can do nothing else but relinquish her 'I's' dominant reign of life, its defences, its identity along with its former view of self, *and* of life. What drops away from her everyday ego is the hoping, wishing, desiring, fearing ... that is, the affective emotional relation to the future: 'I will get better'. What remains is only that which was and is. This 'egocide'[45] occurs in 'the underground psychic soil ... in which the seeds of the true self are embedded and from which they ultimately can germinate'.[46] The 'voluntary death of one's psychic comfort, rightness, and rationality ... allows oneself to be less in order to be more – less nearly perfect, but more nearly whole'.[47] And sometimes, a double death occurs – that of the ego and the body – if not completely, than by degree – impaired, paralyzed, disabled. Like Inanna, she is condemned to death, struck down, for the ways

---

41 Ibid., 169.

42 Enrico Francot, *The Icy Side of the Self: The Role of Cold in the Individuation Process* (Milano, Italy: L'Ossessione Espressa, 2013), Chapter 1.

43 Ibid., 170.

44 Perera, *Descent to the Goddess*, 14.

45 David Rosen, *Transforming Depression: Healing the Soul through Creativity* (York Beach, ME: Nicolas-Hays, 2002), xxvi.

46 Ibid., 34.

47 Edward Edinger, *Anatomy of the Psyche: Alchemical Symbolism in Psychotherapy* (Chicago, IL: Open Court, 1994), 161.

of the underworld must be fulfilled. After all, 'coming to consciousness is a violent act'.[48]

'Nothing but crystallized insights and sharp-edged truths' serve.[49] Anyone who cannot meet her on these terms, or whose 'urge [is] to warm the cold and melt the ice, reflects an effort of one who has not been able to meet the ice at its own level', for there are few who can accompany her, who can witness,[50] like Ereshkigal for Inanna or Hecate for Persephone.[51] Yet, there is a presence, a consciousness that imbues the dark, that bears testament to such events, that witnesses because it is aware of them *a priori*. As Susan Griffin penned: 'At the center of / all my sorrows / I have felt a presence / that was not mine alone'.[52] Of this, Hillman suggests that part of us is not pulled from under but has always already lived there. So when we find ourselves in such dark terrain, a part of us is not surprised. We nod with dread and knowing to the thread that stitches us with our past, with tradition, and with our dead. For the forces that Ereshkigal symbolizes connect not only to active destruction but also to transformation,

> via those slow, cell-by-cell organic processes like decay and gestation, which work [even invasively] upon the passive, stuck recipient ... and reduce her to the primal state of inert animal matter – but matter that undergoes change, in passive submission to the givens.[53]

Analogous to folk and fairy tales' uninhabited forests that inspire a feeling of mystery, the underworld has an integrity of its own. In the structure of oral tales, this knowledge often comes in the form of a talisman or a gift – imbued with a blessing that enables it to function on its own accord. The *mortificatio* process, often brutal and harsh, eventually leads to nothingness, revealed sometimes through the literal, but always 'existential, imaginal, symbolic, and

48 Ronald Schenk, *Dark Light. The Appearance of Death in Everyday Life* (Albany, NY: State University of New York Press, 2001), 137.

49 Hillman, *The Dream and the Underworld,* 170.

50 Pam Morrison and Annie McGregor's chapter, 'Making and Sharing Meaning out of Terminal Illness', in this volume offers a profound account of the power of witnessing. They offer a narrative of sister love and empathy that brings me to tears. As a middle child among five, becoming ill has been the loneliest experience of my life, and despite being in my near tenth year of shattering illness, I remain mostly alone in it. Their gift of co-journaling, 'interleaving our entries to share our daily lives, along with our fears, our hopes, our griefs and joys', offers a way *through* that can certainly heal soul despite the result of the body-mind. Theirs is an account of hope.

51 Ibid., 170.

52 Susan Griffin, *Unremembered Country* (Port Townsend, WA: Copper Canyon Press, 1987), 122–123.

53 Perera, *Descent to the Goddess*, 24.

poetic'.[54] In other words, 'death fertilizes the imaginal and works to open a poetic space that brings depth and meaning to everyday life'.[55] And yet this truth is paradoxical, for the dead must be taken literally – all those who have come before us, personal and collective, familial and archetypal, must be accounted for – as Jung discovered during his descent. This forgotten insight is one of the reasons for retelling old tales and creating new, especially ones that run counter to dominant plot lines. Non-conforming and emergent patterns are necessary for the richness and complexity brought to storying our lives. As in this tale, the 'now' of death is an 'imaginal reality: a dark and pervasive presence and a primordial abyss',[56] 'that obliterates the light of [logos] consciousness even as *it opens up and frees one for the symbolic life*'.[57] 'We need', as Jung advises, 'the coldness of death to see clearly'.[58] We cannot live authentically without that encounter.

8 An Ethic of the Dead

Descending into the depths is not only a descent to the land of the dead, but also a descent to the ancestors, to 'the darkness of humanity', to the echoes of history – to the source of who we are and how we shape and live our lives.[59] Jung discovers through his own disintegration and lament that 'unless we come to terms with the dead[,] we simply cannot live', for they not only animate us, but 'our life is dependent on finding answers to their unanswered questions'.[60] Jung knew this for he evoked his inner figures and let them speak through methods of active imagination, dream interpretation, and imaginal dialogues[61] during his *katabasis* – for they knew what he did not.

Attending to family seeks to recollect all familial members and to honour their membership to the familial soul regardless of the outer world narratives about select persons, thereby abandoning no one. Whether literal or metaphoric, gestures from the ancestors seek to connect us to history – to

54 Marlan, *The Black Sun*, 76.

55 Ibid.

56 Carl Gustav Jung, *Memories, Dreams, Reflections*, trans. Richard and Clara Winston, ed. Aniela Jaffe (New York: Random House, 1961/1989), 128.

57 Marlan, *The Black Sun*, 76.

58 Carl Gustav Jung, *The Red Book: Liber Novas*, ed. Sonu Shamdasani. Philemon Series. (New York: W.W. Norton & Company, 2009), 274.

59 Carl Gustav Jung, *Visions: Notes of the Seminar Given in 1930–1934*, ed. Clare Douglas (Princeton, NJ: Princeton University Press, 1997), 118–119.

60 Hillman and Shamdasani, *Lament of the Dead*, 1.

61 See Stephani Stephens, 'Active Imagination and the Dead', *International Journal of Jungian Studies* 8 2 (2016): 46–59.

'the forms that are neglected, forgotten, and feared'.[62] After all, inheritance of group origin – be it familial, cultural, geographic, or ethnic – is the most common cause of disease. The immune system is said to possess incredible powers of memory; it knows all our secrets, all our sorrows. If choice exists in the creation of illness, it arises from the unconscious strata where the ghosts of memory reside. Most of us have forgotten or deny this system of mutuality, this system of reciprocity between the living and the dead. As with the burden of responsibility that accompanied images for Jung, as well as traditional cultures in the example of cave art, so too recollecting the voices of the dead comes with an ethical obligation. This '*ethic of the dead*', like the ethic of the cultural, social, affective, and political, is bound to our ability to live as fully as possible – to make life meaningful – and that necessitates honouring the past, all of its aspects, not just the good.[63] While the dead for Jung are more than 'spirits of the departed' – his familial eight great-grandparents – we must also understand our personal grandparents, the ostracized uncle, even the stillborn or miscarried children – as ancestors who are no longer present, because they too influence our lives.[64]

This connection to human ancestry comes both in the form of 'unearthed shards and small bones' of our animal ancestors as well as in the 'spirits of the dead'.[65] Recall that protagonists who communicate with the animals typically are found to be wise, for they have not turned against or away from nature. Old tales that place wise ones in relation to the elements and animals embody vital ecological messages of our interconnectivity and interdependence. Traditional African cosmology, for instance, accounts for those who have died alongside those who are living which might be the root of the Haitian belief that

> those who die never *really* die. They undergo a 'translation of state' – not unlike the reconfiguration that befalls those who partake of an underworld descent. Thus, the spirits of the Haitian dead, or 'those we don't see', do not depart, as in many other religions but 'remain extremely close to us', the living.[66]

62 Hillman and Shamdasani, *Lament of the Dead*, 96.

63 Alexandra Fidyk, 'Unconscious Ties That Bind: Attending to Complexes in the Classroom, Part 2', *International Journal of Jungian Studies* 8.3 (2016): 196, emphasis in original.

64 Jung, *Memories, Dreams, Reflection*, 338.

65 Jung, *The Red Book: Liber Novas*; Robin van Löben Sels, 'Ancestors and Spirits of the Dead', *Quadrant: Journal of the C.G. Jung Foundation for Analytical Psychology, xxxx* 2 (2010): 82; Marie-Louise von Franz, *Projection and Re-collection in Jungian Psychology. Reflections of the Soul* (Peru, IL: Open Court Publishing, 1980/1995), 104.

66 van Löben Sels, 'Ancestors and Spirits of the Dead', 82.

In this cultural context, 'the spirits of the dead have not left the living, there they are, *among* the living'.[67] They are 'invisible but *tangible*, and they inhabit a parallel universe on the other side of any mirror, beneath the surfaces of all water, and just behind the veil that divides us from our dreams'.[68] Jungian analyst Robin van Löben Sels elucidates in reference to the terrible wreckage of Port au Prince:

> With families destroyed utterly, lost among the rubble of devastated homes, with 150,000 dead, the traumatized Haitians who remain, the survivors, know that the energy of NOT lost souls can spring back into their living world through the riches of their culture, through visual art and music – much of which is rooted in the rhythms of ceremonial drumming – and through a vivid Haitian literature and an ever-evolving language. So perhaps those who remain in the living Haitian world today are not only suffering; they can expect to and they will find in the depths of suffering riches and treasure.[69]

Comparable to Western religions which place the spirits of the dead and ancestors in another world, in an after-life out of reach from the day to day of this life, Haitians have a taken-for-granted richness in their religious experience, stories, and worldview: the nearness of 'invisible but *tangible*' energies, 'the enormous and impersonal power of archetypal force-fields, and the presence of personified presences – 'those we don't see' – all of whom appear to us in various guises'.[70] Similar richness lies hidden in the West, except perhaps in the remnants of specified events or days such as All Saints Day or All Souls Day, the yearly remembrance of the deceased.

9 Metaphoric and Archetypal Ancestors

Ancestors with a capital A also include our archetypal Grandparents – the great Grizzlies, Bison, and Cranes, as well as the great Whales of every ocean, 'the Big Cats of Asia and the Elephants of Africa and India'.[71] Anthropologist Paul Shepard[72] suggests that originally our human sense of beauty constellated

67 Ibid.
68 Ibid.
69 Ibid., 83.
70 Ibid.
71 Ibid., 82.
72 Paul Shepard, *Coming Home to the Pleistocene* (Washington, DC: Island Press, 1998).

around our Ancestors as they watched the big animals – the mammoth, elephant, eland, and bison – move around in the open world, as illustrated with the development of language. Behind these Grandparents stand the great Sequoia, the desert Baobab, the Pine and Redwood. 'These presently-living ancestral creatures open us to awe', van Löben Sels writes.[73] 'Their struggles and sufferings and demise are teaching us despair. These are the Ancestors who live today *with* us, in the here and now and they are not faring well'.[74] Of these psychological and physical worlds, archetypal and cellular, South African Jungian analyst and wilderness guide, Ian McCallum asks, 'How long is it going to take to acknowledge that there is indeed a menagerie within each of us ... a wolf, a hyena, a lion ... a wild man and a wild woman?'[75] To re-member our ecological kinship is to come home to a more inclusive understanding of self that is always already united with animals, elements, and wild places. He reminds us of relations that were woven into the old oral tales: of our molecular origins, of our geology, of those first cellular membranes and to the eventual expression of a species capable of reflecting upon itself. The relationship of principal cations that the electropositive elements of the blood serum of all animals and human beings is constant, 'calcium : sodium : potassium = 5 : 10 : 160'.[76] This measurement is a close representation of their respective proportions in seawater, differing only by a greater content of magnesium in the oceans of today. McCallum expands:

> The animals, then, are in us and with us; we share their genes and their juices. Made up of countless molecules, cells and complex organs, each one of us is the carrier not only of the pattern of embryonic gill slits and tails, but the entire history of life also. It would appear that the aboriginal 'water of life' still circulates in the blood of every animal, including us.[77]

This molecular pattern joins us all – humankind, human ancestry, all entities – those of our ecological homes and our psychological ones. Our ancestors then comprise 'the entire history of life' pulsating through our veins and calling us from behind the veil of our dreams, felt sensations, and visions. We would fare much better if our cosmology, if our reality was as inclusive – if we found a 'way of finding the return ... to the world ... of bringing ... the depths of the psyche,

73 van Löben Sels, 'Ancestors and Spirits of the Dead', 82.

74 Ibid.

75 Ian McCallum, *Ecological Intelligence: Rediscovering Ourselves in Nature* (Cape Town, SA: Africa Geographic, 2006), 165.

76 McCallum, *Ecological Intelligence,* 64.

77 Ibid., 65.

and the weight of human history back into human life'.[78] This re-membering and re-collecting can be enacted through stories. The infinite, the unconscious, the forgotten, has meaning only when it is linked to consciousness; 'otherwise, it is, as it were, "lost in itself"'.[79] The gifts of transforming the 'lost' into found appears to have 'a positive long-lasting influence' in the 'library' of the collective unconscious – the storehouse of Life.[80]

10 Personal Ancestors and 'Fateful Links'

Shifting from this magnified view of Ancestors back to the personal, I return to Jung who discovered the importance of family to psyche and its fateful weight upon the individual. Although it is one area not fleshed out in his collected work, it is one that he judged as critical to psychotherapy. Such knowing found its place in his auto/biographical writing:

> When I was working on the stone tablets, I became aware of the *fateful links between me and my ancestors…* . I am under the influence of things or questions which were left incomplete and unanswered by my parents and grandparents and more distant ancestors. It often seems as if there were an impersonal karma within a family, which is passed on from parents to children. It has always seemed to me that I had to complete, or perhaps continue, things which previous ages had left unfinished.[81]

And further:

> A collective problem, if not recognized as such, always appears as a personal problem, and in individual cases may give the impression that something is out of order in the realm of the personal psyche. The personal sphere is indeed disturbed, but such disturbances need not be primary; they may well be secondary, the consequence of an insupportable change in the social atmosphere. The cause of disturbance is, therefore, not to be sought in the personal surroundings, but rather in the collective situation [in the family and more distant ancestors]. Psychotherapy has hitherto taken this matter far too little into account.[82]

78 Hillman and Shamdasani, *Lament of the Dead*, 65.
79 von Franz, *On Dreams and Death*, 142.
80 Ibid.
81 Jung, *Memories, Dreams, Reflection*, 233, emphasis added.
82 Ibid., 233–234.

Much healing and psychological development can occur through creative work – writing, drawing, dramatization, activity that integrates the arts and engages the body – each of which operates in consort with material from the unconscious. In living out family traumas, psychiatrist Norman Doidge writes, 'Psychotherapy is often about turning our ghosts into ancestors'. By identifying the source of our generational traumas, our ghosts can 'go from haunting us to becoming simply part of our history'.[83]

The universal urge toward wholeness and unity expressed in oral tales, governs clans and families too.[84] When a problem appeared personal and a life is disturbed, the cause may not be found 'in the personal surroundings, but rather in the collective situation'. As Jung suggests, a family works as a whole, a unit or soul where questions 'left incomplete' in one generation need to be completed by another or 'perhaps continue'. Similarly, 'fateful links' and 'impersonal karma' conjoin familial members often through 'illness or misfortune'. Swiss psychoanalyst Bert Hellinger concurs:

> This loyalty among members of a family and extended family manifests as a need for systemic balance between the benefits enjoyed by one member and the disadvantage suffered by another. It is this systemic urge for balance that leads one member of the group to court misfortune when another is suffering, or that tempts one person into illness or misfortune when another is ill or found guilty, or that makes someone long for death when another member of the system dies.[85]

And further,

> [W]ithin this confined fellowship of fate, loyalty and the need for balance and compensation assure that one member participates in the guilt and illness and fate and death of others; they lead to attempts to bring about someone's well-being through one's own misfortune, someone else's health through one's own illness, someone else's guilt through one's own

83 Norman Doidge, *The Brain That Changes Itself: Stories of Personal Triumph from the Frontiers of Brain Science* (New York: Penguin, 2007), 243.

84 Yomna Saber's chapter, 'Toni Cade Bambara's *The Salt Eaters*: Hearing the Silent Voice of Pain', in this volume challenges discussions of wholeness – what it means to 'being' as well as to 'living'. Her address through Velma's responsibility to herself adds depth that is relevant here.

85 Bert Hellinger, *Love's Own Truths: Bonding and Balancing in Close Relationships*, trans. by M. Oberli-Turner and H. Beaumont (Phoenix, AZ: Zeig, Tucker and Theisen, 2001), 311.

> innocence, or someone else's innocence through one's guilt, and someone else's life through one's own health.[86]

This 'fellowship of fate' burdens us all as every family has its own set of rules, checks, and balances. As Indigenous and 'traditional peoples' knew, the dead must be respected – yet these are not stories often told or heard today in the West and not in relation to illness.

11 Reuniting with the Ancestors, Images, and Darkness

Transgenerational patterns, family constellation systems, and the field of morphic resonance demonstrate that genealogical shadow, and by extension, inherited shame, is encountered most often in families or communities where there are silences, secrets, and unanswered questions surrounding traumatic events from the past, such as suicides, bankruptcies, betrayals, violence, and thefts. In addition, forgotten miscarriages and abortions can impact greatly the quality of life of a family member.[87] Often illness reveals stories of familial, blind or unconscious, love and loyalty.[88] In the images and movements that arise 'invisible and tangible' when conducting a family constellation, for example, what was previously unknown appears and can be brought into consciousness, thus beginning a new story.[89] It can then give voice and form not only to the ancestors but also to their homelands and significant events such as wars, genocides, and famines, along with their effects. Often this latter story subverts the previous autobiographical plot line because it is not influenced by desires, fantasies, or morals. By allowing ourselves to be moved by the new,

86 Ibid.

87 Recording a detailed family genogram accompanied by stories for three or more generations from the respective lineages can conjure up the unconscious as it 'offers itself to us from outside as a fated event, or from inside in the course of our life', von Franz, *On Dreams and Death*, 142.

88 Utilizing Hellinger's method of constructing a constellation is an effective way to bring to light unconscious impulses that underlie a problem nested within a larger tapestry shaped by ancestral familial traumas. It can diffuse familial complexes, expressed as unconscious patterns of thought, attitudes, or behaviour among family members, including what Jung called 'possession' via an 'ancestral soul'. Jung's methods of active imagination and imaginal dialogues are also beneficial ways of supporting mutuality between the living and the dead, especially when used with body and breath work so to prevent fragmentation or dissociation. Carl Gustav Jung, *The Archetypes and the Collective Unconscious, The Collected Works of C.G. Jung*, trans. By R.F.C. Hull (Princeton, NJ: Princeton University Press, 1959/1969), 9i: par. 224.

89 Fidyk, *Unconscious Ties That Bind*, 200–203.

emergent image, and honouring it as the ancestors have taught us, it overruns the old trauma emotions and sensations that have hijacked us from within. When this image is unearthed from the field, it reflects a connection of the Self, both individual soul as well as the family soul, with the numinous. Only a conscious realization of the Beyond which, 'as *spiritus rector* of all biological and psychological occurrences', represents the eventual unity with all archetypes – a unity or whole – which etymologically means to 'heal'.[90] What is made conscious – 'only *that* remains with us in death'.[91] Storying our lives through connection to the unconscious and the unknown releases the potential of 'wondrous transformation'. In this way, the story rises, autonomously, organically, from the depths of our ancestry and activates the power of the archetypal. This narrative differs substantially from most autobiographies and memoirs that are not written *with* or make room *for* the Other. 'Sooner or later', says Jung, 'all the dead become what we also are', alluding to the 'mystery of the Self in which all souls, those of the dead and of the living, are merged into a multiple unity'.[92]

Regardless of how we find our way to the ancestors, this reunion is tantamount for they teach us 'the primacy of the psyche, for that is the one thing which life does not make clear to us'.[93] We are so hemmed in by things and by appearances, that we do not heed the givens. Nor do we revere the dead as the basis of our existence. Illness can wake us. And descent offers the potential to learn another way. When we do, we discover that they are 'bound up with ["things" and] the event', the *what* and the *way*, which reveals the coinciding of 'our own imaginings with what is taking place within the world'.[94] 'There is no longer … a distinction between the lifeless and the living[;] everything is animate and soulless, vigilant and asleep at once'.[95] Their presence, an imageless image, experienced as a felt sense[96] demonstrates the power of body knowing: 'a kind of sixth sense, which perceives with such a profound sense of reality and intensity that no doubt can remain in the

90 von Franz, *On Dreams and Death*, 142.

91 Ibid.

92 Ibid., 143.

93 Carl Gustav Jung, *Psychology and Religion: West and East. The Collected Works of C.G. Jung*, trans. by R.F.C. Hull (Princeton, NJ: Princeton University Press, 1958/1989), 11: par. 841.

94 Shamdasani in Hillman and Shamdasani, *Lament of the Dead*, 130.

95 Walter Otto, *The Homeric Gods: The Spiritual Significance of Greek Religion*, trans. Moses Hadas (New York, NY: Thames and Hudson, 1954), 118–119.

96 'Felt sense' from Gendlin is not a mental experience but a physical one; a bodily awareness of a situation or person or event (which includes brain/mind). Eugene Gendlin, *Focusing* (New York, NY: Bantom Books, 1980).

visionary that [her] experience was real'.[97] Visionary is used here to signal the task of the ones chosen by illness for a *katabasis*. This experience 'must therefore be followed with consciousness and with expression that is appropriate both to the feeling and to the moment in which it is expressed'.[98] As such, the ancestors teach the importance of staying with the thing itself, even when it activates 'chaotic defensive furies, such as rage, [and] greed ... inevitable aspects of the archetypal underworld'.[99] For when we deny, armour, or distance ourselves, in defence against 'the sense of helpless surrender to her impersonal and instinctual forces, seeking to dull the heroic ego's humiliation at being brought so low that we must confront our primal smallness in the cosmos',[100] they are there with us. They teach the centrality of life unfolding: what is *is*, and the secondary place of the conceptual. Its reward is a different kind of knowing – not that which reduces and defines, interprets, and explains. Rather, through the rightness and terrible slowness of the event, we learn to surrender. When all options have been explored and have failed, we know with quiet certainty that there is no other way out or forward or anywhere. It is humbling to be brought so low that the *only way* to be is to agree to the chill of Ereshkigal's impersonal and instinctual forces, and to remain within the inhibiting coldness, surrendering consciously, willingly, fully. 'Only an act of conscious, willing surrender can turn that poisonous side of the dark goddess into life'.[101]

While recognized and appreciated in this tangential tale, darkness is not a phenomenon welcomed by many. Historically, it has not been treated hospitably by psychiatry, medicine, counselling, or education.[102] As such it has remained in the unconscious and viewed 'primarily in its negative aspect', constituting a shadow – 'something to integrate, to move through and beyond'.[103] Its intrinsic importance is bypassed. The innocence that keeps us insulated from the weight and reality of the human condition eventually 'risks a different loneliness and rigidity, one of staying stuck in a surface, or outer role or

97 Jeffrey Raff, 'The Felt Vision', *The Sacred Heritage: The Influence of Shamanism on Analytical Psychology*, eds. Donald F. Sandner and Steven H. Wong (New York, NY: Routledge, 1997), 80.

98 Ibid., 81.

99 Ibid., 23–24.

100 Ibid., 27.

101 Ibid.

102 Alexandra Fidyk, 'A Black Blessing', *On the Pedagogy of Suffering: Hermeneutic and Buddhist Meditations*, eds. David Jardine, Christopher Gilham, and Graham McCaffrey (New York, NY: Peter Lang, 2015), 101–106.

103 Marlan, *The Black Sun*, 12.

identity [that] one has outgrown'.[104] Darkness however 'has its own peculiar intellect and its own logic which should be taken very seriously'.[105] After all Persephone does not become 'Queen of the Underworld *until* she has suffered the descent, the loss, the frozen timeless darkness of the Hadean realm'.[106] Black dissolves meaning and the hope for meaning. It destroys any philosophy, theory, or belief of anything else unfolding. Seeing this way 'shears us of our defences and entails a sacrifice of easy collective understandings; it is crude, chaotic, surprising'.[107] 'It is awful and yet bestows a refined perception of reality to those who can bear it'.[108] As T. S. Eliot aptly wrote, 'wait without hope, for hope would be hope for the wrong thing; ... Wait without thought, for you are not ready for thought'.[109] Only then might the mind begin to recognize what the body *alone* feels, for the mind is forced out of its abstractions, its concretisms. When all defences and mental constructs have dissolved, we eventually let go and discover suffering as a valid part of life's process – a fact of the human condition – a story that must be told. Remember, one is 'suspended out of life, stuck, *until* and *if,* some act of grace with some new wisdom arrives'.[110]

Up until and throughout the Middle Ages, death was understood to be a part of life, not just something that happened at the end of life. This understanding imbued worldviews and was honoured in ritual, ceremony, and story. By welcoming stories of illness – those of heroism *and* those of surrender – the breadth of existence to which we have access and from which we become, is richer, more complex, more whole. Furthermore, the ancestors, metaphoric and literal, return as our constant companions. Although an unfamiliar plotline, this journey to the underworld *can* give rise to patience, empathy, humility, and another kind of knowing.[111] Such experience has been named renewal, rejuvenation, or rebirth. In learning to suffer *through,* healing occurs not only because a new way is found but also because the process of life is attended with an 'empathetic presence and a mirroring that touches it wherever it is'.[112]

104 Jacqueline Feather, 'The Necessity of Sacrifice for Consciousness: Attitude and Meaning', *Psychological Perspectives* 56 (2013): 339.

105 Carl Gustav Jung, *Mysterium Coniunctionis. The Collected Works of C.G. Jung,* trans. by R.F.C. Hull (Princeton, NJ: Princeton University Press, 1963/1989), 11: par. 345.

106 Feather, 'The Necessity of Sacrifice for Consciousness', 339, emphasis added.

107 Perera, *Descent to the Goddess,* 33.

108 Ibid.

109 T.S. Eliot, 'East Coker', in *Four Quartets* (London, UK: Faber and Faber, 1944), 25.

110 Perera, *Descent to the Goddess,* 36.

111 Fidyk, 'A Black Blessing'.

112 Perera, *Descent to the Goddess,* 74.

Healing in this way is for the soul; the body, on the other hand, may well be slowed, riddled, or aged irrevocably.

*****

Stories about home are stories about love of place, including those of exile, longing, and displacement. They are also about suffering – suffering 'the loss of relationship, or at least the most tangible expression of it – the caring, attendant presence of one to the other'.[113] Of this theme, my story is similar.

It takes place in the land of the dead. While no longer resident there, I carry it with me always. Like she who has eaten the red pomegranate, there is no escape. She is not again free to roam the upper world without its weight or gravitas. She is bound to it and the ways of the underworld indefinitely.

'The terrain of the sick, like the underworld ..., is surrounded by the waters of forgetfulness'.[114] *Yet what is washed away is not the memory of comforts, or abilities, but the person I was and how I moved, felt, existed, before becoming ill – the ease of conversation, the grace of balance, the joy of laughter.*

After struggling for ten years with chronic pain, tumours, infections, fatigue, and brain fog, the stress of another international relocation initiated my collapse.[115] *Within weeks of starting a new academic term, I struggled to remember colleagues' names. Within a month, a short drive to campus brought me to tears for I could no longer coordinate thought, body, and vehicle. Within four months, short-term memory, subtle emotions, and cognitive acuity were gone. Then a full decapitation of not only my will, but also my ability to read and write ('generalized brain atrophy'*[116]*), and with it, all capacity to care.*

---

113 James Hollis, *The Eden Project: In Search of the Magical Other* (Toronto, ON: Inner City Books, 1998), 11.

114 Duff, *The Alchemy of Illness*, 17.

115 Years later, when completing Integrated Body Psychodynamic training, I realized that illness inundates. Such inundation for years-on-end overloaded my autonomic nervous system, creating complex trauma. Sudden, unresolved, illness traumatised and my shattering experience of "self" sent me into dorsal vagal complex. That is, my nervous system was under severe threat from my own shock regarding extreme symptomatology and intense medical treatment – the unspoken, but constantly felt, albeit somewhat unconscious, 'I am going to die' – and activation of the sympathetic nervous system. My functioning or lack thereof was compounded by both a freeze and a collapse trauma response. In this way, Saber's thoughtful analysis of trauma and pain, through Bambara's character Velma, echoes aspects akin to my own experience. Too, Debra King's term 'blackpain' is a fitting description for the pain that accompanies the psychological shattering of descent through illness and suffering – there is a parallel here between black in its literal and metaphoric amplifications. Likewise, 'pain is alienating'; 'pain is a disability', and pain silences.

116 Alexandra Fidyk, MRI report December 2009, Edmonton, AB.

Diagnosed with a complex, chronic, neurological disease, not medically recognized in Canada nor supported by healthcare, expensive, radical, and aggressive protocols, by US specialists, dictated the days and years of my life. Confined to a new city without family or friends, on full medical leave, months passed without a visitor or friend. The world as I had known it – international career and travel – collapsed to the space of my kitchen, washroom, bed, and chaise. The resistance felt at the onset of diagnosis was gone. Hours of every day focused on extensive treatments – intramuscular and intravenous injections, antibiotic pulsing, scaffolding 60-plus pills/day, detoxification regiments, supplementation, continuous testing, and so on – often followed by nausea and diarrhea, and always encased in a cold, isolating inhibition. Relationships ended. Debt rose. Plunged into 'blacker than black',[117] *psychologically shattered and physiologically stripped, seven long years passed.*[118]

'Illness', Duff writes, 'is a taste of death, a practice in dying for the living', a temporary residence in the limens and bardos *reserved for the nearly or recently deceased.*[119] *While the diminishment of some symptoms has been experienced, others, such as acute vestibulitis, have come to dominate, prolonging a disengagement from the social fabric of life. Waking to my own motion sickness, sedated for transport by ambulance to hospital, vertigo has become a new norm. Living requires on-going modification to driving, walking, bending, and balancing – movement that was taken-for-granted, a sense of at-homeness that has been lost. Its long-term effect includes a hyper-vigilance where little bodily equilibrium exists. What was thought to be temporary quarters has become a permanent dwelling.*

As modern alchemy or homeopathy teaches, each person has only one disease in the course of a lifetime. It simply assumes different forms or guises as the various illnesses of one's life and death. Each of our illnesses can be construed as an encounter with the part of ourselves that will most likely kill us someday.

The bacteria released by the infected tick that inhabited my body, has multiplied through endless reproduction into millions of tightly coiled spirochete passing from flesh to blood, from blood to organs, from organs to brain. Blood no longer viable for banking; organs no longer acceptable for donation. No part of my body remains untouched, uncontaminated. I am Other. Other as stranger, as foreigner, differentiated only by a memory of difference – and even that has begun to wane. Psychologically, the foreigner, as symptom, signifies the difficulty we have living as an Other and with others, finding a liveable tensionality that

117 Hillman, 'The Seduction of Black', 50.

118 Fidyk, 'A Black Blessing', 105; Fidyk, 'An Ethic of Humility', 313.

119 Donne cited in Duff, *The Alchemy of Illness*, 61.

respects both entities. I am aware that this difference too shall pass for in my current situation memory and being have become precarious.

And yet, I have read, 'symptoms are ways home ... a letting go of the familiar and [an] entering of the unfamiliar.... The symptom acts as a leitmotif, a main theme of a person's life', something that has been beckoned, invited to contribute toward a completion.[120] *It is an invitation to include the whole of life – beyond the personal to the impersonal, the transpersonal. It is 'a way into the whole, to the person's story, to her history, to her "storied" life'.*[121] *In this way, symptoms are for 'wholing, healing, coming home'.*[122]

It must be shared that some time early in this descent, something called me north. Something called me home, back to a place of familiarity and family. I had just relocated from Chicago to California for another academic position, and I was delighted by sun and sea and the shifting direction of my research. Yet within the year, conflicted and unconvinced of current conditions, I surrendered to the urge and moved 'home' – to a locale 3000 kilometres north in the prairies of western Canada, 700 kilometres from my childhood farmland – distance considered 'close' for us who grew up in this terrain.

The Greeks called 'being'; 'presence'; 'arrival' parousia. *Its translation is a cluster of significations comprising 'homestead, at-homeness, a homecoming'. It is to this ground that one must strive to come home – a symbolic 'return to true self', which requires that one 'enter an abyss deeper than hell itself',*[123] *the process and goal of authentic being – of coming home.*[124]

This journey was not a heroine's. There was no egoic striving, no return in better shape for the tasks of life. Rather, suffering through – both psychologically and physiologically – brought about a 'point of view "beyond" and "below" life's concerns'.[125] *That is, the striving for, the desire or acquisition of things, which includes career achievements, marriage, children, financial stability, happiness – the very things that stories are made of.*

A warning must accompany nigredo *for there were times when I sensed that I might succumb to 'the tragic paradox of black'.*[126] *Not necessarily by my own*

---

120 Dianne Connelly, *All Sickness Is Homesickness* (Columbia, ML: Traditional Acupuncture Institute, 1993), xvi.

121 Ibid., 61.

122 Ibid., 61.

123 Carl Gustav Jung, *The Archetypes and the Collective Unconscious. The Collected Works of C.G. Jung*, trans. by R.F.C. Hull (Princeton, NJ: Princeton University Press, 1959/1969), 9i:par. 135.

124 Fidyk, 'An Ethic of Humility', 313.

125 James Hillman, *Revisioning Psychology* (New York, NY: Harper Colophon Books, 1975/1992), 206 207.

126 Hillman, 'The Seduction of Black', 50.

hand but by the act itself – rotting on the meat hook – for there were excruciatingly long periods of time when there was no movement.[127] *Of all alchemical colours, 'black is the most densely inflexible and* [*thus*] *the most oppressive and dangerously literal state of the soul'.*[128] *Like the stickiness of pitch or tar, it holds fast. The task even here is to yield. To wait without waiting … .*[129]

Many years ago, I heard a phrase that stuck with me: 'all sickness is home sickness' and its inversion, 'all healing is coming home'.[130] *Home, for me, literally resonates with the rich, black humus of the Saskatchewan farm. It symbolizes a life lived closely with Nature, its beauty and cruelty. Life lived with the seasons and the moon, attuned to the waxing and waning of light and dark. Life located in family and community, birth and death. I left this place long ago and while I always returned, somewhere I lost its inherent balance.*

Black humus is not just any soil. It refers to rich, organic matter that has reached a point of stability, where it will break down no further. If conditions are maintained, it may remain essentially stable for millennia. Human, humanity, humble, humility – all find their roots in this terrain. It is into this humble terra that I surrendered.

*****

Stories of descent through illness reveal that black darkens and sophisticates the eye. In accepting humiliation, sacrifice, and surrender, one comes to the depths of human ancestry, to psyche – as opposed to a spiritual or material being. Alchemists call this the *caput mortuum*, the death head. The death head is a way of seeing, a way *through* for having lived *with* the dead, the expulsion of light, the cold of isolation, and ways of becoming that are rarely valued. However, in the wisdom of the ancients, this becoming has been called a *hermaion* – a 'godsend', a gift, a blessing for bearing witness to extremity.[131] Like

127 Hans Sternudd's exploration of depression in his chapter, 'Voices of Depression: An Analysis of a Collective Narrative', in this volume gives me pause. While I would not have self-identified as depressed, in hindsight, and through 'Voices of Depression', I admit to living in a depressed state, for chronic illness is depressing. In a strange way, the themes of isolation, concealment, and self-destruction, while not self-caused, are accurate characteristics to describe the descent suffered through and amplified here. In what ways might a discussion of depression inform the descent of a counter-narrative? And further, in what ways might depression be a call toward a different kind of soul movement?

128 Ibid., 51.

129 Fidyk, 'A Black Blessing', 106.

130 Connelly, *All Sickness Is Home Sickness*, 61.

131 Lewis Hyde, *Trickster Makes This World: Mischief, Myth, and Art.* (New York, NY: North Point Press, 1998), 132.

the power of the spell carried forth by the old tales, this gift too carries the seeds of transformation.

Bibliography

Abram, David. *The Spell of the Sensuous: Perception and Language in a More-than-Human World.* New York, NY: Vintage Books, 1996.

Bacchilega, Cristina. *Postmodern Fairy Tales: Gender and Narrative Strategies.* Philadelphia: University of Pennsylvania Press, 1997.

Campbell, Joseph. *The Hero with a Thousand Faces.* Princeton, NJ: Princeton University Press, 1949/1968.

Connelly, Dianne M. *All Sickness Is Homesickness.* Columbia, ML: Traditional Acupuncture Institute, 1993.

Dillard, Annie. *The Writing Life.* New York, NY: Harper & Row, 1989.

Doidge, Norman. *The Brain That Changes Itself: Stories of Personal Triumph from the Frontiers of Brain Science.* New York: Penguin, 2007.

Duff, Kat. *The Alchemy of Illness.* New York, NY: Bell Tower, 1993.

Edinger, Edward. *Anatomy of the Psyche: Alchemical Symbolism in Psychotherapy.* Chicago, IL: Open Court, 1994.

Edinger, Edward. *Melville's Moby Dick: A Jungian Commentary: An American Nekyia.* New York, NY: New Directions, 1975.

Eliot, T.S. 'East Coker' *Four Quartets*, 21–27. London, UK: Faber & Faber, 1944.

Feather, Jaqueline. 'The Necessity of Sacrifice for Consciousness: Attitude and Meaning'. *Psychological Perspectives* 56 (2013): 334–341.

Fidyk, Alexandra. 'Unconscious Ties That Bind: Attending to Complexes in the Classroom, Part 2'. *International Journal of Jungian Studies* 8 3 (2016): 195–210.

Fidyk, Alexandra. 'An Aesthetic of Black'. *Psychological Perspectives* 59 2 (2016): 177–190.

Fidyk, Alexandra. 'A Black Blessing'. *On the Pedagogy of Suffering: Hermeneutic and Buddhist Meditations*, edited by David Jardine, Christopher Gilham and Graham McCaffrey, 101–106. New York, NY: Peter Lang, 2015.

Fidyk, Alexandra. 'An Ethics of Humility'. *A Heart of Wisdom: Life Writing as Empathetic Inquiry*, edited by Cynthia M. Chambers, Erika Hasebe-Ludt, Carl Leggo, and Anita Sinner, 306–315. New York, NY: Peter Lang, 2012.

Francot, Enrico. *The Icy Side of the Self: The Role of Cold in the Individuation Process.* Milano, Italy: L'Ossessione Espressa, 2013.

Griffin, Susan. *Unremembered Country.* Port Townsend, WA: Copper Canyon Press, 1987.

Heidegger, Martin. *What Is Called Thinking?* New York, NY: Harper and Row, 1968.

Hellinger, Bert. *Love's Own Truths: Bonding and Balancing in Close Relationships.* Translated by M. Oberli-Turner & Hunter Beaumont. Phoenix, AZ: Zeig, Tucker and Theisen, 2001.

Hillman, James. 'The Seduction of Black'. *Fire in the Stone: The Alchemy of Desire*, edited by Stanton Marlan, 42–53. Wilmette, IL: Chiron, 1997.

Hillman, James. *The Dream and the Underworld.* New York, NY: Avon, 1979.

Hillman, James. *Revisioning Psychology.* New York, NY: Harper Colophon Books, 1975/1992.

Hillman, James and Sonu Shamdasani *Lament of the Dead. Psychology after Jung's* Red Book. New York, NY: W.W. Norton and Company, 2013.

Hopper, Stanley R. 'Once More: The Cavern beneath the Cave'. *Archetypal Process: Self and Divine in Whitehead, Jung, and Hillman*, edited by David Ray Griffin, 107–124. Chicago: Northwestern University Press, 1989.

Hyde, Lewis. *Trickster Makes This World: Mischief, Myth, and Art.* New York, NY: North Point Press, 1998.

Jung, Carl Gustav. *The Red Book: Liber Novas* edited by Sonu Shamdasani. Philemon Series. New York: W.W. Norton & Company, 2009.

Jung, Carl Gustav. *Visions: Notes of the Seminar Given in 1930–1934*, edited by Clare Douglas. Princeton, NJ: Princeton University Press, 1997.

Jung, Carl Gustav. *The Spirit in Man, Art, and Literature. The Collected Works of C.G. Jung*, Vol. 15. Translated by R.F.C. Hull. Princeton, NJ: Princeton University Press, 1966/1978.

Jung, Carl Gustav. *Mysterium Coniunctionis. The Collected Works of C.G. Jung*, Vol. 14. Translated by R.F.C. Hull. Princeton, NJ: Princeton University Press, 1963/1989.

Jung, Carl Gustav. *Memories, Dreams, Reflections.* Translated by Richard and Clara Winston. Edited by Aniela Jaffe. New York: Random House, 1961/1989.

Jung, Carl Gustav. *The Archetypes and the Collective Unconscious, The Collected Works of C.G. Jung*, Vol. 9i. Translated by R.F.C. Hull. Princeton, NJ: Princeton University Press, 1959/1969.

Jung, Carl Gustav. *Psychology and Religion: West and East. The Collected Works of C.G. Jung*, Vol. 11. Translated by R.F.C. Hull. Princeton, NJ: Princeton University Press, 1958/1989.

Marlan, Stanton. *The Black Sun.* College Station, TX: Texas A&M University Press, 2005.

McCallum, Ian. *Ecological Intelligence: Rediscovering Ourselves in Nature* Cape Town, SA: Africa Geographic, 2006.

McConeghey, Howard. *Art and Soul.* Putnam, CT: Spring Publications, 2003.

Otto, Walter. *The Homeric Gods: The Spiritual Significance of Greek Religion.* Translated by Moses Hadas. New York, NY: Thames and Hudson, 1954.

Parkington, John. *Cederberg Rock Paintings.* Cape Town, SA: Creda Communications, 2008.

Perera, Silvia Brinton. *Descent to the Goddess: A Way of Initiation for Women*. Toronto: Inner City Books, 1981.

Raff, Jeffrey. 'The Felt Vision'. *The Sacred Heritage: The Influence of Shamanism on Analytical Psychology*, edited by Donald F. Sandner and Steven H. Wong, 79–90. New York, NY: Routledge, 2013.

Rosen, David. *Transforming Depression: Healing the Soul through Creativity*. York Beach, ME: Nicolas-Hays, 2002.

Schenk, Ronald. *Dark Light. The Appearance of Death in Everyday Life*. Albany, NY: State University of New York Press, 2001.

Stephens, Stephani. 'Active Imagination and the Dead'. *International Journal of Jungian Studies* 8 2 (2016): 46–59.

van Löben Sels, Robin. 'Ancestors and Spirits of the Dead'. *Quadrant: Journal of the C.G. Jung Foundation for Analytical Psychology, xxxx* 2 (2010): 81–94.

von Franz, Marie-Louise. *On Dreams & Death*. Boston, MA: Shambhala, 1987.

von Franz, Marie-Louise. *Projection and Re-collection in Jungian Psychology. Reflections of the Soul*. Peru, IL: Open Court Publishing, 1980/1995.

Zipes, Jack. *The Oxford Companion to Fairy Tales*. Oxford, UK: Oxford University Press, 2015.

CHAPTER 6

Making and Sharing Meaning out of Terminal Illness

Pam Morrison and Annie McGregor

Abstract

In my roles as supervisor in a person-centred counselling programme and a counsellor in private practice, I have a long-held professional and personal interest in formation of coherent narrative. My interest in the nature and impact of storying and voice took a deeply personal turn when my only sister was diagnosed with terminal secondary liver cancer in 2003, and I came face to face with the terror of loss. I was also confronted with my own loss of voice as I struggled to make sense of news that threatened not only our future lives together, but our current relationship. How do we stay real with ourselves and authentically connected with each other? Our solution was to co-journal, interleaving our entries to share our daily lives, along with our fears, our hopes, our griefs and joys. We found a way to capture not only the precious time-limited narrative that could be articulated, but also a place to hold the questions that had no answers. Our own decision to co-journal arose out of our love of words – I was a former journalist, and my sister was a lecturer in communication – and we were taken by surprise at the depth of intimacy and therapeutic invitation that it offered to us both. But while the journaling was deeply personal, it wasn't private, and our entries became a shared conversation, firstly with family through readings and the distribution of written copies and then with a widening circle. Annie was clear that she wanted others to hear our writings, but what of her wish that the writings be published to a wider audience after her death? My chapter follows the journey of our two voices.

Key Words

Voice – co-journaling – cancer – sisters – intimacy – separation – connection – ritual – story – audience

*****

 | DOI:10.1163/9789004396067_008

1 Introduction

I learnt that my only sister had terminal cancer by email.

Annie had written to close family after her specialist appointment to get results from a test which had shown abnormalities in her liver function.

'Alas, not a good morning…' Her message is poignant, careful, factual. The outlook is grim. She signs off: 'I may need your blessings. I'm counting mine and there are heaps. Will that cure me?'

Reeling from words displayed on my computer, I rang her and left a long message on her home phone. Later that day she called me. She loved the message. She planned to type it up and place it into a treasure box.

Amidst the bewildering array of feelings, I was surprised to find a powerful reaction coming to the surface. My words were going to be taken down in writing and boxed in a container. The idea appalled me, and it haunted me in the hours that followed.

Where was my voice? What was my voice? The box became a vivid, suffocating metaphor as I felt locked up and silenced by news of something too terrible to contemplate.

I open my chapter with these fearful memories about the written word with some fascination. For it was the written experiences that were to follow that offered both me and Annie an open door to a richer encounter than we could ever have imagined spanning the final year of her life.

In this chapter I will first describe and display the process by which Annie and I created a way to tell our own story to the other. With the use of selected excerpts in chronological order, I will outline the gifts and challenges that were captured by our co-journaling and the ways that our voices framed the worlds we now inhabited.

My chapter will then examine ways that we used metaphor to find our own voices and mark our separate and shared journeys. I will also explore the impact of this process on our relationship as we navigated our way towards inevitable, impending loss.

My decision-making process, as I grappled with the question of sharing the conversation, is the focus of my final section. Should there be an audience and what value might our story hold for others? How do I determine the 'rightness' of sharing a personal story with an unknown public, and what impact does that have on me as the 'storyteller' and on the essence of our story?

2 How It Began

The two events occurred within days of each other. I turned 49, and my sister Annie, five years older than me, learned that she had advanced secondary cancer, with no primaries detected.

Details of the birthday, three days prior, are lost to me, nearly all my memories eclipsed by the news of Annie's cancer. What I do remember is the birthday present of a journal, given by an artist friend who had created an artwork for the cover, called 'Walking with Pam'.

My response to the large landscape journal was one of awe: how could I put my mark on something so pristine and so beautiful? Then came the news.

During the days that followed my voice remained strangled. I recall turning in circles, a creature in distress. The shocking intrusion of cancer had unleashed a primal response and I struggled to find a way to give any shape to this new reality – too big, too crazy, too unthinkable to absorb.

I turned to my new journal, and picked up a pencil. Unsure what scrawl could make sense of my distress, I discovered an unexpected clarity as I began writing.

> (Pam Monday 17 March)
> For two days the pain has been growing, and now I'm clear. I must enter this fully and take my place alongside Annie – not for my sake or for her sake, but that third strand – for our sake.[1]

Annie lived in a different city, and the journal, with its now multiple entries, came with me when I visited her a few days later. Within three days, after reading my entries to her, she asked to join in and we decided this would become our shared repository.

> (Annie Sunday 23 March)
> Here we are – Pam and me – both in bed together, again. I've got my lolly pink and white cheer-up pyjamas on. Outside it's still and grey. A perfect day. I find myself lying in this beautiful bedroom listening to my breath; with the in-breath I follow the cradling of my soul from my left foot up into my head and with my out-breath it goes down again, the other side. And with an easy rhythm, I connect with my essential soul. It seems to be cradling this mischievous body. After I've slept I always wake regenerated, and ready for a good time. So now I'm going to practice the simple

1 Annie McGregor and Pam Morrison, *Fields of Gold* (New Zealand: Rosa Mira, 2014).

> rhythms and know that the simplicity of resting does not mean I am dying or being a slob. Last night when Pam read what is now our shared journal, it was one of the sweetest gifts I've been offered. Graham had lit the candles and it felt like yet another perfect way to begin this journey – not a test but a path.[2]

This was Annie's first entry. A ritual had begun. I was the scribe of her spoken words and Annie would book me in when she was ready – on her bed or at either end of her generous couch when together; on my large bed at home, with phone and pencil, if we were apart. Between her entries, I would write my own, and these would be read to Annie when we next spoke on the phone. We had entered a form of slow uninterrupted dialogue, and in so doing, created a container for shaping and sharing our stories.

> (Pam Tuesday 25 March, Dunedin)
> 6:20 am. I have been awake since 3 o'clock or so. Waiting for dawn to turn on the light and re-enter this journal. I thought as I travelled south that this book is like a pair of hands, able to hold whatever is placed in them. Also bare of its cover and so a little vulnerable without its clothing – good to think of (the cover) now in Annie's bedroom and breaking into the new day with her.[3]

The journal process of capturing the moment created room for the multiple threads in Annie's new reality: sadness in company with gratitude; the mundane merging with the sublime.

> (Annie Sunday 20 April)
> Last night, the kids were here. There was music playing, the sounds of whistling and chopping, cooking noises, recipes being changed. I was in front of the fire under the red mohair rug. I tell you what. I was in heaven, or pretty close, about 5km away. Sometimes I wonder: why didn't I come to this place earlier? Then I remember – oh that's right!
>
> Graham says he's noticed some frailty in me. And there is, at times. Then I think: It's only ten days since I had the radiation treatment into my liver. I was told I would feel terrible. I haven't been trampled by an elephant; I've been trampled by a sheepdog.[4]

2 Ibid., 19.

3 Ibid., 22.

4 Ibid., 31.

Increasingly it seemed that journaling was offering us a 'way in' to dilemma where there were no clear pathways; no immediate answers. Example? How does someone like Annie, with her exuberant love of life, also embrace her own illness?

> (Annie Monday 28 July)
> I've been married for 15 days. We're so proud. I listened to an Eastern meditation last night and it asked me to identify a time that I was really happy. It was wonderful. I immediately thought of standing beside Graham at our wedding ceremony bursting with love…
>
> However I'm struggling with the changes. I can't believe that I haven't written anywhere about the details of our wedding. But going to the specialist the day after the wedding and learning then about intravenous chemo was a big lurch. The lung cancers had doubled. There's a part of us that's just so naïve. We cried and cried. How could we not think it was a possibility?
>
> I think someone else is in my skin. And I'm waiting to meet her. I'm quite sure the secret is rest – serious rest, and the more I stop and breathe the better I feel. Not exactly contented, but in the present, and that's where we need to live. Quite hard for a spirit like mine. Of course there are rewards, and I'm learning about those too. I'm not frightened.[5]

Annie loved ritual, and it was ritual that she returned to, creatively and wholeheartedly, to meet oncoming shocks, such as the start of hair loss after chemotherapy treatment.

> (Annie Wednesday 13 August)
> What a rich night we've had… Graham and Janion and I shared warm chicken salad, followed up by summer pudding with redcurrants, blackcurrants and loganberries from the garden. Then the hair. We put a sheet on the ground to pick up every hair, and had another sheet around me. As Graham cut my hair with the smooth pulsating rhythm of the clippers, Janion held my hand tightly and read Leunig's poem about hair.[6]
>
> Afterwards, we all gathered up the hair and put it in one of Graham's precious green bowls I love so much. The hair was very soft. Each day we have decided to put some under the little pear tree where the birds gather and they may take it away to help them build their nests. Or it may

5 Ibid., 43–44.

6 Michael Leunig, *When I Talk to You: A Cartoonist Talks to God* (East Melbourne: HarperCollins Publishers, 2004).

> blow into the garden, and that's fine too... Graham brought in his large wooden mirror for me to see the finished product. I looked like myself, but prouder and braver. It felt like a dignified and respectful process. I felt like a Buddhist novice – although without my saffron. I'm ready for the next part of the journey.[7]

Friends also created ritual – including 'a gentle wishing for Annie's wellbeing', for Annie to connect with friends and family around the world at a set time each week. Annie drew strength from this – and not only from those still living.

> (Annie Tuesday 26 August)
> Sunday was the first of gentle wishing for my well being. I was surprised to find myself really excited – like meeting a boyfriend for a date.
>
> I lit the candles and the oil burner with lavender, and before I got in I felt my tummy and said to Graham, 'this tumour feels enormous. I want to feel my body and the shape of what's happening'.
>
> I climbed into the bath and stayed there for an hour. I invoked the spirits of my grandparents. Bill's gentleness and patience, Nana Molly's fortitude with cancer, Grandma Annie's courage with her daughter's handicaps for 30 years, and Andrew's sense of adventure with whatever came his way.[8]

Days later, a different theme, as I grapple with a now familiar impasse. How do I stay honest – both with myself and with my sister? What do I do with the responses that feel like they've let both of us down? A new journal entry gives me back my voice.

> (Pam Monday 1 September)
> I'm almost scared to begin writing today. I'm experiencing something new – I am feeling afraid. Annie spoke to me last night about her despair when she discovered two more hard lumps under her skin – more cancer... "I tell myself all will be well", she said – "and I believe it. Then I realise that I don't want to die and I'm a liar". The same is true of me. I am resolutely in the present. There is so much now that is sweet and satisfying. And now, suddenly, with the image of the black ugly knot inside Annie's body, I feel shocked and afraid. I recall speaking so mystically and calmly last night, and today it feels like a crock of shit. It's like my emotions are on slow release, and 12 hours after the conversation they

7 Ibid., 46–47.
8 Ibid., 52–53.

> catch up with me. I want to call her, to apologise for something I can't name. For being healthy. For not having to face what she does. For pouring out words and ideas to give breathing space to my feelings, and imagining that they would give solace; – when I know she is afraid. And what I want, I want to do is sit with her and say: I am afraid too.[9]

Celebrations also thread through the story. Annie's wedding in July is followed by the birth of her first grandchild in early November. It's now eight months since diagnosis, and the reality that she might die had remained unthinkable.

> (Annie Saturday 29 November)
> Yesterday I was told that our consultant would definitely not offer me top-up chemo next year, if I needed it. I heard the sound of a very heavy solid wooden door drop from an upper lintel and hit the ground. He looked at me squarely and said 'Annie, you will have a good life after chemo. There are tools with which we can help you, like hospice and palliative care'. We were speechless. Dying is off the agenda. I said to Graham, it felt like the leering face of a jack-in-the-box springing out and wobbling, when we thought we had secured the lid and put the box to one side.[10]

Making meaning out of love, intimacy and imminent death, I find myself in new realms as I attempt to describe what concrete ideas can't capture.

> (Pam Friday 19 December)
> Sometimes I see a pool of light ahead of me – shaped like an oval. And altering in size. Beyond its edges – nothing. Absence of knowing, of colour, of light. My joy has been and is in occupying the light pool. And yet I know it cannot continue…[11]

Finding words had been a salvation, but there came a time when I was struck with fear that even these would fail me.

> (Pam Sunday 11 January)
> What if I can't find words? It frightens me. I'm afraid that if I have no means to build, there'll be nothing for me to inhabit.[12]

9 Ibid., 54.
10 Ibid., 64–65.
11 Ibid., 70.
12 Ibid., 74.

Amidst that fear of being unable to create any pattern of meaning, was the ongoing question. How do I stay true to my own experience, while managing the tensions of our differing griefs?

> (Pam Sunday 18 January)
> Life has been far from straightforward. At times I feel like I'm in a paper-boat, bobbing on a current, which takes me anywhere it pleases. At other times it's felt like I'm under an ever-changing sky. I look up and find there's been a dramatic shift. I've been wrestling with the question of how to give expression to my own needs and feelings when I'm with Annie. A week ago I was feeling dismantled and distant from her and me. Lots of crying. Now, three days on, I think there is no place for any of this while Annie is alive. I was almost appalled that I would take any measure of sorrow into my interaction with her. And now, as I write that, the pendulum has swung again. How could sorrow not be present? And so the sky changes. My boat sails on.[13]

Terror of separation would rise up at times, again almost too big to name. What if I say it? What if she hears it?

> (Pam Sunday 25 January)
> I've been sitting here in bed, journal and pencil at hand, ready to record Annie's chapter as planned. But when Annie phoned, she was very uncertain about putting anything into the journal... I truly hadn't considered that this might happen... I hadn't imagined that this book would not continue to receive her. Not just this book. That I would no longer be given entry to her. And that the precious, slow process we have put in place to meet one another would end – like a book shutting.[14]

This I am able to read to Annie. And Annie is able to reply.

> (Annie Wednesday 28 January)
> Finally, we're together again. I think I've put off four conversations – always too tired. But tonight, it's a priority. Pam has just read me some of her reflections about this journey and wasn't sure I wanted to hear them. I do. I do. I do. One of the things I've learnt in the last two weeks... is that I am not the only one in turmoil. My underlying optimism serves me well,

13 Ibid., 74–75.
14 Ibid., 19.

> but sometimes I have a deep sadness and disbelief that sits in my belly. And when we're all honest together, that load is so much lighter.[15]

And so to the final leg of the journey.

> (Annie Friday 20 February)
> Pam is here. I've been longing for her. We tuck into one another's bodies and cry and then laugh and then cry more. I feel so safe. She's been here for 23 hours and we've just started to journal, and I'm reminded how precious this process is. Amongst other things, she gave me a beautiful t-shirt and we sat in bed until quarter to 12 looking like fashion boffins, hanging onto one another and whispering personal and sacred details about my dying process. Anointing, sacred time just for our family. Some if it was a bit of a laugh really. Like whipping off my favourite red skirt before the lid goes on the coffin at home so that the skirt can go in the dress up box. But of course the irony is that it's not a laugh. And frequently, like now, tears roll out. And with Pam they are safely wrapped.[16]

> (Pam Friday 12 March)
> Annie died today at 2:07pm.[17]

And here, returning to our familiar place of the shared book, I describe how as a family, we farewelled Annie, and Annie, us.

Over the next five days I continue to journal alone, and yet not alone. In my final entry, a letter written to Annie from my bed, I conclude with these words:

> Darling Annie, I don't know anything about my future. It holds almost as much mystery as your own. But right now, it's 1:16pm and as I have dipped in and out of this journal through the morning, I am in a different place from where I began. I can trust that movement will continue. That's all I know. I'm ready now to get up.[18]

2.1 *Finding Voice through Metaphor*

And so the two of us, each in our own way, found our voices, allowing us to weave our narrative through the final chapter of life together. We had

15 Ibid., 79.
16 Ibid., 90–91.
17 Ibid., 109.
18 Ibid., 115.

discovered a way to honour the everyday events, now laden with meaning, and to give form to the questions without answers. Even more, we had created a 'room' where aspects of our experiences could be shared with each other to a depth that spoken conversation may never have allowed.

What was it about co-journaling – a collaborative reflective dialogue that we had never encountered elsewhere – that enabled us to capture and articulate our story?

The discovery, like many births, was delivered following a period of anguish. News of Annie's cancer had cast us into what Sontag calls 'the nightside of life'[19] where there was, for me, the sense not only of stumbling in the dark, but of losing the facility of language. What could I possibly say or write that would make any meaning of this madness?

As someone who had made sense of life through using words, this experience of being struck dumb was confounding and scary. I had written personal journals interspersed with poetry for years, weaving thoughts onto paper to make meaning of my experience. Words had been my salvation and my bread and butter – I had spent more than two decades years working as a journalist, and gained satisfaction in wielding words to capture meaning and impact.

In this new terrain without handholds or known markers, what did remain was a muscle memory process. Reaching for the empty journal was a reflex towards something familiar, even without any clear sense of what I wanted or needed to say. I took a pencil, and as I wrote my first entry I saw a metaphor was taking shape – one that over time would become an undergirding concept, enabling me to find my way back to the centring reality of our relationship. There was not just an Annie and a me, there was an us.

This presented itself in my mind as a braided path – the path itself another useful image that we would both return to again and again. We didn't know where we going, but we knew we were on our way. 'The image of a journey is so appropriate… In the face of an unimaginable future my faith lies in this: we walk where we must'.[20]

In my ongoing search for a language, the metaphors emerged like stepping stones – a pathway that presented itself as I wrote my way through the new landscape. This experience of metaphor, as 'a creative force which creates and reflects reality',[21] allowed something to be birthed that would offer shape and give meaning to the terror and beauty of this time.

19 Susan Sontag, *Illness as Metaphor and Aids and Its Metaphors* (London: Penguin, 1991).

20 McGregor and Morrison, *Fields of Gold*, 70.

21 Katherine Froggatt, 'The Place of Metaphor and Language In Exploring Nurses' Emotional Work', *Journal of Advanced Nursing* 28.2 (1998): 332–338.

Even more than providing descriptive form, it brought something into being that would offer us both a place to stand and a space to inhabit. Charon puts it this way:

> Once the experience has a form conferred on it ... the writer can, in effect, walk around the representation, seeing aspects around its back or over to the side that were (previously) unavailable to the subject.[22]

3 Our Metaphorical Language

While military imagery, incorporating metaphors such as battle, enemy and triumph or defeat, is frequently identified in literature citing people's experience of cancer,[23] it had almost no place in our ongoing exchange. By contrast, two repeating motifs emerged in my writing of sound and woven fabric or garments, both of which had scope to capture the vastly differing experiences of the time.

Sound first made its appearance as an expression of joy, six weeks after diagnosis.

> I'm amazed how much this cup of life can hold... All going well, Annie will be holding her (first) grandchild in seven months' time. I said to Annie, I can hear the harmonics pinging inside my body; my own bells pealing for joy.[24]

Much later it would become the means of understanding the dissonance and distress of feeling disconnected from each other:

> For all Annie's positivity, I'm finding this a sombre and confusing time. A picture comes to me of her vivacity starting to echo and bounce off walls, as if the room were becoming empty. Is this what happens when the trappings and padding of 'normal' life are stripped away? Or am I feeling this way because of things we haven't been able to say to each other.

22 Rita Charon, 'Narrative Medicine: Attention, Representation, Affiliation', *Narrative* 13.3 (2005): 261–270.

23 Catherine A. Czechmeister, 'Metaphor in Illness and Nursing: A Two-Edged Sword. A Discussion of the Social Use of Metaphor in Everyday Language, and Implications of Nursing and Nursing Education', *Journal of Advanced Nursing* 19 (1994): 1226–1233; Carola Skott, 'Expressive Metaphors in Cancer Narratives', *Cancer Nursing* 25.2 (2002): 230–235.

24 McGregor and Morrison, *Fields of Gold*, 32.

> Perhaps when we can both give voice to what is scary – each in our own way – then the echo will go; true notes will sound.[25]

As Annie's physical self became weaker and our physical lives together came under threat, I found myself turning to the metaphor of sound to express how I experienced her life in me, and to examine my own notions of spirit.

> I've been pondering the idea of spirit as sound. ... I realised that the resonance of Annie that I carried within me could be silenced, and it terrified me... I can go anywhere this journey takes me. But how can I live with that absence of sound. And yet as I think of Annie's body losing its vigour and health, I know that her resonance doesn't and won't dim. I heard once that earth emits a sound, out of our detection range. Our beings surely do the same.[26]

Three weeks later the same sound motif appeared in the writing.

> It seems to me that all that spills out from spirit – melody, harmony, dissonance, vibration – can never be contained. They take their place. Some notes will be out of audible range. But they are no less real for evading capture. Like aspects of this experienced that can't be plumbed or articulated.[27]

Metaphors of fabric and garments also found their way into the entries, calling up images to evoke softness and to portray covering.

Early on in our journaling, the metaphor was used to express the inadequacy of language.

> How strange it is to put words to this experience. It's as if the words – the garments we make to show the shape of it – have turned to threads. They lie over it. But they cannot cover it. Or define it.[28]

Three months later, the metaphor presented itself as welcome wisdom, passed on. 'Someone said to me once that... grief was a cloak – sometimes an unbearable weight, sometimes silken – but always present'.[29]

25 Ibid., 76.
26 Ibid., 77.
27 Ibid., 89.
28 Ibid., 27.
29 Ibid., 37.

The journal as a whole was represented as holding the story by weaving together chosen articulated moments of time. 'I want to gather some of the threads of recent time, put them on the loom again'.[30]

As Annie started approaching the end of her life, fabric as metaphor appeared in my writing to express a growing sense of the ineffable and sacred, amidst the harsh physical trials.

> I have the book in my hands again to spin my spider strand. This book keeps altering its weight and shape. (Just now) it seemed like a heavy angular object, too heavy for the soft intricate weave of these times. I've wondered too if writing it is something of an idolatrous practice – a substitute for the terrifying and holy and beautiful thing that is taking place here.[31]

And in one of the final communications with Annie, written in the form of a letter shortly before she died, fabric became the symbol of the love in our relationship, and of all that would remain.

> You talked about gossamer in our journal… I have this sense of it as something exquisitely woven, so the warp and weft are no longer visible; and something that has no weight. And I've decided that it's also as strong as life, and love, and death. That is what I see and sense, as your body gets frailer…and you get ready to disrobe and move on. A love that remains that has strong, subtle and perfect substance.[32]

4 Finding Connection through Voice

In the context of knowledge that life will be ending, intimacy and separation take on a particular potency. The meaning of 'connection' is intensified. 'People are constantly reconciling the experiential and the existential, as they seek and create meaning in their situations'. says Czechmeister.[33]

The present and the future were unutterably altered at the point of diagnosis. The journal offered a vehicle for a new construct. Annie and I entered a

30 Ibid., 60.
31 Ibid., 93.
32 Ibid., 99.
33 Czechmeister, 'Metaphor in Illness and Nursing'.

'relational process of co-construction',[34] and in so doing, generated a story that spoke truth to the new reality.

Our process and the journal itself provided a container, capable of holding and communicating our separate responses to all that mortality was inviting. How do you live well when you are dying? How do you love and let go? How do you maintain authentic, honest relationship when you are experiencing singular and differing griefs?

My first entry in the journal led me to an insight, referred to earlier in the chapter that would provide a key to this exquisite dilemma. Beyond me and Annie there was also the *us*.

The gift of this concept was immediate. I felt my own paralysis unlock as I recognised the presence of the relationship, almost as a third entity. The year to come would add further depth and richness to this awareness as we gave voice to our stories, weaving a dialogue that both inhabited and represented the space that was *us*.

I experienced a deepening appreciation of what Martin Buber calls, in translation, 'the between'. 'Meaning is to be found neither in one of the two partners nor in both together, but only in their dialogue itself, in this "between" which they live together'.[35] Samoan has a word with similar meaning: *va* – the space that connects one person to another.

These links are echoed by psychotherapist and author Irvin Yalom:

> It is the synergy between ideas and intimate connection with other people that is most effective both in diminishing death anxiety and in harnessing the awakening experience to effect personal change.[36]

5 Inviting Others to Share the Conversation

Our journal offered us a secure holding place by co-creating a relational space not dissimilar to a therapeutic encounter. Our stories could be slowly and reflectively shaped, captured wholly without interruptions, then spoken aloud

34 Stuij, Elling, Tramper and Abma, 'Developing a Relational Narrative about Diabetes: Towards a Polyphonic Story', in this volume.

35 Martin Buber and Judith Buber Agassi, *On Psychology and Psychotherapy: Essays, Letters, and Dialogue* (New York: Syracuse University Press, 1999), 75.

36 Irvin D. Yalom, *Staring at the Sun: Overcoming the Terror of Death* (San Francisco: Jossey-Bass, 2009), 119.

and heard. The complexity of our experiences, which at times could have silenced us or separated us, instead became a potent, connecting narrative.

It was a deeply intimate process and yet from the outset Annie was clear that she wanted our entries to be shared. Before she started writing into the journal herself, she asked for my entries to be read aloud at a family gathering, and this took place again on later occasions.

Towards the end of her life she wanted the journal typed and collated so that everyone in the close circle could have a copy. My two older children typed up all of the pencil-scribed entries, and five weeks before she died the journal to date was sent out to family.

Annie had another wish with regard to the journal which she voiced to me on two or three occasions. If there were an opportunity to do so, could the journal be published as a book?

Five days after Annie's death the journal was completed but never closed. Over subsequent months friends and extended family were given copies, and in the years following, our writing was read by an ever-widening circle of people.

Meanwhile Annie's request remained vivid yet unaddressed: could I, should I publish the writing as a book?

My only conviction after Annie had died was that I would not look at the question of publishing while clouded by my own grief. I knew that proceeding with the idea could only take place when I was free of any invested need for personal healing or the desire to transform the experience of others.

This was in fact the only clarity I had. The journal's title *Fields of Gold*, when shorthanded to FoG, became an apt metaphor itself for the 'unknowing' I had around making our writing available to the wider public.

The emergence of voice for each of us through this vehicle for sharing our lives had provided meaning and connection. Others who had read our story were touched by the legacy that Annie had left, and inspired by the rituals and the co-journaling process that allowed these to be shared.

But should the writing be taken further as Annie wanted? What should guide my process around opening our lives to an unknown audience? As I said in the published book's conclusion, written as a letter to Annie:

> You told me more than once that you were happy for the journal to be shared and published. You were clear about that but then again you were getting ready to leave. For me (still here) the process has been more gradual.[37]

37 McGregor and Morrison, *Fields of Gold*, 116.

Exploring the question of sharing one's life experience and opening one's personal story to strangers seems pertinent in this era when popularity of memoires as a genre is burgeoning, personal blogs are proliferating and autoethnography has become a recognised research methodology.

Using the autoethnographic lens, I will trace my own process, drawing on the personal journal entries that I wrote over the three year period before publishing as I visited and re-visited Annie's request.

These reflections and questions began in earnest when the offer came in 2010 from Rosa Mira Publishers for the journals to be published as an eBook. It was a proposal that made sense to me. I could conceive of the journal being 'out there' if it were to remain in the ether rather than sitting on bookshop shelves as another item for thumbing through. People who were interested in our story could seek it out via the internet rather than stumbling upon it. It was a comforting thought.

I said a tentative 'yes', and late the following year, publisher and editor Penelope Todd and I had our first meeting to discuss the way forward. I was full of questions and aware of my need for reassurance.

> (15 November 2011)
> I am just home from my breakfast meeting with (publisher) Penelope – our first meeting proper to talk about the publishing of Annie's and my journal, *Fields of Gold*, by Rosa Mira Books.
>
> My head was full on the trip into town. Why was I doing this, again? Two comments have landed with weight over the years, and I keep returning to them. One came from author and former Burns Fellow Paddy Richardson who said: "Pam, I don't think you *should* publish. I think you *must* publish. This is a universal story". The other is an image from academic and sociologist Martin Tolich, passed on recently by my colleague Margaret McKenzie, when considering the idea of published research based on the journal: Think of autoethnography as an ink tattoo. Once published, it is indelible.
>
> Driving in the early morning traffic, I asked for Annie to be present. What do I need to consider? There was an immediate thought: do family and close friends still support this project? They said yes some years ago to the idea of publication. Now it is a potential reality. Are they still ok with this?
>
> Why publish? This was the alive question when I parked – and the first one that I put to Penelope when we took our seats at the café. She said this: (as close as I can recall). "I love the premise. I love both voices – yours and Annie's. I love that you've captured your own stories through

to the very end of this tender process, and that you were bold enough to see it through. And this journal fits my ethos of publishing – I'm looking for books that touch here and here". With that she gestured to her head and her heart.

She also talked about the journal's more particular potential readership as she saw it – those who are experiencing grief or loss; those considering the impact of dying from the standpoint of supporter or medic or academic. Not to be promoted through the New Zealand Womens Weekly magazine, she added.

So yes – she wants to publish, and she's clear about why. Somehow it's enough. I know she's not doing it to support me. To fulfil a need of mine – conscious or unconscious. It is in itself, a story that has independent validity, credibility, to be out there in the public arena.

Then, at the wrought iron table on the upper deck of the café, we talked through the steps. This is how the contract will look – or possibly like that. (Depending on the available dollars in each of our bank accounts at the time.) Whichever way we took, the outcome was the same and was fair. Such ease. We are not stumbling to look after each other's or our own interests. She's done this a number of times with many authors. Of course this can be straight forward…and I am relieved.[38]

Straight forward? I discover that my own process is only just beginning, as the meaning and impact of story its widest sense call me to deeper introspection.

(28 January 2012)
I feel like I've slipped my moorings. This has brought up feelings and perspectives that are unfamiliar and unsettling. I'm slowing down as I write – wondering how to capture this, but I'll let it flow, and see how it emerges.

As I made my cup of tea, just now, my question was framed up as: does my (life) story shape me or do I shape myself – am I the ongoing product of it, forever in its thrall, or am I the body under the garment of my story?

It seems to me that I have it in my power to shape myself. To choose, in its largest sense, my posture and gait, to know and own my own body. Can it be said that the story itself is ultimately irrelevant? That the potency is in the transfer of power back to myself – from whatever the 'seen covering' might be.[39]

38 Fragments from personal journal.

39 Ibid.

Meanwhile the process of preparation for publishing had different traction and was heading towards our agreed outcome. Coming face to face with this reality called me up short, and I was suddenly confronted with my conviction: I was *not* ready to publish.

> (17 March 2012)
> On Wednesday I received an email from Penelope to say she had completed her edits on *Fields of Gold*. Just minutes later another one arrived – she had written the draft post of a blog for the Rosa Mira book site to say that this book would be the next one launched.
>
> It's crystallised what's been forming in me over the past few days – perhaps weeks. I'm not ready for the manuscript to be published. It's more than not ready. I've lost sight of why I'm putting it out for the public to access. And it seems like a vital question that I need to have entered and understood, even if some corners are not easily articulated. I must visit them, and fully process this before it goes the next step.
>
> I've been wondering what my impulse is. Yes, Annie gave it her blessing – by raising the idea and even expressing her own wish; others have given encouragement that this is a worthwhile, even important thing to do. I'm aware in all of this how often I've sought the reassurance of others – is this wise / appropriate / or is it the opposite? Grasping for something substantial enough to guide my decision.
>
> All the while, my own sure voice was missing. It feels ironic. That I have a voice so clearly in the journal itself – an avenue to speak my own experience and have it heard. Yet there is no clarity, no voice in me around who should hear that experience.[40]

I was consumed with the notion that I must be able to answer the 'why?' question, before moving ahead. I felt sure that I needed a cogent, formulated rationale to explain (to myself and others) the reason I was telling our story publicly. Less than a month later, I express the seed of an idea that would ultimately release me from this roadblock of uncertainty.

> (6 April 2012)
> I've been reading the introduction to a book of ethnographic articles on music. The ideas that resonate with me are these. Firstly that expression of ideas can be expressed like music – with melody, dissonance and harmony, counterpoint, pulse, cadence. There's something important there

40 Ibid.

> that I 'get' and love, that feels like it could both release and carry my writing. (I'm also aware that these terms were often present in Annie's and my journal writing.)
>
> Secondly, and this is important, that writing is intended to touch, move, inspire a reader, in the same way that music does. That writer and reader enter a dance together, in which self-consciousness or ego of the writer has no place – in fact can only get in the way. It's hard to describe my new insight on this. It's like I'm saying to myself – just give voice to this, and people will engage with it (or not) as they will. It is not about judging the work – myself or others (though some will do that); it's about letting the ideas or story 'sing', and allowing whatever happens to happen in response.[41]

I discovered in the months to follow that I was no longer compelled to find answers. The 'why' question and the need for my own response to it had slowly yet simply evaporated. In August 2013 I attended and presented at a conference on attentive writing in health contexts at Glasgow University where I shared our process of co-journaling in a more public forum. I discovered that the academics, practitioners and writers who attended were receptive and curious about what we had done.

Furthermore, I realised, like Simpson-Gervin, that by sharing my story, 'others may be able to create their own stories in order to make sense of a traumatic experience'.[42]

Three months later I identify that a distinct shift has taken place which is enabling the story to have its own separate life.

> (11 November 2013)
> As I look back now I can see that an intriguing journey has taken place. There is now a story about the story – one that can be told. I'm no longer assailed by multiple questions about my motivations. I am simply ready. It will 'sail out' as an eBook. Where it goes, who it reaches, is as it is.[43]

In March 2014, almost ten years to the day after Annie's death, *Fields of Gold* is published and launched as an eBook. I arrange for a limited number of hard copy books to be available for friends and wider family to purchase.

---

41 Ibid.

42 Simpson-Gervin, 'Narrative Medicine and Storytelling: An Alternative Method for Healing', in this volume.

43 Ibid.

The next leg of the journey is complete.

Bibliography

Buber, Martin and Judith Buber Agassi. *On Psychology and Psychotherapy: Essays, Letters and Dialogue*. New York: Syracuse University Press, 1999.

Charon, Rita. 'Narrative Medicine: Attention, Representation, Affiliation'. *Narrative* 13.3 (2005): 261–270.

Czechmeister, Catherine A. 'Metaphor in Illness and Nursing: A Two-Edged Sword. A Discussion of the Social Use of Metaphor in Everyday Language, and Implications of Nursing and Nursing Education'. *Journal of Advanced Nursing* 19 (1994): 1226–1233.

Frank, Arthur W. 'The Rhetoric of Self-Change: Illness Experience as Narrative'. *The Sociological Quarterly* 34.1 (1993): 39–52.

Frank, Arthur W. *The Wounded Storyteller*. Chicago: University of Chicago Press, 2013.

Froggatt, Katherine. 'The Place of Metaphor and Language in Exploring Nurses' Emotional Work'. *Journal of Advanced Nursing* 28.2 (1998): 332–338.

Hyden, Laer-Christer. 'Illness and Narrative'. *Sociology of Health and Illness* 19.1 (1997): 48–69.

Leunig, Michael. *When I Talk to You: A Cartoonist Talks to God*. East Melbourne: Harper Collins Publishers, 2004.

McGregor, Annie and Pam Morrison. *Fields of Gold*. New Zealand, Dunedin: Rosa Mira Books, 2014.

Rimmon-Kenan, Schlomith. 'Illness and Narrative Identity'. *Narrative* 10.1 (2002): 9–27.

Scott, Carola. 'Expressive Metaphors in Cancer Narratives'. *Cancer Nursing* 25.3 (2002): 230–235.

Sontag, Susan. *Illness as Metaphor and Aids and Its Metaphors*. London: Penguin, 1991.

Yalom, Irvin. D. *Staring at the Sun: Overcoming the Terror of Death*. San Francisco: Jossey-Bass, 2009.

CHAPTER 7

Toni Cade Bambara's *The Salt Eaters*: Hearing the Silent Voice of Pain

Yomna Saber

Abstract

The African American discourse has frequently converged with that of disability studies as both seem to have much in common. However, the intersection of race, gender and disability is not additive, it points to forging multi-layered identities that endure marginalization, pain and stigma on myriad levels. African Americans have been linked historically to disability since the time of slavery to justify racial oppression. The black canon continued to display disabled characters whose physical impairments symbolized the violence and institutionalized the exclusion blacks have been subject to. Throughout the 20th century, disability in African American literature became a politicized metaphor for victimization and isolation, and grew into another oppressive social construction like race and gender. Published in 1980, Toni Cade Bambara's *The Salt Eaters* delineates a silent protagonist suffering from a number of disabilities and the attempt of her healer to recuperate her voice. This chapter addresses the following questions: how can pain emanating from disability be expressed, and is it possible to hear the silent voice of pain? Is Minnie healing Velma by listening to her silent voice or is she speaking on her behalf? Is it just Velma's mental condition that renders her disabled, or is the experience of pain equally disabling? Is the novel a narrative of overcoming or an expression of the protagonist's alterity and otherness as a literary invalid? Is Velma's disability oppressive or liberating? Hegemonic systems of representation have featured a lot of mad women in the attic who are deleteriously pitiable and stereotypically undesirable. How does Bambara conceptualize and negotiate disability in her novel for an African American woman? Is she racializing and gendering disability or does she conceive race and gender themselves as disabilities? And how does the black woman handle her disability and express her pain?

Key Words

Disability – pain – stigma – trauma – healing – storytelling – Toni Cade Bambara – African American

 | DOI:10.1163/9789004396067_009

*****

'Are you sure sweetheart that you want to be well?'[1] is the intriguing question with which Toni Cade Bambara's *The Salt Eaters* starts introducing the traumatized protagonist Velma Henry and her healer Minnie Ransom. The question instantaneously points to Velma's disability and focuses on making choices and shouldering responsibilities. Trauma theorists, such as Elaine Scarry,[2] Dori Laub and Shoshana Felman,[3] Cathy Caruth,[4] and Judith Herman,[5] contend that language fails to vociferously express pain. Where such language is usually pigeonholed as insufficient, fractured and disintegrated, Bambara takes it a step further in her text by creating a domain of silence and muting the voice of her protagonist. Voice is a slippery term to define and it is even more difficult to specify in African American literature since the hermeneutics of voice in this context is laden with diverse connotations. Voice can refer to the conflict between orality and literacy in black writings, or it can allude to the use of the black dialect as a cultural token in black art. It is possible to use it in a post-structuralist context as in the theory of signifyin(g) in Henry Louis Gates' *The Signifying Monkey*[6] in which he argues that the voice of African American writers is all the time signifying upon their predecessors in the canon. And it can also point to Audre Lorde's "The Master's Tools Will Never Dismantle the Master's House"[7] in which she calls for a true black voice that does not mimic the voice of the white master. However, the premise of voice in this chapter is principally concerned with the notion of agency. I am not referring to the linguistic agency as a means of expression, but philosophically to agency as it denotes human will and independence in making choices in life against society and totalitarian systems. Bambara's novel is a narrative of suffering told in the silent voice of pain, in which Minnie, the district healer,

1 Toni Cade Bambara, *The Salt Eaters* (New York: Vintage Contemporaries, 1980), Kindle edition.
2 Elaine Scarry's *The Body in Pain: The Making and Unmaking of the World* (New York: Oxford University Press, 1987).
3 Dori Laub and Shoshana Felman's *Testimony: Crises of Witnessing in Literature, Psychoanalysis, and History* (New York: Routledge, 1992).
4 Cathy Caruth's *Trauma: Explorations in Memory Front Cover* (Maryland: The Johns Hopkins University Press, 1995).
5 Judith Herman's *Trauma and Recovery The Aftermath of Violence – From Domestic Abuse to Political Terror* (New York: Basic Books, 2015).
6 Henry Louis Gates' *The Signifying Monkey* (New York: Oxford University Press, 1988).
7 Audre Lorde's article was published in *Sister Outsider: Essays and Speeches* (New York: Ten Speed Press, 1984).

painstakingly tries to recuperate Velma's voice in their two-hour healing session.

Hegemonic systems of representation have featured a lot of mad women in the attic who are deleteriously pitiable and stereotypically undesirable.[8] This chapter tries to answer the following questions: How does Bambara conceptualize and negotiate disability in her novel for an African American woman? Is she racializing and gendering disability or does she conceive race and gender themselves as disabilities? And how does the black woman, who had long been seen as 'de mule uh de world', to borrow the phrase of Zora Neale Hurston, handle her disability and express her pain?[9]

The chapter first contextualizes Bambara in the black canon of writing and draws upon the significance of historicizing her work to understand it. I then examine the convergence of the discourses of race and gender with that of disability and I argue that the term disability has crossed the boundaries of physical abnormalities to embrace such disabling social notions, with special reference to African American and feminist discourses. Next, I contend that pain could also be categorized as a disability and this argument is anchored by Debra King's *African Americans and the Culture of Pain,* and what she calls 'blackpain',[10] trying to examine how pain emanating from disability can be expressed and whether it is possible to hear the silent voice of pain. Finally, I am interested to know if it is just Velma's mental condition that renders her disabled or if the experience of pain is equally disabling, and whether the novel is a narrative of overcoming or an expression of the protagonist's alterity and otherness as a literary invalid. To this end I examine Velma's story in two main sections: narrating her tale in the silent voice of pain in the context of the healing session and within her intruding memories. The second section is concerned with her healer Minnie Ransom and her strategy for curing Velma from her metaphorical and physical disabilities and examines if Minnie is healing Velma by listening to her silent voice or by speaking on her behalf.

8 This is an allusion to Mr. Rochester's wife, hidden from public scrutiny in the attic of his house because of her insanity. Charlotte Brontë, *Jane Eyre* (Hertfordshire: Wordsworth Editions, 1847, 1992).

9 Zora Neale Hurston's famous quotation has been praised as one of the best descriptions of the plight of the black woman who endures racism, sexism and prejudice, and suffers from ostracization. Zora Neale Hurston, *Their Eyes Were Watching God* (New York: Virago Press, 1937, 1986).

10 Debra Walker King, *African Americans and the Culture of Pain: Cultural Frames, Framing Culture* (Charlottesville: University of Virginia Press, 2008), 11.

1 Bambara and Disabling Race and Gender

Bambara's fiction is multifarious as it delves into the profound recesses of African American life, dreams, frustrations, cultural traditions, vernacular, politics, feminisms, and history. Bambara's work was not limited to one genre; she published literary works, screenplays and anthologies. She was also among the prominent activists of the Black Arts Movement that took place in the 1970s. She states that the

> novel grew out of [her] attempt to fuse the seemingly separate frames of reference of the camps; it grew out of an interest in identifying bridges; it grew out of a compulsion to understand how energies of this period will manifest themselves in the next decade.[11]

The period she refers to is post-Civil Rights Movement, an epoch characterized primarily by disillusionment and frustration. Although the Civil Rights Movement adopted a non-violent civil disobedient strategy and succeeded in issuing new federal legislations that ended segregation based on colour, race and sex, the racist discrimination did not end and African Americans in northern urban ghettoes, as well as in the South, were still suffering as before. The epoch Bambara depicts in her novel is mainly concerned with the disillusionment that characterized this time and how African Americans felt frustrated and angry. However, reading Bambara's novel is not an easy job. The disintegration of this world for African Americans is conspicuously reflected through Bambara's technique to disintegrate the structure of the novel, allowing nobody and nothing to occupy the centre of the narrative. Janelle Collins explains that her novel

> adapts a non-mimetic form of representation, rejects linear history in favor of a flattened, one dimensional chronology of events, displays multiple angles of vision rather than either a first person or omniscient perspective, presents a "decentered" subject rather than unified subjectivity in the character of Velma Henry, offers a labyrinth of events instead of a plot to follow, and rejects closure in favor of open-ended meaning.[12]

---

11 Janet Sternburg, ed., *The Writer on Her Work* (New York: W.W. Norton and Co., 1980), 165.

12 Janell Collins, 'Generating Power: Fission, Fusion, and Postmodern Politics in Bambara's *The Salt Eaters*', *MELUS* 21.2 (1996): 36.

No specific borders are to be found in the text as the narrative re-produces the personal history of Velma and the collective history of African Americans at that crucial time. Both histories are primarily marked by an agonizing disillusionment. Intricate questions of subjectivity and representation are further complicated since the protagonist's voice is inaudible. As disabled and silent Velma sits on her stool, her consciousness is split between her current surroundings in which Minnie occupies centre stage, and the flood of disconnected memories of people and events.

In addition to the broken structure, what also makes the novel difficult as Jane Duran argues is that 'it is unclear which take on reality is something like an "actual" take, and in many cases it is unclear whose take is being presented'.[13] The realms of the imagined and the real in the narrative overlap many times which renders it hard for the reader to establish clear-cut boundaries between them in the plot. The mythical intertwines with the real, the tragic with the comic, the dead with the living, the sane with the insane, and Velma's voice maintains its silence as all those realms get tangled. Bambara deliberately forces her readers to embark upon a tough journey to put the fragmented pieces together in order to grasp how Velma ends up as a disabled character and to scrutinize the tormenting itinerary of her healing process.

Disability poetics has featured characters as bed-ridden, hysterical, psychotic, neurotic, or suffering from cognitive disability, body impairment or nervous prostration. It has also delineated much of the alleged pathology of the black race and other marginalized groups. The works of Douglas C. Baynton,[14] and David R. Roediger and Elizabeth D. Esch[15] thoroughly examine the justifications that were claimed to create a false bond between black slaves and disability. Examples of disabled black characters abound in nineteenth-century American literature such as scarred Prue and crippled Hager in Harriet Beecher Stowe's *Uncle Tom's Cabin,*[16] insane Pip in Herman Melville's *Moby Dick,*[17] the exchanged twins in Mark Twain's *Pudd'nhead Wilson,*[18] and the mentally

13 Jane Duran, *Women, Philosophy and Literature* (Hampshire: Ashgate Publishing Limited, 2007), 133.

14 Douglas C. Baynton's 'Disability and the Justification of Inequality in American History' in *The New Disability History: American Perspectives* (New York: New York University Press, 2001).

15 David R. Roediger and Elizabeth D. Esch's *The Production of Difference: Race and the Management of Labor in US History* (New York: Oxford University Press, 2002).

16 Harriet Beecher Stowe's *Uncle Tom's Cabin* (London: Wordsworth Editions Ltd, 1999).

17 Herman Melville's *Moby Dick* (New York: Bantam Classics, 1981).

18 Mark Twain's *Pudd'nhead Wilson* (New York: Dover Publications, 1999).

disabled Jupiter in Edgar Allan Poe's "The Gold Bug".[19] However, there seems to be no consensus on defining disability studies. Simi Linton contends that

> [t]he term *disability*, as it has been used in general parlance, appears to signify something material or concrete, a physical or psychological condition considered to have predominantly medical significance. [However], [a] project of *disability* studies scholars and the disability rights movement has been to bring into sharp relief the process by which *disability* has been imbued with the meaning(s) it has and to assign a meaning that is consistent with a sociopolitical analysis of *disability*.[20]

From this perspective, disability crosses the boundaries of physical abnormality; it is an umbrella term that embraces a lot of deviations from the norm including social, economic, political and racial deviations. Political ideologies and social structures tend to shun deviants and hence such people become tagged as representationally disabled persons who fail to achieve utter normalcy. Thus, a disability can be physical, emotional or cognitive. Rosemarie Thomson also takes disability beyond medical definitions and points to other dimensions in its hermeneutics. She argues that disability is a

> pervasive, often unarticulated, ideology informing our cultural notions of self and other [...] Disability – like gender – is a concept that pervades all aspects of culture: its structuring institutions, social identities, cultural practices, political positions, historical communities, and the shared human experience of embodiment.[21]

The cultural facet of disability is not to be ignored for it is a founding pillar of the term. According to Thomson, the disabled are truly the deformed, the debilitated, the insane and the abnormal. But disability as marker of otherness can also be for the ugly, the old, the feeble, the marginalized, the oppressed and the silenced.

Owing to the intricate webs of identity markers women find themselves entangled in, disability studies and feminist schools congregate at multiple points. A surge of interest in bringing together the schools of feminism and

19 Edgar Allan Poe's *The Gold Bug* (North Charleston: BookSurge Classics, 2004).

20 Simi Linton, 'Reassigning Meaning', *The Disability Studies Reader*, ed. Lennard J. Davis (New York: Routledge, 2006), 162.

21 Rosemarie Garland-Thomson, 'Integrating Disability, Transforming Feminist Theory', *The Disability Studies Reader*, 259.

disabilities studies has been noticeable lately in the works of Susan Wendell,[22] Rosemarie Garland Thomson,[23] and Barbara Fawcett.[24] Thomson, for example, contends that

> [m]any parallels exist between the social meanings attributed to female bodies and those assigned to disabled bodies. Both the female and the disabled body are cast as deviant and inferior; both are excluded from full participation in public as well as in economic life; both are defined in opposition to a norm that is assumed to possess natural physical superiority. Indeed the discursive equation of femaleness with disability is common.[25]

The patriarchal discourse has pushed women further into the peripheries of normalcy by persistently depicting women as physically weaker and intellectually inferior, both categories which fall under the rubric of disability. Normal women are socially disabled by chauvinism, which makes it much worse for women who are physically disabled. This should not indicate that every woman suffers from a disability by virtue of her gender, but it contends that, like gender, disability is a social formulation, and both similarly create barriers that deprive their bearers of many opportunities. As Susan Wendell points out: '[d]isabled women struggle with both the oppressions of being women in male-dominated societies and the oppressions of being disabled in societies dominated by the able-bodied'.[26] Such two-fold struggle poses a threat upon a disabled woman's agency; being cornered in such positionality, she is likely to become a hostage in the hands of silence and her voice is lost as she battles on so many fronts. Her gender intensifies her physical disability as she bears a double stigma of being inferior. Hence, curing her wounds involves hearing this taciturn voice, which was once resonant but has been deliberately muffled.

---

22 Susan Wendell's *The Rejected Body: Feminist Philosophical Reflections on Disability* (1997) and 'Toward a Feminist Theory of Disability', in *Hypatia*, 4.2, 1989, 104–124.

23 Rosemarie Garland Thomson, *Extraordinary Bodies: Figuring Physical Disability in American Culture and Literature* (New York: Routledge, 1997), and in *Disabilities Studies Quarterly* 34.2 (2014), which were published under the themes: 'Disability Is a Feminist Issue: Bringing Together Women's and Gender Studies and Disability Studies', and *Feminist Disability Studies*, ed. Kim Q. Hall (Bloomington, Indiana: Indiana University Press, 2011),

24 Barbara Fawcett's *Feminist Perspectives on Disability* (New York: Routledge, 2000).

25 Rosemarie Garland-Thomson, *Extraordinary Bodies: Figuring Physical Disability in American Literature and Culture* (New York: Columbia University Press, 1997), 19.

26 Susan Wendell, 'Toward a Feminist Theory of Disability', *The Disability Studies Reader* (New York: Routledge, 2013), 244.

In addition to disabling gender, there is disabling race. African American discourse has frequently converged with that of disability studies as both seem to have much in common. The link between disability and slaves originated on slave ships and created the association between race and disability, and American literature fortified this concept in eighteenth – and nineteenth-century writings.[27] African Americans have been linked historically to disability since that time to justify their racial oppression, and 19th century slave narratives teem with such disabled characters. For example: in *The History of Mary Prince, a West Indian Slave*[28] Mary was crippled; Mr. Ruggles in *A Narrative of the Life of Frederick Douglass, an American Slave*[29] was blind; Page in *Narrative of William Wells Brown*[30] was crippled for life; in *Twelve Years a Slave, Narrative of Solomon Northup*[31] Solomon fell blind for three days; and, in *Incidents in the Life of a Slave Girl*[32] Harriet's grandmother was badly ill and so was her little son. The African American canon continued to display disabled characters whose physical impairments symbolized the violence and institutionalized exclusion blacks have been subject to. Such examples of disabled characters include: the ever-sick Frado in Harriet E. Wilson's *Our Nig: Sketches from the Life of a Free Black*;[33] Earl the disabled son in Zora Neale Hurston's *Seraph on the Suwanee*;[34] Miss Thomson with ulcerous on her foot in Paule Marshall's *Brown Girls, Brownstones*;[35] Uncle Willie who walks with the help of a cane, his left hand is atrophied and the left side of his face suffers from paralysis in Maya Angelou's *I Know Why The Caged Bird Sings*;[36] Maggie the crippled

27 George Gordon-Smith, "Constrained Bodies: Representing Slavery and Disability in American Literature and Culture", (Dissertation, Emory University, 2015).

28 Mary Prince, *The History of Mary Prince, a West Indian Slave* (New York: Penguin Classics, 1831, 2001).

29 Frederick Douglass, *A Narrative of the Life of Frederick Douglass, an American Slave* (New York: Dover Publications, 1845, 1995).

30 Willaim Wells Brown, *Narrative of William Wells Brown, a Fugitive Slave* (New York: Reada-Classic, 1847, 2010).

31 Solomon Northup, *Twelve Years a Slave, Narrative of Solomon Northup* (Connecticut: Martino Fine Books, 1853, 2010).

32 Harriet Jackobs, *Incidents in the Life of a Slave Girl* (New York: Dover Publications, 1861, 2012).

33 Harriet E. Wilson, *Our Nig: Sketches from the Life of a Free Black* (New York: Dover Publications, 1859, 2005).

34 Zora Neale Hurston, *Seraph on the Suwanee* (New York: Harper Perennial Modern Classics, 1948, 2008).

35 Paule Marshall, *Brown Girls, Brownstones* (New York: Dover Publications, 1959, 2009).

36 Maya Angelou, *I Know Why The Caged Bird Sings* (New York: Ballantine Books, 1969, 2009).

sister in Alice Walker's "Everyday Use";[37] and, Audre Lorde as herself in *The Cancer Journals*.[38] Toni Morrison's oeuvre, in particular, is a startling example on how African American writers delineate disabled figures such as scarred Seth, one-armed Nan and limping Baby Suggs in *Beloved*,[39] mad Shadrack and one-legged Eva Peace in *Sula*,[40] blind Marie Therese Foucault in *Tar Baby*,[41] Pauline Breedlove with her disabled foot in *The Bluest Eye*,[42] and Pilate Dead, who has no navel, in *Song of Solomon* (1977).[43]

Throughout the 20th century, disability in African American literature became a politicized metaphor for victimization and isolation, and grew into another oppressive social construction like race and gender. Lennard Davis draws a coherent analogy between disability and race that still exists in modern times, concurring that the disabled is 'an icon that needs to be excluded in a similar way to the body marked as differently pigmented'.[44] The pain of exclusion is equal and so is the biased social gaze on both. Race and disability continue to relegate people to a position of victimization and subject them to disenfranchisement while enforcing negative stereotypes and multi-faceted oppressions upon blacks.[45] In the pervasive historical web of discrimination in the United States, race has developed into a social disability that bears the stigma of difference and places non-whites in an inferior position in the social hierarchy, which brings race closer to disability. Race in this case might not be a disability *per se*, but it is categorically disabling. Therefore, the intersection of race, gender and disability is not additive, it forges multi-layered identities that must endure marginalization, pain and stigma on many levels.

Establishing links among those three mantras proves that a disabled woman of colour like Velma Henry is definitely not at a comfortable intersection, but a figure who suffers immensely from oppressive racism, sexism and exclusion; a figure who is victimized by the pain that enforces unwelcome alterations while imposing a re-negotiation of one's identity. Velma's trauma is her physical

---

37 Alice Walker's story was published in *In Love and Trouble* (New York: Mariner Books, 1973, 2003).

38 Audre Lorde, *The Cancer Journals* (San Francisco: Aunt Lute Books, 1980, 2006).

39 Toni Morrison's *Beloved* (New York: Vintage, 1987).

40 Toni Morrison's *Sula* (New York: Vintage, 1973, 2004).

41 Toni Morrison's *Tar Baby* (New York: Signet, 1983).

42 Toni Morrison's *The Bluest Eye* (New York: Vintage, 1970, 2007).

43 Toni Morrison's *Song of Solomon* (New York: Vintage, 1977, 2004).

44 Lennard J. Davis, *Enforcing Normalcy: Disability, Deafness, and the Body* (London: Verso, 1995), 80.

45 Chris Bell, *Blackness and Disability* (Michigan: Michigan State University Press, 2012), in which he draws attention to the absence of blacks in disability studies and scrutinizes the historical association between African Americans and disability discourse.

disability, but her race and gender are her metaphorical social ones. However, there is another dimension to her disability, namely the dimension of pain as it holds within the repercussions of all her disabling ailments. The pain stemming from her condition is immense, it hits hard and as it gradually metamorphoses into an additional disability, it embraces all the other disabilities she bears. Pain becomes the true embodiment of her status and the main reason behind her oppressively enforced silence as it envelops her race, gender and physical trauma. It iconizes her disability both historically, socially, politically and also physically. In the following sections, I will focus on the pain in Velma's story and argue that despite everything she is suffering from, pain stands out as the biggest impediment and the most tormenting disability from which her voice withers and her agency sinks.

2 Narrating Pain in Silence

'What is your story?' Minnie asks Velma and Velma's story is indeed one of pain.[46] Disability entails much pain, be it physical, emotional, psychological or social. Velma's pain transcends the threshold of the physical pain of her trauma and enters the domain of another kind of agonizing pain related to her race. Pain in African American history plays such a crucial role that it has become part and parcel of being black in America. King points out that

> [a]s much as we might like to deny it, sometimes when we see black skin, we assume the presence of pain. It is there either as a history embedded in the tones and texture of the flesh or as a mythology accepted as truth. This kind of image-reading allows the black body to function as a metaphor for suffering, injury, and pain.[47]

Black bodies bear a legacy of pain that has developed into some kind of disability which stands in the way of being accepted as normal. Instead, one is socially castigated and negatively imaged. King coins the term 'blackpain' to refer to the 'visual and verbal representation of the pained black bodies that function as rhetorical devices, as instruments of socialization, and as sociopolitical strategy in American popular culture and literature'.[48] Blackpain trespasses the allusion to the physical pain historically inflicted upon black bodies in slavery,

46 Bambara, *Salt*.
47 King, *Pain*, 48.
48 Ibid., 16.

lynching, rape, torture, and other racist practices; it is a prevailing part of being African American. Blackpain is also a political means of segregating blacks and pushing them to the periphery. Since they fail to fall under the mythological rubric of pain-free American identity, blacks become 'outsiders who can never be "let in", the ones who do not belong but who, by virtue of their pain, are failed Americans'.[49] Blackpain is a socio-political hindrance in the lives of blacks that bears witness to various forms of oppression. The holistic structuring of this kind of pain makes it an integral part of the African American identity and defines it as a disabling trait. After all, disability is not only a physical deviance. King argues further that the

> symbolic implications of blackpain are built upon the assumption that racially biased political dogma cannot be conceived as distinct from the bodies they segregate, define, and mark as "Other". Such dogma is intimately tied to those bodies, and in fact, it depends on them for sustainability and justification.[50]

Blackpain maintains the racial hierarchy and keeps blacks in an inferior position by inflicting a social disability that excludes them from mainstream culture. Thus, it becomes a political, racial, and social disability that African Americans have to endure. It defines them, marks their struggle on myriad fronts, and renders them as *others*. In addition to the physical ache of her trauma, Velma's story palpably embraces this kind of pain.

Bambara paints Velma's character with a brush of silence as she hardly utters a word and her voice is almost totally absent. She is physically silent as she says nothing, and emblematically silent as she takes no actions and makes no choices during the entire session with Minnie. Her interior monologue of memories, which is the only voice that Bambara gives her, is overloaded with pain in all its sporadic intrusions upon the narrative. Most of her memories are incomplete and they only become comprehensible through the memories of other characters such as Obie and Sophie, which weakens this voice more and renders it unreliable. Velma's silent voice therefore entails dissociation between the body and the self. Her silence iconizes non-sovereignty over her life and lack of agency. Pain targets the individual's agency since it is always out of control; it is present albeit unspoken, and hence silence becomes its best language. Elaine Scarry draws a connection between pain and silence and

49 Ibid., 17.
50 Ibid., 16.

explains that 'pain does not simply resist language but actively destroys it'.[51] Such destruction inevitably results in silence, for pain surpasses words that fail to express the feeling unreservedly. As alienation, rejection and fear join hands, Velma falls prey to the exclusionist paradigm of disability and becomes the Other. She is ensnared in tenuous positions. Her introduction in the novel reminds one of Franz Kafka's "Hunger Artist".[52] Kafka's story follows the declining career of a Hunger Artist who performed in a cage his art of fasting for an audience that suspected him and never understood the quality of his art. He is also victimized by his impresario who never allowed him to fast for more than forty days for fear of losing the sympathy of his audience. The Hunger Artist, however, loses the interest of his audience and is left to die in a cage lamenting the art that nobody was ever able to appreciate. He loses his humanity and becomes a mere prop in a farcical show performed to an unknowing audience; a postmodern freak show.[53] Velma enters the text as an insane woman who failed in her suicide attempt and is now held in the Southeast Infirmary Community where the local healer tries to help her in the presence of a bored audience. She is delineated as a silent, estranged and detached patient who

> clutched the stool. She felt faint, too faint to ask for a decent chair to sit in. She felt like she was in the back room of some precinct, or in the interrogation room of terrorist kidnappers, or in the walnut-paneled office of Transchemical being asked about an error. She cut that short. She hadn't the strength. She felt her eyes rolling away.[54]

Her pain steals away her voice and she is not even given the privilege of groaning or screaming. In addition to her mental disability, she is the spectacle of blackpain and could be identified as one of 'those who are innocent of the stories their bodies tell'.[55] Velma bears the burden of too many pains; she suffers the rifts of being a woman, a black, and an activist who fails to achieve anything she has ever dreamt of. Losing her voice implies losing the will to

---

51 Scarry, *The Body in Pain*, 4.

52 Kafka's short story was published in *A Hunger Artist and Other Stories* (New York: Oxford University Press, 1922, 2012).

53 Freak shows (16th–19th centuries) depended on physical deformities and visible diseases for entertainment. However, they declined in the twentieth century as science developed and such deformities were medically explained, and the new waves of disability rights also attacked their lack of respect for humanity.

54 Bambara, *Salt*.

55 King, *Pain*, 12.

craft authority over her life. As her entire world tumbles down before her, she collapses, loses her mind, and attempts suicide.

From the beginning, Bambara creates two realms: the healing scene and that of the retrospective memories that intrude to bring about many oppressions. In both realms Velma resides in a landscape of pain and silence where, as Derek Alwes points out, even her memories are 'crippling'.[56] Her pain is both physical and psychological and so is her silence. Her husband Obie wonders 'It's got to be costing you something to hang on to old pains ... It takes something out of you, Velma, to keep them all dead moments alive'.[57] But those moments never died for Velma and they still return with the same flood of pain. King defines pain 'as a boundless perception woven intricately from experiences of physical, mental, and emotional wounding and trauma that threaten one's ability to move "safely" into survival and wholeness'.[58] Velma's corporeal and emotional pain falls within the premises set by King and it is a part of all her memories. She recalls a sickly memory of menstruation as she marches in a protest with other women, which is juxtaposed with the arrival of the black political leader they are supporting, in the company of a woman dressed in silk as 'wasted blood and rage'.[59] She vividly remembers the infidelity of Obie 'You are sleeping around, Obie, and not very discreetly'[60] and her revengeful affair 'And then a stupid affair with a man she wasn't certain she even liked, certainly didn't trust'.[61] She goes back to bitter recollections on the plant when she was falsely accused of leaking information against the benefit of the entire black community, 'remember last time she leaked some material?[62]' Velma is not only oppressed by hegemonic institutions; she is let down by everything and everyone and hence pain hits her on all levels, and silence becomes her last refuge. She is not an enslaved girl who is raped, tortured or lynched, nor is she a black pauper who lives in the socioeconomic nadir of a black ghetto, yet she is painfully oppressed and her disabling pain results from the symbolic violence she experiences that almost murders her voice. King argues that

56 Derek Alwes, 'The Burden of Liberty: Choice in Toni Morrison's *Jazz* and Toni Cade Bambara's *The Salt Eaters*', *African American Review* 30.3 (1996): 361.
57 Bambara, *Salt*.
58 King, *Pain*, 16.
59 Bambara, *Salt*.
60 Ibid.
61 Ibid.
62 Ibid.

> [v]iolence against the black body does not end with overt acts of injury and murder, however. The lessons of racially motivated violation inform moments of symbolic violence [which] is not the same as the brutal exploitation and overt violence of lynching, yet both types of violence yield similar regulatory and disciplinary effects. Both are sources for racial hurt, psychological wounding, and, ultimately, soul murder.[63]

The damage incurred by this symbolic violence is an assault on Velma's sense of self; her dignity is compromised and her world is shattered. This pain turns Velma from being a subject into becoming an object and hence she loses her agency and consequently her sense of wholeness and her voice. Pain disables Velma and becomes the real cause of destroying her sanity.

A disabling world inexorably creates disabled people; Velma's reminiscing is overflowing with images of pain and disability and even in her memories she is ever silent. Bambara introduces blacks in her novel as people who

> wore their crippleness or blindness like a badge of honor, as though it meant they'd been singled out for some special punishment, were special. Or as though it meant they'd paid some heavy dues and knew, then, what there was to know, and therefore had a right to certain privileges, or were exempt from certain charges, or ought to be listened to at meetings. But way down under knowing "special" was a lie, knowing better all along and feeling the cost of the lie, of the self-betrayal in the joints, in the lungs, in the eyes.[64]

Velma is not the only disabled character in the narrative for her memories are inhabited by other disabled and ill black persons in pain. As Carter Mathes argues, her memory 'moves between layers of temporality and psychic space' in which those characters appear sporadically to emphasize that oppression can eventually lead to disability, as much as disability can lead to oppression.[65] Sophie, Velma's godmother, suffers from 'a wave of nausea' and 'the buzzing throb in her temples and the lift and drop in her stomach'.[66] Fred Holt is the traumatized bus driver who is haunted by his dead friend Porter because he is unable to let go of his memory or to release his pain. He agonizingly recalls:

---

63 King, *Pain*, 34.

64 Bambara, *Salt*.

65 Carter Mathes, 'Scratching the Threshold: Textual Sound and Political Form in Toni Cade Bambara's *The Salt Eaters*', *Contemporary Literature* 50.2 (2009): 382.

66 Bambara, *Salt*.

> Porter. Had to bribe a doctor to get his papers through and get the job with the bus company. Some kind of wasting disease was eating him up. [...] Hospitalized, discharged, no compensation, no records. Not service-connected they said goodbye, get lost buddy, drop dead. She stabbed him, they said, in the side of his neck as he leaned into his '133' cup, lips pursed, hot coffee. He fell, they said, like cattle fall in the stockyards.[67]

He gets lost in his reminiscing while all the passengers on his bus are talking about beating, diseases and hospitals. Velma's first lover Smitty, while trying to blow up a Confederate Statue in a protest during the Vietnam War, is crippled by the beatings of the police forces:

> Smitty pulled down against the cement pedestal, slammed against the horses' hooves, dragged on his stomach to the van. A boot in the neck. Child. Four knees in his back. Son. The package ripped from his grip. The policeman racing on his own path and none other's.[68]

Pain does not stop with her memories. Her ultimate collapse also involves much pain as she attempts suicide by putting her head in the oven and then cutting her veins. Velma's past and present conspire against her and deprive her of establishing an agentic positionality and silence her voice.

Bambara intends to depict the disability of Velma as the status of the African American activists after the Civil Rights Movement when almost everything failed them and they were left with nothing but pain, and hence the socio-political dimension in her story is quite significant. Her politics of representation is distinguished; Velma is not a literary invalid[69] being the character who is chronically ill or disabled and hence is portrayed as helpless, nor is she a pathetic sick person as Helen Burns[70] and Beth March.[71] In Charlotte Brontë's *Jane Eyre*, Helen Burns is the pious friend of Jane that she meets during her stay at Lowood School. Helen is a meek Christian who is willing to accept injustice all the time unlike Jane. She dies of consumption and tells Jane that she bears her physical pain patiently and is happy to leave this world. Beth

67 Ibid.

68 Ibid.

69 For a more detailed analysis for such characters and their association with female figures in American literature, Diane Price Herndl, *Invalid Women: Figuring Feminine Illness in American Fiction and Culture, 1840–1940* (Chapel Hill, North Carolina: University of North Carolina Press, 1993).

70 Brontë, *Jane Eyre*.

71 Louisa May Alcott's *Little Women* (New York: Maplewood Books, 1868–69, 2015).

March, on the other hand, appears in Louisa May Alcott's *Little Women*. Beth is the selfless and gentle sister; she develops scarlet fever and although she is cured, her health becomes too weak and she eventually dies at a young age. Her death is the most tragic blow that hits the family and she is delineated in the text as rather pathetic and very different from all her sisters as she lacks ambition and is too shy and kind. Velma's narrative of suffering is told differently; it is told in silence. Hers is not an everywoman story because her mental disability makes her different from any disabled African American woman who is archetypally oppressed by race, gender, and class such as Maggie in Toni Morrison's "Recitatif".[72] In Morrison's story, a black and a white girl are sent for four months to an orphanage. The racial identities of both girls are never revealed and the story traces their four encounters at four different decades in America in which they disagree in their memories on Maggie the coloured and disabled cook at the orphanage who was kicked down and humiliated by the bigger girls. Maggie stands for a woman who is coerced by class, race, gender and disability. Although she is delineated as a pathetic character, her memory haunts the two girls as an icon of guilt and hatred for their two mothers who abandoned them. Velma is not solely a disabled woman; she is a human wreck silenced by pain. Tobian Siebers argues that pain 'is a subjective phenomenon, perhaps the most subjective of phenomena'.[73] He explicates that the disabled is a distinct Other who deviates from the norm, yet disability remains a discrete experience, for being deaf and being blind are definitely not the same. What makes every disability unique is the individuality of its pain. Velma's blackpain, as Duran emphasizes, shows 'how the alienation imposed on black women, in particular, meshes with general existential concerns, and pushes individuals out of their trajectories'.[74] Velma is pushed into the private territory where the weak, the ill, the disabled, the silenced and the pained often reside. Blackpain is prolonged and recurring in Velma's life to the extent that she somehow becomes too perilously comfortable in her pain and becomes disconnected from her surroundings. Thus, her disability is not portrayed as an advantage because of the amount of pain she has to bear and because of her silent voice and absent agency. Despite not hearing her voice, Velma's story is not too hard to decipher. Healing her, however, imposes a lot of grim challenges.

---

72 Toni Morrison's story was published in *Confirmation: An Anthology of African American Women*, eds. Imamu Amiri Baraka and Amina Baraka (New York: William Morrow, 1983).

73 Tobian Siebers, 'Disability in Theory: From Social Constructionism to the New Realism of the Body', *The Disability Studies Reader*: 176.

74 Duran, *Philosophy*, 147.

3 Healing the Wounds

Pain crushes Velma's soul and hence it demolishes her sense of existence. King emphasizes that blackpain murders the soul which is 'the death of personal will, everyday living, and, consequently, life'.[75] This is the disability of pain that Velma suffers from and Minnie understands, not only the disability of her trauma. Minnie Ransom, 'the fabled healer of the district', knows that the price of healing is dear and her inaugurating question for Velma poses challenges and opens the door to choices and decisions; she understands that Velma needs her voice back to regain her stolen agency.[76] Minnie does not impose a voice upon Velma and does not attempt to speak on her behalf either, as she tells her: 'Choose your cure, sweetheart. Decide what you want to do with wholeness', and then she assures Velma: 'The source of health is never outside, sweetheart'.[77] According to Scarry, the healer 'can hear the fragmentary language of pain, coax it into clarity, and interpret it'.[78] Bambara believes that realising the pain of African Americans might help in healing them and this is the strategy Minnie uses in healing Velma; she listens to her silent voice and sees through it to help her get back her sanity and her sense of being. Minnie's mission is made more difficult since Velma's language is not fragmented; it is simply absent altogether, but Minnie comprehends that it is not dead yet and that she can still save Velma's voice.

Being well and being whole both entail a big responsibility. Minnie knows that getting a voice back necessitates vision and hence she endeavours to help Velma step out of her domain of false consciousness to attain such a vision when she asks her: 'Can you afford to be whole?'[79] James Charlton explains that disability creates a false consciousness that

> isolates individuals. Most people with disabilities actually come to believe they are less normal, less capable than others. Self-pity, self-hate, shame, and other manifestations of this process are devastating for they prevent people with disabilities from knowing their real selves, their real needs, and their real capabilities and from recognizing the options they in fact have. False consciousness and alienation also obscure the source of their oppression. They cannot recognize that their self-perceived pitiful lives are simply a perverse mirroring of a pitiful world order. In this regard

75 King, *Pain*, 16.
76 Bambara, *Salt*.
77 Ibid.
78 Scarry, *The Body in Pain*, 6.
79 Bambara, *Salt*.

> people with disabilities have much in common with others who also have internalized their own oppression.[80]

Velma is trapped in the painful vortex of false consciousness and seclusion; pain makes her shut people out. Her disability is a trope which is reduced to exclude her and Minnie's healing process attempts to include Velma back in the circle of the sane and the whole. King argues that oppression can result in 'a broken spirit. Pain emanating from such brokenness weakens the will, makes courage volatile, overwhelms confidence, fuels anger; and yes, it can *kill*'.[81] Minnie sees through that breach and does not target Velma's insanity but rather her pain, telling her: 'got to give it all up, the pain, the hurt, the anger and make room for lovely things to rush in and fill you full'.[82] Minnie tries to break the chain of silence that Velma incarcerates herself in. Giving Velma her voice back involves moving her from the realm of self-rejection to that of self-acceptance; '"Answer me now", Minnie insisted'.[83] Velma needs to make the choice to be healed; to speak up and to make her voice resonantly heard so that she is ontologically present and not absent. Minnie puts the broken pieces of her spirit back together by listening to her silent voice and pulling it back to life.

'Not all dying is the physical self' says Sophie to Velma.[84] Velma's death is spiritual and her pain also bears a similar nature. Minnie feels Velma's spiritual pain and identifies with her. Velma's voice becomes coterminous with what King calls soul power which she defines as 'will power on fire – a combination of hope and self-determination that influences how woundedness, pain, and injury are read internally, as well as how fully their negative potential is manifested externally'.[85] Soul power is significant since it allows one to maintain control over varied reactions and overcome pain. However, King warns that it

> is not fatigable. It cannot be taken away or conquered, but it can be killed or given away. Consequently, it diminishes only if those suffering symbolic and overt violence collaborate with pain and its champion to the point of being consumed.[86]

80 James Charlton, 'The Dimensions of Disability Oppression: An Overview', *The Disability Studies Reader*: 220.
81 King, *Pain*, 39. (italics in the original).
82 Bambara, *Salt*.
83 Ibid.
84 Ibid.
85 King, *Pain*, 39.
86 Ibid.

Velma has reached that point and Minnie's mission is to win her back to regain her 'soul power' and voice. Minnie's healing involves the presence of the Old Wife who serves as a mythological presence in the narrative, since Minnie seems to be suffering from similar spiritual pain; the Old Wife becomes the healer of the healer and Minnie pleads with her 'I'm gonna lose the patient [...] if you don't give me some directions. She's lost a lot of blood and her system's still full of gas. I just can't seem to generate the energy to bring her back and restore her'.[87] The missing voice of Velma renders her unable to master her narrative of pain; hence it is replaced by that of the Old Wife who warns Minnie: 'You and that gal on the stool cut from the same cloth'.[88] Throughout their conversations, the Old Wife can also be seen as Minnie's alter ego especially when Minnie wonders:

> What is wrong with the women? If they ain't sticking their head in ovens and opening up their veins like this gal, or jumping off roofs, drinking charcoal lighter, pumping rat poisons in their arms, and ramming cars into walls, they looking for some men to tear his head off. What is wrong, Old Wife?[89]

The Old Wife helps Minnie through the healing process, as much as the latter helps Velma in recovering, by showing Minnie the border lines that she needs to acknowledge if she really wants to save her life. The Old Wife provides answers to Minnie's questions and emphasises to her that she has endured the same amount of pain that Velma is going through, and hence she is the only one capable of curing her.

Minnie is not detached as a healer; she is pulled into the centre with Velma.[90] She fails to maintain a distance from her patient as the Old Wife observes 'Love, Min. Love won't let you let her go. I'm not the leastways worried'.[91] Establishing a spiritual bond based on love with Velma, Minnie maps out a terrain for her outside her false consciousness and beyond her pain and interlacing cycles of oppression; a terrain to find her lost voice in as she compels her to: 'Quit wrasslin, sweetheart, or you may go under. I'm throwing you the

87 Bambara, *Salt.*

88 Ibid.

89 Ibid.

90 To know more about how going through a similarly painful experience helps in a better understanding of mental distress, Hans T. Sternudd, 'Voices of Depression: An Analysis of a Collective Narrative', in this volume.

91 Ibid.

life line. Don't be too proud to live'.[92] Pain remains a personal experience, but Minnie cures Velma because she shares her pain, especially when she urges Velma: 'Hold my hand daughter [...] Let me share your pain'.[93] King explains that 'sharing encourages sympathetic engagement and sometimes helps those involved in the event of sharing to not only claim their own pain but also claim responsibility for healing the pain of others'.[94] Although Minnie is emotionally involved in the healing process, she is not patronizing her patient. Minnie turns the lens inward to let Velma see her inner voids and fill them up to get over her disability. She shows Velma through her recurrent questions on whether she wants to become whole again that she needs to face the situation, instead of escaping from it by living in the past. Throughout her conversations with the Old Wife it becomes obvious that Minnie went through similar painful experiences herself and was able to get over them with the help of the Old Wife. The lesson that she learnt from her personal pain is that healing is a decision that must be made, and this is her message to Velma.

Minnie's crucial technique in healing Velma relies on clearing the blurred contours for her and showing her that being well is a matter of choice, a matter of agency: 'Just so's you're sure, sweetheart, and ready to be healed, cause wholeness is no trifling matter. A lot of weight when you're well'.[95] Ann Folwell Stanford points out that 'Minnie is no self-effacing stranger eager to "fix" Velma. She offers a question fraught with risks, one that shifts the location of healing from external sources to Velma herself'.[96] The interrogative tone in Minnie's words asserts that she does not try to put words into Velma's mouth but to persuade her to speak up and act as she explicitly asks her 'Sweetheart, what's the matter?'[97] Being, or not being, whole is Velma's decision and Velma's responsibility; it is Velma's salt. The titular motif is manipulated to create a metaphor of equilibrium in Velma's story for

> [t]he body needs to throw off its excess salt for balance. Too little salt and wounds can't heal. Remember Napoleon's army? Those frogs were dropping dead from scratches because their bodies were deprived of salt. But too much –.[98]

92 Ibid.

93 Ibid.

94 King, *Pain*, 137.

95 Bambara, *Salt*.

96 Ann Folwell Stanford, 'He Speaks for Whom?: Inscription and Reinscription of Women in *Invisible Man* and *The Salt Eaters*', *MELUS* 18.2 (1993): 25.

97 Bambara, *Salt*.

98 Ibid.

Too much salt can still be more detrimental than too little because it iconizes a sense of defeat owing to the 'difference between eating salt as an antidote to the snakebite and turning into salt, succumbing to the serpent'.[99] A big amount of salt then is an undignified way of accepting victimization. The narrative also alludes to Lot's wife who got solidified as a punishment for looking back to denote that Velma needs to stop living in the past when Sophie wonders: 'Wasn't that what happened to Lot's Wife? A loyalty to old things, a fear of the new, a fear to change, to look ahead?'[100] Salt in this biblical allusion clearly points to a penalty, not balance. According to Esther Jones, during the time of slavery salt 'was used as an instrument of punishment, to "season" the enslaved, when masters enforced submission by literally rubbing salt into the slaves' bleeding wounds as an additional punitive measure'.[101] Salt, in this sense, *is* black-pain and when Bambara says that people in the black community 'have eaten salt together', she is actually referring to the myriad pains and the accompanying bitterness they had to share and endure.[102] In an interview, Bambara states that

> [w]e got grounded because we ate too much salt, but some folks say it, we got grounded because we opened ourselves up to horror – invited it onto the continent – that created tears. And it was that salt that drowned our wings and made us earth-bound.[103]

If African Americans want to get back their wings, they need to get rid of the excess salt in their blood, as Minnie pleads with Velma: 'Release, sweetheart. Give it all up. Forgive everyone everything. Free them. Free self'.[104] Velma needs to free herself from the extra disabling salt in order to restore balance and become whole again and find her voice. She equally needs to refuse being punished for ever and anon for deviating from the social norm enforced by her community and accept herself for what she is. However, for this to happen she has to act and be an agent, not an object in her story.

99 Ibid.
100 Ibid.
101 Esther L. Jones, *Medicine and Ethics in Black Women's Speculative Fiction* (New York: Palgrave Macmillan, 2015), 3.
102 Bambara, *Salt*.
103 Bambara, 'An Interview with Toni Cade Bambara', *Conversations with Toni Cade Bambara*, ed., Thabiti Lewis (Jackson: University Press of Mississippi, 2012), 49.
104 Bambara, *Salt*.

4 Inconclusive Conclusions

Velma's story closes ambiguously; it is hard to categorize it under the rubric of a typical narrative of overcoming since there are no promises of a better future for her. Velma rises up and it is spring time with a joyful festival outside the window,

> [n]o need of Minnie's hands now. This is clear. Velma's glow aglow and two yards wide of clear and unstreaked white and yellow. Her eyes scanning the air surrounding Minnie, then examining her own hands, fingers stretched and radiant. No need of Minnie's hands now so the healer withdraws them, drops them in her lap just as Velma, rising on steady legs, throws off the shawl that drops down on her stool a burst cocoon.[105]

Bambara delineates a black disabled woman who handles her pain bravely and survives: 'Of course she would fight it, Velma was a fighter'.[106] But her contending silence is a warning sign. King argues that many blacks believe that 'silence is a mechanism of surviving racial and gender hurt – even when silence fails to subvert threats of fatal physical injury' and she calls this 'silent mobility' in which

> inert silence dissolves into a liberatory movement, an energy that allows the subjects of racial and gender hurt to redefine for themselves, their families, and their community the presence of weakness and the unsayable within painful experiences.[107]

Silence becomes intertwined with blackpain since the latter is unutterable. It helps pained subjects to re-conceptualize the implications of their oppression and the enforced impediments that stand in their way of being whole. Pain is alienating, personal and tacit, but as King explains

> [t]his silent mobility allows the individual to endure painful, difficult, and unjust atrocities with an uncompromised sense of dignity. It is a movement beyond suffering that acknowledges racial hurt without public expressions or personal submission to the limitations pain imposes.[108]

---

105 Ibid.
106 Ibid.
107 King, *Pain*, 19.
108 Ibid.

However, Velma's silence is not as liberating as King argues since her voice is unwillingly taken away from her which does not render this silent mobility as her disposed choice. Physical silence might allow Velma to contain her pain by creating space for her intruding memories to renegotiate her past. However, refraining from action and losing her voice metaphorically add more shackles to her because they restrict her agency and hence she fails to reach the stage King talks about. Silence in Velma's case denotes absence not liberation; she is not present in her own story and her hushed voice risks her very subjectivity. As the story ends with Velma rising up from her chair, silence winds up the scene and presages that pain will still be part of her future; she displays agency without mastery. Her agency remains incomplete because she says nothing and leaves all the exigent questions that Minnie had been imposing upon her in their healing session unanswered. The symbolic significance of not granting Velma her voice till the end points to the missing parts in the big puzzle of her life and also the life of African Americans at the time Bambara depicts in her novel. The picture remains unfinished and Velma's enduring silence draws a heavy shadow upon her brave act of rising up and leaving her chair.

Bambara says that 'In *Salt* [...] the question is: do we intend to have a future as a sane, whole, governing people?'[109] The answer to her question is as ambiguous as the ending of the novel. Disabled women in other narratives reach conclusive endings. Bertha Mason, Mr. Rochester's mad wife that he hid in the attic in Charlotte Brontë's *Jane Eyre,* is portrayed in the Victorian novel as a repulsive character and her presence is marked by much Gothicism. Mr. Rochester claims that she is a drunkard and disgusting wife and that he was fooled into marrying her by her rich family in the Caribbean islands. Bertha Mason loses her mind completely and ends up burning Thornfield and causing blindness in one eye and crippleness to Mr. Rochester as he tries to save her, yet she dies. Charlotte Perkins Gilman's "The Yellow Wallpaper",[110] on the other hand, portrays a woman's descent into psychosis. At the beginning she is diagnosed with depression and her husband rents a mansion to spend the summer at and give her time and space to relax and recover. However, she completely loses her mind by the end of the story and becomes obsessed by the yellow wallpaper of the nursery where she sees other women like her creeping on the walls behind its pattern. Unlike Bertha Mason and the unnamed protagonist of "The Yellow Wallpaper", Velma rises up again and recovers eventually, but is there

109 Bambara, 'Salvation is the Issue', *Black Women Writers (1950–1980): A Critical Evaluation*, ed., Marie Evans (New York: Anchor Books/Doubleday, 1984), 47.

110 Charlotte Perkins Gilman's *The Yellow Wallpaper* (Ballingslöv: Wisehouse Classics, 1892, 2016).

any promise of eliminating her blackpain with all its connotations and denotations? Velma's world remains tainted with racism, sexism and oppression. It is indeed a disabling dystopia for a black woman like her and also for many African Americans. Furthermore, Bambara does not show how long Velma would be capable of maintaining her newly-acquired ableism and whether she will be capable of conquering her non-physical vulnerabilities. Stanford points out that 'healing is a release from bondage' which is what Velma acquires by looking forward instead of living in her past, yet this release does not promise to take the pain away since everything in Velma's world remains intact and the readers are still incapable of hearing her voice.[111] Bambara emphasizes that the answer to the simple question that Minnie broaches at the beginning of the novel 'tends to be "no!" To be whole – politically, psychologically, spiritually, culturally, intellectually, aesthetically, physically, and economically whole – is of profound significance'.[112]

Velma stands up, puts the broken pieces back together, clutches to hope instead of her stool, is independent of Minnie's hands, however, her pain is still there and her voice is still silent. The ending of the novel might apocalyptically create a ray of hope that salt can, after all, be balanced and blacks can restore their wings and seek their voices. Velma remains silent and pained, but at least she conquers her insanity and decides not to give in. The novel does not close upon utter despair. Velma does take the decision and makes the choice to be whole and sane; and although Bambara speculates that the answer to her question is most probably not in the affirmative, she leaves the door ajar in ending her novel by implying that, like Velma, African Americans have to take matters in hand and rise up if they genuinely want to recuperate their voice and restore their agency but they should seek to make it agency *with* mastery.

Bibliography

Alwes, Derek. 'The Burden of Liberty: Choice in Toni Morrison's *Jazz* and Toni Cade Bambara's *The Salt Eaters*'. *African American Review* 30.3 (1996): 353–365.

Bambara, Toni Cade. *The Salt Eaters*. New York: Vintage Contemporaries, 1980. Kindle edition.

111 Stanford, 'He Speaks for Whom?', 28.

112 Bambara, 'Voices beyond the Veil: An Interview with Toni Cade Bambara and Sonia Sanchez', *Wild Women in the Whirlwind: Afro-American Culture and the Contemporary Literary Renaissance*, eds., Joanne M. Braxton and Andree Nicola McLaughlin (New Jersey: Rutgers University Press, 1990), 348.

Bambara, Toni Cade. 'Salvation is the Issue'. *Black Women Writers (1950–1980): A Critical Evaluation*, edited by Marie Evans, 41–47. New York: Anchor Books/Doubleday, 1984.

Bambara, Toni Cade. 'Voices beyond the Veil: An Interview with Toni Cade Bambara and Sonia Sanchez'. *Wild Women in the Whirlwind: Afro-American Culture and the Contemporary Literary Renaissance*, edited by Joanne M. Braxton and Andree Nicola McLaughlin, 342–362. New Jersey: Rutgers University Press, 1990.

Charlton, James. 'The Dimensions of Disability Oppression: An Overview'. *The Disability Studies Reader*, edited by Lennard J. Davis, 217–230. New York: Routledge, 2006.

Collins, Janell. 'Generating Power: Fission, Fusion, and Postmodern Politics in Bambara's *The Salt Eaters*'. *MELUS* 21.2 (1996): 35–47.

Davis, Lennard J. *Enforcing Normalcy: Disability, Deafness, and the Body*. London: Verso, 1995.

Duran, Jane. *Women, Philosophy and Literature*. Hampshire: Ashgate Publishing Limited, 2007.

Garland-Thomson, Rosemarie. *Extraordinary Bodies: Figuring Physical Disability in American Literature and Culture*. New York: Columbia University Press, 1997.

Garland-Thomson, Rosemarie. 'Integrating Disability, Transforming Feminist Theory'. *The Disability Studies Reader*, edited by Lennard J. Davis, 257–274. New York: Routledge, 2006.

Jones, Esther L. *Medicine and Ethics in Black Women's Speculative Fiction*. New York: Palgrave Macmillan, 2015.

King, Debra Walker. *African Americans and the Culture of Pain: Cultural Frames, Framing Culture*. Charlottesville: University of Virginia Press, 2008.

Linton, Simi. 'Reassigning Meaning'. *The Disability Studies Reader*, edited by Lennard J. Davis, 161–172. New York: Routledge, 2006.

Mathes, Carter. 'Scratching the Threshold: Textual Sound and Political Form in Toni Cade Bambara's *The Salt Eaters*'. *Contemporary Literature* 50.2 (2009): 363–396.

Scarry, Elaine. *The Body in Pain: The Making and Unmaking of the World*. New York: Oxford University Press, 1985.

Siebers, Tobian. 'Disability in Theory: From Social Constructionism to the New Realism of the Body'. *The Disability Studies Reader*, edited by Lennard J. Davis, 173–184. New York: Routledge, 2006.

Stanford, Ann Folwell. 'He Speaks for Whom?: Inscription and Reinscription of Women in *Invisible Man* and *The Salt Eaters*'. *MELUS* 18.2 (1993): 17–31.

Sternburg, Janet, ed. *The Writer on Her Work*. New York: W.W. Norton and Co., 1980.

Wendell, Susan. 'Toward a Feminist Theory of Disability', *The Disability Studies Reader*, edited by Lennard J. Davis, 243–256. New York: Routledge, 2006.

CHAPTER 8

Voices of Depression: An Analysis of a Collective Narrative

Hans T. Sternudd

Abstract

In this chapter the articulations of mental distress among young people are analysed. The main part of the material for the study was collected from the comments section of an autobiographical YouTube video about depression. Additional material emanated from comments on and references to other YouTube videos and media. The material was analysed using a content analytic method and the result was interpreted using a discourse theoretical framework. In line with this discursive approach, a constructive perspective on illness was emphasised in the analysis and interpretation. The study showed how the video is part of a YouTube genre of videos produced by young people that addresses depression and other types of mental distress. The study shows how collective and supportive groups can evolve in internet milieus, like the analysed comments sections. Important features that were needed for creation of the analysed group were a communal autobiographical storytelling about mental distress in general and depression specifically. Through these stories a narrative evolved that articulated the illness and the subjects' suffering from it. The characterisation of the latter could be summed up in the themes of isolation, concealment and self-destruction. They often apprehended themselves as mistreated and neglected, and their suffering was sometimes described as predetermined. This articulation also relied on the constitution of an outside world inhabited by grown-ups, parents and professionals that did not understand and deprived them of help. The outcome of the study indicated a reinforcing aspect of these communities: communicating with their peers shows individuals that they are not alone. At the same time, dwelling on the problem can create an atmosphere that reinforces social deviancy and possible destructive behaviours.

Key Words

Mental distress – depression – content analysis – discourse analysis – storytelling – pathography – YouTube

*****

 | DOI:10.30965/9789004396067_010

1 Introduction

Mental distress among Western youth has attracted an increasing interest from the media since the 1990's. A number of reports have described a particular group of young people who suffer from depression and other mental problems.[1] As young people today are often active in interactive internet milieus, the web reflects these kinds of issues. YouTube is one of the places for these articulations of mental distress and it therefore attracts the interest of many scholars.[2] This chapter focuses on how single utterances, conversations and storytelling on YouTube create a collective narrative about, and for, young people with depression.

The point of departure for this study is the same as that for my previous article 'Having the Voice of Depression', in which *How Depression Effects Someone's Daily Life* (hereafter *HDE*),[3] a YouTube video made by Saraphine Stanier, and published online in 2015, was scrutinised. Although the focus was on *HDE*, the influence of the context, i.e. the YouTube page on which Stanier published the video, was discussed. I concluded that for 'a broader discursive understanding of Stanier's work, the context, YouTube, needs to be thoroughly analysed'.[4] In an attempt to follow this suggestion, this article will analyse the comments section, a supplementary resource on all YouTube pages, and also some of the links and other media mentioned in the comments. An overarching concept

1 See, Leslie Morrison Gutman et al., *Children of the New Century: Mental Health Findings from the Millennium Cohort Study* (London: Centre for Mental Health, 2015), viewed on 20 June 2018, http://cdn.basw.co.uk/upload/basw_120221-1.pdf; Center for Behavioral Health Statistics and Quality, Behavioral Health, *Trends in the United States: Results from the 2014 National Survey on Drug Use and Health* (HHS Publication No. SMA 15–4927, NSDUH Series H-50, 2015), on 20 June 2018, http://www.samhsa.gov/data/sites/default/files/NSDUH-FRR1-2014/NSDUH-FRR1-2014.pdf.

2 See, Anna Johansson, 'Hybrid Embodiment: Doing Respectable Bodies on YouTube', *Hybrid Media Culture: Sensing Place in a World of Flows*, ed. Simon Lindgren (London, Routledge 2013), 34–50; Hans T Sternudd and Anna Johansson, 'The Girl in the Corner: Aesthetics of Suffering in a Digitalized Space', *Narratives of Suffering: Meaning and Experience in a Digitalized Space*, ed. Lolita Guimarães Guerra and Jose A. Nicdao (Oxford: Inter-Disciplinary Press, 2015), 105–115; Anna Johansson and Hans T Sternudd, 'Iconography of Suffering in Social Media: Images of Sitting Girls', *World Suffering and Quality of Life*, ed. Ronald E. Anderson (Dordrecht: Springer, 2015), 341–355.

3 Hans T Sternudd, 'Having the Voice of Depression: An Example of Pathographic Film Narratives on YouTube', *Narrating Illness: Prospects and Constraints*, eds. Joanna Davidson and Yomna Saber (Oxford: Inter-Disciplinary Press, 2016), 221–234; Saraphine Stanier, *How Depression Effects Someone's Daily Life-Short Film*, YouTube, 2015. Viewed on 20 June 2018. https://www.youtube.com/watch?v=203pnN95zHY.

4 Sternudd, 'Having the Voice', 227.

for this study is that meaning is socially and collectively produced – it is a product of many voices.

2 How Depression Effects

This section begins with a summary of *HDE*. Stanier's video is one of a number of autobiographic YouTube videos on depression produced by young individuals. Stanier acts as herself in the video, but to be able to analytically differentiate between the producer of the video and its protagonist, her surname will be used for the former and her first name, Stephanie, for the latter. The plot in *HDE* follows Saraphine's morning routines in six scenes. (1) It begins in the bedroom when an alarm wakes her up and she gets out of bed. (2) In the second scene she starts eating breakfast, but stops after briefly chewing on some food. After breakfast (3) she goes into the bathroom, brushes her teeth and takes a bath. These activities are interrupted by self-destructive actions: Saraphine swallows a handful of pills and cuts herself. In the following scene (4) Saraphine dresses and after trying on and rejecting two outfits she settles for a third and (5) walks out of the house. After a few steps she turns around, goes back inside and (6) returns to bed (see Figure 3).

During these scenes a voice is heard. It comments on Saraphine's actions and also on her external appearance. Often it takes an active role, persuading and commanding Saraphine. As the voice has a vocal pitch that denotes a female older than Saraphine, it probably represents somebody else, talking from an outside position or as a superego. When Saraphine is looking at herself in mirrors (scenes 3 and 4) the voice makes comments and remarks on Saraphine's bodily features. It says things like, 'You realise how fat you are? Why would somebody want to look at you …?' In scene 4 this voice stops Saraphine from choosing clothes that reveal her stomach or show her 'armpit fat'. The 'outside' position of this voice makes it clear that what troubles Saraphine is this imagined or real view of others. The voice intervenes in the storytelling by trying to make Saraphine stay in bed and stop her eating sweets, saying, 'You are already fat enough.' In the bathroom scene the voice orders Saraphine to swallow lots of pills. When she is leaving for school, she is guided by the voice and goes back to bed. The voice says, 'Come lay down in bed. You'll feel so much better.' Saraphine obeys.

Two themes that are at the centre of Stanier's story are important in the analysis in this study: bodily features and self-harming activities, understood here as including a variety of self-destructive behaviours. Saraphine's body is not only the main target for the voice; it is also, through an intimate use of

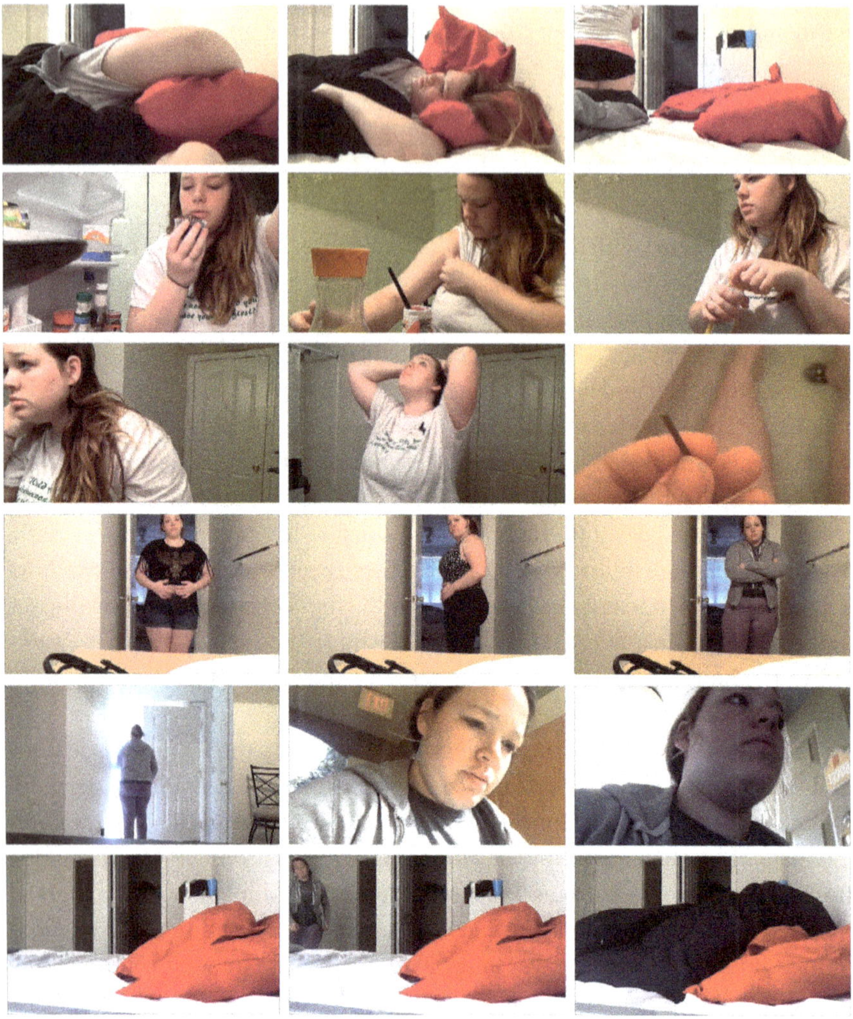

FIGURE 3 Screenshots from *How Depression Effects Someone's Daily Life*. Each row represents one scene as referred to in the text.

close-ups and other means, the central visual element in the video's different shots. Her performance also often addresses her body, for instance when she critically examines it by posing before a mirror and when she pinches her skin under her arm when the voice says, 'Look at yourself … You are disgusting.' How Saraphine's bodily features are valued is the single most pronounced aspect of the video that relates to her mental state. Saraphine's body is also physically under attack through the self-harming activities.

3 Points of Departure

The aim of this study is to analyse the context in which *HDE* was produced. Stanier's video has become a focus point around which other media evolve, and links are established to them through intertextual references or hypertexts. Given that this situation creates an infinite number of sources, only some of these links are followed. Instead of undertaking an extensive study of data, the approach is more qualitative in this study. It will look briefly at some of the media products that are mentioned in the video that were produced before and after *HDE*. In this way, Stanier's video is placed in a discursive context and is understood as something produced in, and by, a discursive field. The study has been guided by the following question: how is mental distress articulated among young people active on social media? This is specified further in the question, how is meaning constructed through affirmations, negotiations and conflicts in comments sections on YouTube? How does the context in which these comments are made contribute to a meaning-making process? YouTube has been chosen as a source because of its dominant position among social media today. Previously, the type of discussions described in this chapter more often took place on special, closed forums rather than on open platforms like YouTube, Facebook or Tumblr.[5]

The study of illness narratives has become quite an extensive field,[6] but only a few studies focus on first-hand narratives on depression.[7] In a recent study, Issakainen and Hänninen examined young people's 'depression narratives'.[8] They found that their informants predominantly understood that the reason behind their depression was 'problems in their life'.[9] Scholars from different disciplines have been interested in internet phenomena since its inception.

5 My impression is that the type of discussions on serious matters like mental distress and self-harm during the last five years have moved more and more from closed secure forums, which require a special id and password, to open comments sections on YouTube, as in this case, or easily accessible Facebook groups. If so, the consequences have to be further investigated. On the decline of forums see Patricia A. Adler and Peter Adler, *The Tender Cut: Inside the Hidden World of Self-injury* (New York: New York University Press, 2011), 49–50.

6 For an overview of 'illness narratives' see e. g. Amy Chandler, 'Narrating the Self-injured Body', *Medical Humanities* 40 (2014): 111–116.

7 Cf. Leeat Granek, 'What's Love Got to do with It? The Relational Nature of Depressive Experiences', *Journal of Humanistic Psychology* 46.2 (2006): 191–208; Mervi Issakainen and Vilma Hänninen, 'Young People's Narratives', *Journal of Youth Studies* 19.2 (2016): 237–250; John L. Oliffe, et al., 'Connecting Masculinity and Depression Among International Male University Students', *Qualitative Health Research* 20.7(2010): 987–998.

8 Issakainen and Hänninen, 'Young People's Narratives': 238.

9 Ibid.: 241.

Questions about the internet's potential to constitute a multitude of identities were discussed by academics during the 1990s.[10] This concept fitted well with a postmodern view of a shattered subject. Later studies showed, however, that this prediction could not be verified; instead, users of social media and online game players more often than not were honest when revealing their identities.[11] The early years of the internet saw a growth of Usenet support groups, forums and other places where members could discuss and share their experiences of different subjects. For this study, research on the communities that attracted young individuals dealing with subjects related to mental illness in combination with eating disorders or other potential self-destructive behaviours is relevant.[12] These communities seem to have had their heydays during the 1990s and up to the late 2000s. Research on the communities often highlighted positive aspects of them, like the possibility of exploring behaviour that in other places were seen as deviant or abnormal.[13] This contact with peers in online communities could be empowering but could also reinforce and normalise potentially dangerous behaviours, as an example self-injury could become an identity instead of a habit.[14] YouTube has been an object of studies right from the start; three years after the first video was uploaded on the site came the comprehensive volume *The YouTube Reader*.[15] Johansson's study 'Hybrid Embodiment', on the construction of the self-injured body in

10 Cf. Sherry Turkle, 'Construction and reconstruction of the self in virtual reality: Playing in the MUDS', *Mind, Culture, and Activity* 1.3 (1994): 158–167.

11 Cf. Diane J. Schiano and Sean White, 'The First Noble Truth of CyberSpace: People are People (even when they MOO)' (Los Angeles: *Proceedings of the SIGCHI Conference on Human Factors in computing systems,* 1998): 352–359; Michael W. Ross, *Typing, Doing and Being: A Study of Men who have Sex with Men and Sexuality on the Internet* (Malmö: Faculty of Health and Society, Malmö University, 2006); Olle Findahl and Sheila Zimic, *Unga svenskar och Internet 2008* [Young Swedes and Internet 2008] (Hudiksvall: World Internet Institute, 2008).

12 Cf. Patricia A. Adler and Peter Adler, 'The Cyber Worlds of Self-Injurers: Deviant Communities, Relationships, and Selves', *Symbolic Interaction* 31.1 (2008): 33–56; Adler and Adler *The Tender Cut*; Anna Johansson, *Självskada: En etnologisk studie av mening och identitet i berättelser om skärande* [Self-injury: A ethnological study of meaning and identity in narratives about cutting] (Doctoral dissertation) (Umeå: h:ström – Text & kultur 2010).

13 Katelyn Y.A. McKenna and John A. Bargh, 'Plan 9 From Cyberspace: The Implications of the Internet for Personality and Social Psychology', *Personality and Social Psychology Review* 4.1. (2000): 57–75; Janis L. Whitlock, Jane L. Powers and John Eckenrode, 'The Virtual Cutting Edge: The Internet and Adolescent Self-Injury', *Developmental Psychology* 42.3 (2006): 2.

14 Adler and Adler, 'The Cyber Worlds', 41.

15 Pelle Snickars and Vonderau, Patrick (eds.), *The YouTube Reader* (Stockholm: National Library of Sweden, 2009).

vlogs and videos, and her collaborative projects with the author of this chapter should also be mentioned.[16]

This chapter is grounded on the discursive understanding that meaning is constituted by *articulations*, which are contagious and shifting fixations of meaning in a certain *domain*,[17] in this case one that deals with youth and mental health. Illness and diseases are understood as concepts constructed in a cultural context.[18] From this it follows that experiences of depression must be communicated in a culturally recognisable way to be understood in a certain socio-historical context. *HDE* is seen as an example of a media product, a proposition shaped by, and part of, a mental health discourses on YouTube. Stanier uses her own experience to enlighten 'people' about how depression 'affects everything that that person does', as she writes in a supplementary statement to the video. *HDE* is an example of testimonies or confessions that have been recognised as an important part of the so-called therapeutic culture.[19] The role of witnesses, that is, those suffering from or who have survived mental distress has been discussed as a powerful element in self-help communities, which are founded on the members' knowledge gained through their own experiences.[20] In line with this, Stanier explains that she based *HDE* on her 'daily life dealing with depression'.[21] In line with discourse theory, Stanier's story is one 'utterance' in a speech choir that includes many voices and is constituted by a collection of utterances, personal stories and conflicting argumentations. Together these voices generate a fairly coherent articulation of mental distress among young people in general and depression specifically. In line with the

16 Johansson, 'Hybrid Embodiment', 16–33.

17 Theoretical and terminology grounded in Ernesto Laclau and Chantal Mouffe, *Hegemony and Socialist Strategy: Towards a Radical Democratic Politics* (London and New York: Verso, (1985) 2001); and, Marianne Winther Jørgensen and Louise Phillips, *Discourse Analysis as Theory and Method* (London: Sage, 2002).

18 See, Joan Busfield, 'Introduction: Rethinking the Sociology of Mental Health', *Sociology of Health & Illness* 22.5 (2000): 543–558; Jane M. Ussher, *The Madness of Women: Myth and Experience* (London: Routledge, 2011).

19 An important theoretical ground in this concept is Michel Foucault, *The History of Sexuality, Vol. 1: The Will to Knowledge* (Harmondsworth: Penguin, 1990). On cultural significance of confessions see Frank Füredi, *Cultivating Vulnerability in an Uncertain Age* (London: Routledge, 2004), 40–43.

20 Mark Cresswell, 'Psychiatric "Survivors" and Testimonies of Self-harm', *Social Science & Medicine* 61.8 (2005): 1668–1677, viewed on 20 June 2018, http://dx.doi.org/10.1016/j.socscimed.2005.03.033. In previous studies on photographs of self-injuries I have recognised the witnessing aspect of publishing them, see Hans T Sternudd, 'Photographs of Self-Injury: Production and Reception in a Group of Self-Injurers', *Journal of Youth Studies* 15.4 (2012): 421–436.

21 Stanier, *How Depression Effects*.

discursive perspective in this study, the constructive character of the narrative is emphasised. The structure of narration is understood as an articulatory resource that is necessary to access 'reality'.[22]

In the following paragraphs this collection of voices is seen as a collective pathographic narrative. According to Hawkins, storytelling follows certain rules, for instance using certain mythological themes.[23] Here these themes are understood as constituted by the discourse created in a cooperative process. These themes and other elements of the storytelling can create a much-needed order for those suffering from mental distress. As these stories can also convey emotions, they, as Riessman argues, allow 'a search for meaning and enabling connection with others'.[24] The 'speech choir' analysed in this chapter resembles in some aspects the 'collaborate reflective dialogue' of Morrison and McGregor in this volume.[25] In a similar way the many short entries in the comments section make meaning of inner shared experiences through a writing process that create a collective 'us' that have an ability to handle the situation.[26]

Even if illness narratives necessarily reflect inner experiences,[27] a mediation of an inner turmoil through the framework of a narrative structure is part of knowledge production – something that all mediation does, according to Säljö.[28] Riessman's and Säljö's concepts harmonises well with Tomkin's theory that affect, as an inner, intense, chaotic sensation, needs to find its form in feelings and/or emotions, which are communicable social qualities.[29]

In this study, different mediations and transmediations of mental distress will be discussed. Elleström's theory on transmediation states that different media have different capacities to convey meaning, which is an important concept in relation to the different media representations of depression presented in this study. According to Elleström, transmediation that is grounded

22 Jens Brockmeier and Donal A. Carbaugh, 'Introduction', in *Narrative and Identity: Studies in Autobiography, Self and Culture*, eds. Jens Brockmeier and Donal A. Carbaugh (Benjamin, Philadelphia, Pa., 2001), 15.

23 Anne Hunsaker Hawkins, *Reconstructing Illness: Studies in Pathography*, 2. ed. (West Lafayette, Ind.: Purdue University Press, 1999).

24 Catherine Kohler Riessman, *Narrative Methods for the Human Sciences* (London: SAGE, 2008), 10.

25 Pam Morrison and Annie McGregor, 'Making and Sharing Meaning Out of Terminal Illness', in this volume.

26 Ibid.

27 Chandler, 'Narrating', 111.

28 Roger Säljö, *Lärande i praktiken: ett sociokulturellt perspektiv* [Practice of Learning: A Sociocultural Perspective] 3rd ed. (Studentlitteratur, Lund, 2014), 82.

29 Anneli Brännström Öhman, Maria Jönsson and Ingeborg Svensson, 'Inledning' [Introduction], *Att känna sig fram: Känslor i humanistisk genusforskning* [To feel ones way: Feelings in Humanistic Gender Studies] eds. Anneli Brännström Öhman, Maria Jönsson, and Ingeborg Svensson (Umeå: Bokförlaget H: ström 2011), 11.

on central aspects of one medium is recognised by the perceiver of the new medium.[30] A technical medium is the physical object or body that realises the medium,[31] for instance a painting, a video or a dance. Each medium has its own special capacities that are apprehended by the perceiver. Media product refers to a concrete work of art, for instance *HDE*.[32]

The analysis is based on over three hundred comments that had been made in the comments section of *HDE* up to 20 October 2016. Using a content analysis method, themes were identified in the posts,[33] and usually several themes were identified in a single post. The method was used primarily to identify dominating themes and not to quantify the material, but numbers will be used occasionally to show how frequently some of the themes occurred. Links to media products that were suggested, introduced or indicated by the participants in the posts and threads were followed in a way that could mimic the manner, both determined and casual, in which an internet user manoeuvres her/his way around the web. Most of the new sites presented here originate from YouTube and have not been systematically scrutinised. Instead their content is compared to the findings on Stanier's site and resemblance or differences are indicated.

Ethical questions must be considered when sensitive matters like mental distress are studied, especially when individuals can be identified, as in this case. The reason for naming Stanier is that she has chosen to reveal her real name. Arguably, personal exposure such as that enabled by *HDE* on a worldwide scale is potentially more harmful than being mentioned in an academic text. Furthermore, it would be questionable not to give Stanier credit for her work.

4 The Collective Voice

HDE is only one of many utterances in a genre of videos that mediates experiences of depression on YouTube. Searches on YouTube for the phrases 'live

30 Lars Elleström, *Media Transformation: The Transfer of Media Characteristics Among Media* (Houndsmill, Basingstoke, Hampshire: Palgrave Macmillan, 2014).

31 Lars Elleström, 'The Modalities of Media: A Model for Understanding Intermedial Relations', in *Media Borders, Multimodality and Intermediality*, ed. Lars Elleström (Houndmills: Palgrave Macmillan 2010), 12.

32 Elleström, *Media transformation*, 24.

33 The analysis followed Ulla Hällgren Graneheim and Berit Lundman, 'Qualitative Content Analysis in Nursing Research: Concepts, Procedures and Measures to Achieve Trustworthiness', *Nurse Education Today* 24 (2003): 105–112; Hsiu-Fang Hsieh and Sarah E. Shannon, 'Three Approaches to Qualitative Content Analysis,' *Qualitative Health Research* 15 (2005): 1277–1288.

with depression' and 'living with depression' generated over six thousand and nearly one hundred thousand results respectively.[34] Videos represented in these results were produced before and after *HDE* and often use a set of similar images and stories. Stanier's video was not made in a vacuum and thus it is quite natural that *HDE* has similarities with other videos. Its likeness to *What It's like Living with Depression*,[35] a video produced by the internet media company BuzzFeed[36] and published two weeks before Stanier's,[37] is mentioned in a comment. Even if Stanier denies seeing BuzzFeed's video, the two videos have some similarities. The opening scene in BuzzFeed's version has the protagonist waking up when the alarm on a mobile phone goes off, which is similar to Saraphine being woken up by the sound of an alarm clock. A quick search on YouTube provides more examples of this way of starting a story about a day in someone's life. BuzzFeed's waking-up shot repeats nearly exactly the opening of the YouTube video *A Depression PSA* (*Short Film*), a school project created by Alex Yawata in 2014.[38] Another more specific similarity between *HDE* and *What It's Like Living with Depression* is the personification of depression. Instead of representing the thoughts that break the protagonist with a voice-over, the producers of BuzzFeed's video use an actor for this part. In a similar way to the voice in *HDE*, she tries to persuade the protagonist to stay in bed and criticises her choice of clothing because it makes her 'look fat'. This takes on another meaning here because the body features of the character in the BuzzFeed video are in line with normal weight and size ideals – for 'normal' read thin. Using a voice or a character that the viewer understands is in the head of the protagonist is not unique in these videos. It was, for instance, used by Owen McCall in 2014 in *The Voice of Depression*.[39] Further examples can certainly be found in extended searches, but this study only aimed to show how the videos on YouTube are interwoven with each other in an intertextual meaning-making process where formal traits, concepts and ideas are shared, used and reformulated. This is in line with postmodern critiques of the concept of a single authentic author.

---

34 Search on YouTube made 11 November 2016.

35 Throughout the chapter the titles of YouTube videos are using the original spelling and use of upper – and lowercase letters.

36 BuzzFeed, *What It's Like Living With Depression*, YouTube 2015. Viewed on 20 June 2018. https://www.youtube.com/watch?v=Ps8RcOdfHT4.

37 BuzzFeed video publish 23 Feb 2015 Stanier's 13 Mars 2015.

38 Alex Yawata, *A Depression PSA* (*Short Film*), YouTube 2014. Viewed on 30 November 2016. https://www.youtube.com/watch?v=ompcDVq_noU. Since the research for this article was done, this video been removed from YouTube.

39 Owen McColl, *The Voice Of Depression*, YouTube 2014. Viewed on 20 June 2018. https://www.youtube.com/watch?v=hBs6BPT50G8.

Returning to *HDE*, two new types of media are introduced at the end of the video that up to that point consist of moving images and verbal text. A black screen is seen, and while a visual text scrolls up from the bottom of the screen, like the closing credits of a film, a song is heard, starting with the line, 'And she lies tonight.' This song will be considered later, but at this point the focus is on the text emerging on the screen:

> And by the end of the day, or maybe even in the beginning ... you already feel defeated.
>
> Depression is a serious issue and not many people understand it ... I hope this helped even in the slightest.
>
> You can make it through this.

Messages like this, displayed with music, are quite common at the end of YouTube videos. Stanier's text has three different functions. The first sentence alludes to the story in the video, reinforcing its character of hopelessness; the following two lines seem to describe the reason behind making the video, which is a didactic and informative intention; and the last line appears to be a personal, reassuring message to the viewer, who through this is identified as someone suffering from depression. Using this kind of approach probably creates an atmosphere that lowers the threshold for interacting with a comment. This brings us to the comments section.

The impact of *HDE* is quite strong; in June 2018 it has had more than hundred twenty-five thousand views. In an entry on Facebook 2015 Stanier wrote that she was

> amazed and touch that this could reach so many people. There are multiple comments saying how they can relate to or even have depression and I just want everyone to know that in time it gets better.[40]

The following section will take a closer look at these 'multiple comments'. The comments are analysed as part of a collective discourse, but the nicknames of the posters are not usually included in the analysis. This is in line with overarching concept in this study, which states that many utterances contribute to the articulation of depression. This study also strives to give a voice to many of these utterances through a generous use of quotes.

Through the content analysis of the comments, five different groups of topics were identified. 1) The largest group includes posts that discuss the *content*

40 Saraphine Stanier, Status update, *Facebook*. 2015, viewed 1 February 2016, https://www.facebook.com/Saraphine13/timeline.

of the video. *Appearance* is the most frequent subject – around every third post addresses appearance. Usually these posts include comments on Saraphine's bodily features and the different costumes she wears in scene 4, and are usually complimentary. Almost as frequent were posts in which the writer *recognises* and/or *compares* his/her experience with how Stanier describes her experience. This subgroup also includes those who *confirm* that the description is correct. Quite a few posters comment on and discuss whether the condition that the video describes really is depression; this *definition* topic often includes comments on *self-harm*. Nearly every fifth comment includes longer or shorter autobiographical accounts; these *stories* relate in different ways to the content of Stanier's video. 2) The second group includes *social* interactions and posts that address the producer of the video or other posters. *Compliments* dominate this group. This group also includes the topics *advice*, *empowerment* and *comforting*, as well as posters offering *help* to Stanier and *thanking* her. 3) With more focus on the posters themselves, a third group contains posts that describe *emotional* reactions that arose when they were watching the video. 4) The content of posts that negatively comment on the video or other posts/posters constitute a smaller group. This group includes posts that do not affirm the underlying message in *HDE* or the positive atmosphere in the comments section.

The starting point is a discussion of the comments on the content of *HDE*, i.e. those that allude to what is represented in the video. In my article 'Having the Voice of Depression' I described how Stanier's video can be seen as challenging what kind of bodies it is possible to expose in a mass media context. The conclusion was that even if the protagonist Saraphine was defeated by the voice, *HDE* could be seen as a comment that fits into a body activism discourse.[41] Given that this themes appearance is emphasised in *HDE*, it is not surprising that it also dominates the comments in the posts. There is an overwhelming response from posters, with statements like 'wow your really beautiful' and 'woa she's really pretty'. These statements become part of an opposition to the bullying voice in Stanier's video.[42] This dominance is indicated by the frequency of the word 'beautiful', which appears in more than thirteen per cent of the posts. A few posts question other commentaters' preoccupation with beauty; one poster stresses that '[p]retty isn't everything. It's not always the issue'. Another wonders why 'everyone [is] commenting on her physical appearance?', a question that is answered like this: 'Because in this day and age what you look like is

41 Sternudd, 'Having the voice', 228.

42 Language irregularities in the quotes from the comments section are not commented upon (with sic) or corrected, as this could be considered a pejorative action or remove the special character of the interaction.

the most important topic.' This is in line with the impression that a beautiful or pretty appearance is important. This impression is strengthened as repetition of the positive remarks on Saraphine's appearance becomes like a ritual. The posters suppress what is probably understood as hegemonic ideals of weight and body. Several posters defend Saraphine's choice of clothes in scene 4, stating that 'she looked great wearing the polka dot top and black pants?!?! i loved that outfit!!!' Body-weight ideals are negotiated and cultural differences and differences in personal taste are underlined. Even so, the impression is that Stephanie's body is scrutinised by the comments in posts like, 'She's not *that* overweight' (my emphasis) and 'you are not fat your a perfect size and don't let anyone tell u [you] wrong'.

Pronouncing *HDE* as a legitimate representation of depression is a reoccurring subject in many comments. The most prominent proof for this 'consecration' are the posters' own experiences of depression. Compare comments like 'i know this video. its relatable. i have chronic depression and its hard' and 'This is very true. I have suffered from depression for as long as I can remember.' Having a personal experience of depression seems an important position here which gives posters credibility and 'permission' to nominate true candidates. To 'relate' and understand through personal experiences is characteristic of milieus like this and the self-help forums that were so important earlier.[43] Comments including notions of recognition are common: one describes how the video is 'exactly the way my life is'. Often the recognition becomes so total that it is expressed in terms indicating identification: 'this is totally me', 'this is me', 'my life' and so forth. This is somehow contrary to a parallel emphasis on an 'everybody is different' discourse, expressed for instance like this: 'there is only one of you', even if the poster 'know[s] how [she] feel[s]' as 'only people who went through it understand you'. Posters also describe how 'scenes' in their life correspond to scenes in the video: 'every time I look in the mirror xD ive been like OK IMA gonna [wear] shorts and then I look in the mirror and its like … look at all that fat'. The mirrors in *HDE* that, like this comment, allude to the poster's own experience are a reoccurring and important sign in utterances that are part of articulations of mental distress. Looking in the mirror in this domain not only includes an evaluation of physical features but often also an introspective conversation with oneself.

As described above, an interpretative prerogative for defining depression seemed to a large extent to be connected to a situated knowledge, a knowledge

43 See Adler and Adler *The Tender Cut*; Darren Baker and Sarah Fortune, 'Understanding Self-Harm and Suicide Websites: A Qualitative Interview Study of Young Adult Website Users' *Crisis* 29.3 (2008): 118–22; Cresswell, 'Psychiatric "Survivors"'; Johansson, *Självskada*.

gained through self-experience. Even if many posters acknowledge *HDE* as a valid description, which in turn validates Stanier as a representative of someone suffering from the condition, others compare their own experience with those depicted in *HDE*. Usually these posts start by declaring what diagnosis or diagnoses they had, e.g. depression that is specified as a 'chronic' or 'situational' type. To have a diagnosis is important in contexts like this because somebody without one can be accused of being a wannabee or a poser.[44] The posts described above can be understood as negotiations of what constitutes depression and part of a calibration of its definition. Critical posters often direct their critique to how depression is represented in the video and in the description given by Stanier.[45] Disagreements usually question the relationship between depression and body-related problems. 'Depression isn't body shaming', one poster states; others agree with this and suggest that Saraphine's condition should more correctly be labelled an eating disorder, such as 'binge eating' or 'anorexia'. Others defend Stanier's terminology, however, by highlighting individual differences, arguing that 'everybody deals with it differently'.

Regardless of whether posters agree on Stanier's representations of depression, they often add their own experiences: Depression 'feels like a overwhelming sadness mixed with happiness and 100 other emotions', says one poster. Sadness reoccurs in these posts, together with feeling 'mad and worthless, and lonely', as another poster adds. One of the posters blames the 'brain' for the condition. The brain

> makes you see everything differently, especially yourself. I hate my body, even though others tell me I look fine. My stupid brain tells me otherwise, and makes me not believe what others say.

Descriptions of what a depressed person does varies: s/he is likely to 'cry almost every day', is 'always thinking about something' and has a hard time concentrating 'in class'. These examples can be understood as a negotiation of how depression could be manifested in activities and cognitively experienced.

On one occasion a small 'flame war' breaks out around who has the right to diagnose the condition.[46] It starts with the post quoted above, which involves

---

44 See Anna Johansson, 'Constituting "Real" Cutters: A Discourse Theoretical Analysis of Self-harm and Identity', in *Tracking Discourses: Politics, Identity and Social Change*, eds. Annika Egan Sjölander and Jenny Gunnarsson Payne (Lund: Nordic Academic Press, 2011), 197–224.

45 Supplement statement when publishing *HDE*, Stanier, *How Depression Effects*.

46 "A flame war is a heated argument between two individuals, that results in those involved posting personal attacks on each other during or instead of debating the topic at

descriptions of someone who cries every day and also expresses feelings of sadness and thoughts of 'how easy it would be to just not be here ...'. 'Is this normal?' the poster asks. When someone answers, '-Yeah you have depression I do too it's not normal', the claimed situated knowledge is not accepted by some commentators: '[J]ust because someone is sad doesn't mean they're depressed.'

Self-harm is an issue that appears in quite a few comments, more than one in ten. It becomes a relevant subject because of the staged cutting and the revealing of scars in HDE's bathroom scene. Scars are seen on Stephanie's thigh when she steps out of the bath. The question of whether the scars are real is raised and confirmed by Stanier. One poster seems offended by Stanier's exposure of them and questions whether it was necessary to get her 'point across'. The subject also opens up a comparison between Saraphine's actions and the posters' own experiences, such as in the following comments, which could be interpreted as competitive: 'I have cut my self really bad I forgot how many times but I try to stop but it don't work', and 'i cut everywhere, not the [thigh] only'. Personal accounts like these appear in almost every fifth comment. These can be quite short, such as mentioning the age when the poster was diagnosed or what s/he has done in terms of behaviour such as the self-harm mentioned above.

A friendly and supportive atmosphere is created by the tone of the posts. Aggressive, ironic or derogatory comments represent only a small fraction of all the posts. Stanier is often addressed in the comments. When the protagonist in the video is mentioned, the personal pronoun 'you' is more than three times more common than the distancing 'she'. The comments section has a potential for intimacy, it is a place where it is possible to talk 'girl to girl'. If the praising of appearance described above is understood as a social activity it is easier to understand. The ritual distribution of flattering remarks should probably be understood as compliments expressing solidarity and friendship.[47] Stanier also participates in the flow of comments, with eleven posts in which she expresses thanks for the compliments, makes comments on posts and gives encouraging words to posters. Compliments are not only concerned with appearance; Stanier is also commended for her courage in publishing the video with its revealing subject. She is described as brave, strong and inspiring, an 'amazing person' who 'built up the strength to stop and to help others'. In the

---

hand". Marcus, 'flame war', *Urban Dictionary* 2004. Viewed on 8 June 2018. https://www.urbandictionary.com/define.php?term=flame%20war.

47 The social dimension of praising is discussed in Ira Glass's enlightening interview with Julia, Jane and Ella in *This American Life*, '573: Status Update', 2015. Viewed on 20 June 2018. https://www.thisamericanlife.org/radio-archives/episode/573/status-update.

social setting that is created in the comments section, a distribution of gratitude takes place. Posters thank Stanier for making the video and for being so honest, and she thanks them for watching. Her insight into the condition of depression is praised. This is important as '[n]o one truly understands what it is like until they have been through it'. One poster sees the didactic possibilities of *HDE*: 'my family doesn't understand me when I tell them what I feel. I can show my family this! I'm so thankful for people like u.' Posters also share emotional reactions on viewing *HDE*. The video is described as 'sad' and 'moving', and some posters report responding with 'crying' and 'sobbing'. Often a digital lingua with emoticons and acronyms is used, for example: ((, 😰😭, 😭, omg this, I am sorry =(, and so forth.

Empowering messages are also an important part of the socialising rituals of benevolent posters in a comments section like this. Negative and hostile posts are rare and are seldom directed against Stanier or her video. The positive atmosphere is maintained by interactions between posters. Referring to Saraphine's plain costume and approved by the voice, for example, the post 'Lolll last outfit was like Walmart shopper' (which is apprehended as sarcastic), is immediately criticised by a poster: 'And you have to be rude why?' In this and other ways, posters create an inclusive and embracing we, a group that loves Stanier and assures her that she is 'not alone'. Other posters emphasise that 'we need to stay strong, we need to stick together'. These types of empowering utterances use what Hawkins calls a myth of battle – that 'we' are fighting together.[48] Comments giving advice like 'don't give a crap what people think' also contribute to the notion that we who suffer from depression stand together against the world. More specific advice is seldom given, but several posters offer help. This can be unspecified, such as 'i want u to know if u need help in here for u', but it is also specified as 'talk'. This is exemplified in these posts: 'If anybody needs to talk my kik is [poster's kik-id]'[49] or 'Do you want to talk about it?', directed to another poster on a different thread of comments. The supportive atmosphere encourage posters to ask questions that often are answered by other posters.

The analysis has revealed a few important themes and ideas so far. First of all, it can be seen that there is a strong dichotomy between two groups, those who understand, often described as 'we', and those who do not understand or are malicious, often called 'they'. The latter are represented by the 'look' of others and the comments made by them. By constituting an objectifying Mulveyan gaze, the cause of depression becomes a socially caused condition.

---

48 Hawkins, *Reconstructing Illness*, 61–90.

49 KIK is an instant messenger software for mobile phones.

Posters construct a 'we' as members of a group who understand each other through a common experience, a situated knowledge that gives them the right to speak. Inside this group, negotiations can be made regarding the right way to define the individuals' suffering, but an emotional solidarity and friendship based on recognition is the fundament for most of the social interaction. Through this a discourse evolves that positions young people with depression as a group (we) that stands together *against the world.*

4.1 *Stories of Depression*

Through the socialising routines described above, a seemingly safe place takes shape. It is a place that appears to invite participants to tell their own story. Within the discursive understanding of personal experience as a ground for truth claims, these stories give credibility to the poster and provide a position from which s/he can speak. Listed below are some of the reoccurring themes that emerged through the analysis. For the purpose of this study, a selection of thirteen stories was scrutinised. As a literary genre, a comments section by default invites short posts. The stories analysed, often appearing in between other subjects, ranged from slightly over twenty words to over one hundred and fifty. In the analysis, the stories are treated as collectively told and thus become more of a mutual narrative than individual accounts.

Isolation, concealment and *self-destruction* are three themes that are used to characterise the situation for the individuals who tell these stories. Some stories describe how the person no longer goes outside: 'I used to ... I used to ride my bike..play with friends ... Walk around..But now all I do is lay in bed.' One poster describes her/himself as being 'a social butterfly and as of lately not anymore'. The condition and its effects are kept hidden; parents do not know about it and fears are concealed: 'i wear sweaters all the time and the bad part is my dad he knows nothing about it'. Self-harming activities are a reoccurring element in the stories. Its use is sometimes specified as a way of coping with awful feelings, and at other times it is described as a collective act: 'Slicing our skin, holding lots and lots of pills.' The vulnerable situation of these posters is sometimes connected with a notion of *determination*. Posters compare their situation with that of their parents; one describes her condition as similar to her mum's and another says that she fears becoming 'like her [mother] someday'. Posters are *not getting helped* by 'people' or through 'counselling'. The only way to get help is to 'search on the internet to read other people's experiences', as one poster states.

Mistreatment, negligence and *diagnosis* are three themes that reoccur in relation to others. Usually they describe a power relation in which the subject in the story occupies a subordinate position. Posters describe how they are abused by their parents or caregivers or how they get 'bullied everyday'. In some stories, age is the factor that creates the subordinate position. The young person's problem is dismissed: 'If I told anyone they would say it's just a phase, but it's always been here.' Doctors make fun of the patient, saying the person is too young to have depression. Posters describe how their mothers do not understand their depression. A couple of posters elevate the issue to a social level, saying that depression is 'unrecognized in society that it's a big killer in the States' and people 'in our society push it aside as if it doesn't exist anymore'. Together these conditions raise obstacles for individuals who need recognition, such as a diagnosis, to receive help.

Through these stories, an articulation of the subject of depression evolves. It is a subject that is characterised by living disconnected from social life and being subordinated and misunderstood by the world outside. Often this world is inhabited by persons referred to as 'they'. Who are they? Looking through the stories selected here, 'they' are doctors, parents, caregivers, counsellors and grown-ups. This definition of 'they' is necessary to constitute 'we', and it is an act that creates a powerless subject that is young and without a platform from which to operate. At the same time, by constituting 'they', a border is created against the others, those who do not understand, which can be the ground for a solidarity that strengthens and empowers the group and provides a possible platform.

4.2 *Additional Voices*

As YouTube is a resource that in several ways opens up for other media products, additional utterances on topics are always at hand. On the page where HDE is published, a multitude of videos is suggested. In this context it is natural that other media are mentioned in the comments section. Several posts suggest alternative versions, or transmediations, of HDE. In one post, Stanier is asked if it would be okay to make a version with a boy as the leading character. Stanier in another post is asked if she, as the maker of an 'incredibly accurate' video, would like to participate as a guest speaker on a YouTube channel dealing with mental health issues. As mentioned above, the similarities between HDE and a BuzzFeed video is noted by one poster. Commentators also 'contribute' with more random references to other media, such as invitations to subscribe to YouTube channels.

As discussed above, HDE ends with a written text and a song. The song is 'Another Empty Bottle', performed and written by Katy McAllister.[50] Stanier uses a sample from the song's refrain that includes lyrics that fit well with the last clip,

50 The song appears on McAllister's second EP *Throwbacks* released in 2012.

in which Stephanie has returned to bed: 'And she lies tonight underneath a caving roof/And she cries tonight wondering what she can do/And she tries …'.[51] Stanier lets the song fade away in the middle of the third line, probably due to the lines that follow: 'tonight remembering who she once knew/But they've died inside/Another empty bottle takes a life.' These lines allude to the theme of the song, a family situation characterised by domestic violence, abuse and alcoholism. In this respect, the topic of the song does not correspond to that of *HDE* – at least this is not indicated by the storyline. However, many features and concepts in the lyrics of 'Another Empty Bottle' fit rather well with the stories told in the comments section described above. The protagonist in the song, called 'she', is isolated, hiding 'away behind a door she kept locked', and she is 'trapped in her mind'. The miserable life of her parents – 'her father live in regret' and 'her mother cry in an empty bed' – is also comparable to some of the stories from *HDE*'s site. As well as the underlying fear of the protagonist that she may become like them, 'this is the best life gets/And she dies inside'. Similar to the themes in the stories from the *HDE* site, McAllister's lyrics describe a mistreated girl with fighting parents who neglect her. The girl in McAllister's song is trapped and is described with a claustrophobic metaphor: she lies 'underneath a caving roof'. Something that is emphasized even more in 'Another Empty Bottle' than in the stories analysed above is how vulnerable the protagonist is; she is living 'as a broken tool' that 'she believes she's unable to fix'. At the end of the song she takes her own life:

> And she's wondering/What's beyond the sky, could she see the light if she falls asleep/Cause she feels more alive in her own dreams/So tonight she lies, lifted up through her own roof.

The song also describes how she is mourned by her parents when it is too late. This is something that is quite common in stories about suicide: 'And they cry tonight, a daughter that they hardly knew/And she's lost in time.' Although suicide is indicated a couple of times by posters in HDE's comments section, as in this post, 'just thinking how easy it would be to just not be here…', McAllister's song opens up a route for a more destructive way of dealing with mental distress.

A search for 'Another Empty Bottle' on YouTube resulted in 67,700 hits.[52] Most watched, with over 3.5 million views, was *Katy McAllister – Another*

51 Lyrics from *AZ*, Katy Mcallister Lyrics, Viewed on 20 June 2018. http://www.azlyrics.com/lyrics/katymcallister/anotheremptybottle.html.

52 Search made on the 2 November 2016.

Empty Bottle – Lyrics, uploaded by Sammy Rose.[53] The video consists of the lyrics displayed on dialogue intertitles as the song is heard. In her comment about the video, Rose explains:

> I'm always here for anyone who needs someone to talk to! Or if you need to vent. Suicide isn't the answer! Trust me, I know. I love you all! You're all BEAUTIFUL. xx.

A quick glance at the comments section, with its over three thousand posts, gave the impression that the posts are quite similar to those on Stanier's site. Comments are also made here on the subject of the song. This means that comments on suicide and the family situation, such as issues with parents, are quite common. Here it can also be seen that the video gives posters the opportunity to describe their own experience and to compare it to and relate it to the story in the song. In addition, with the aim of giving other posters advice, depression is addressed in posts and the criteria of diagnoses are discussed.

The second most viewed video was *Another Empty Bottle*, performed by Emmacore,[54] a Dutch artist who produces nightcore covers that are played to a backdrop of manga-style images.[55] The image in this case depicts a young girl on her knees, crying with her hands against her ears. Behind her is a cloudy dark-blue sky full of cracks, like a wall that is about to fall into pieces. The nightcore version changes the character of the song from McAllister's acoustic singer-songwriter style to electronic pop. As in the previous examples, the comments section, with slightly over a thousand comments, is full of posters who write that they can relate to the video and describe how they were emotionally affected by it. Personal stories are told and posters give each other advice. Some of the most recent comments stand out. For example one poster writes, 'I want to shatter the bottle and slice my neck and wrists open', which generates

53 Sammy Rose, *Katy McAllister – Another Empty Bottle – Lyrics*, YouTube, 2012. Viewed on 20 June 2018, https://www.youtube.com/watch?v=Cqv9ZHveNbk.

54 Emmacore, *Nightcore~ Another Empty bottle*, YouTube, 2015. Viewed on 20 June 2018, https://www.youtube.com/watch?v=ClVY_X_a7HA.

55 Nightcore is 'a subgenre of trance' and is 'characterized by a sped-up melody (sometimes), fast rhythmic beat (usually), and ALWAYS higher than normal pitch. Almost all nightcore music are original songs nightcored (remixed into nightcore) by nightcore fans./Very popular is a belief that nightcore is a nickname of a person who remixes the songs. In reality anyone who knows how to use a computer can nightcore a song and upload it on Youtube.' nightcore_fan, 'Nightcore', *Urban Dictionary*, 2010. Viewed on 2 November 2016, http://www.urbandictionary.com/define.php?term=nightcore&defid=5043157.

replies from posters who try to talk her/him out of it. Issues of bullying and being used and also of 'feeling invisible and broken' are brought up. One poster reaches out for help in a dramatic post: 'I really need someone to text/talk to ... So please, if anyone could text me on Hangouts or just send a mail on Google, I'd really appreciate it ... Please...'. Compared to *HDE*, the subject of suicide is also raised more frequently on Emmacore's site, although in other aspects the style of the site is very like that of Stanier's YouTube site. As Emmacore's video brings in another aesthetic with the visual style of manga and the electronic music, it gives the song another character. Maybe the dramatic posts reflect the different style?

McAllister's own video of 'Another Empty Bottle' is a playback version performed by the artist.[56] The majority of the shots in the video show McAllister sitting in her bed, which has black bed linen, as in Stanier's video, often crouching with her arms crossed over her waist or embracing her knees. These bodily poses are representations of mental distress commonly used in many YouTube videos.[57] McAllister alternates between looking at the camera, and thus establishing contact with the viewer, and looking away as if she is overwhelmed by her feelings. There are some interesting aspects worth mentioning in relation to the YouTube site with McAllister's video. First, the original song has fewer viewers compared to the later versions, even though it is more professional and performed by the original artist. The comments section differs to some degree from those for the other videos. Many comments quite naturally praise the song and show appreciation of McAllister's work. Posters also are thankful because the song has helped them, and some write that it describes what they have been going through. Some specify how different parts of the lyrics fit so well with their own experience. In the same way as in the comments sections described previously, empowering messages can be found here: 'your not alone! your worthy never forget that. its a temporary situation it will get better. keep on going, you can do it!' But these are not as frequent as on Stanier's site. Different transmediations of depression, because of their specific capacities, probably make different articulation of the condition possible and this is reflected in the comments.

The last example is one of the YouTube channels that are mentioned on the *HDE* page. Lydiisadinosaur writes:

56 A video with the title *Another Empty Bottle* by the artist Shady Boy came third place in the search results. For the purposes of this study this video was not considered relevant as it is not related to McAllister's or the subject of this chapter.

57 Johansson and Sternudd. 'Iconography of Suffering'.

> I doubt you will see this but your channel is awsome and this video is incredibly accurate, I make mental health videos on my channel and I'm currently trying to get some guest speakers on my channel, let me know if you are interested.

The channel the poster is referring to is *Life With Lydi*,[58] a channel with just over twelve hundred subscribers created by Lydia, a 'British teenager who happens to make videos on the internet'.[59] *Life With Lydi* deals with Lydia's life in general but especially about sharing her 'mental health experience',[60] according to her own description. *Life With Lydi* is just one example of over one hundred thousand channels on YouTube that were dealing with mental health issues as at the end of October 2016.

Anorexia is the subject of Lydia's two most popular videos. For the purpose of this study *What Depression Feels Like*, one of her lesser watched videos, is more interesting here. The video is built up of cuts between eight different black and white shots, most of them repeated several times. It is quite short, under two minutes, with a structure and style that is very reminiscent of McAllister's, even though Lydia uses a voice-over to comment on the images. But in the same way as Stanier and McAllister, she uses herself as an embodiment of the condition. The viewer who has watched her other videos and vlogs on the channel will recognise her from those. Lydia's and McAllister's videos are more aesthetically staged than Stanier's. In *What Depression Feels Like*, Lydia displays herself in poses and creates a tableau for each shot: her head against a wall, sitting in a corner, looking out of a window (shot from behind), holding her head in her hands (rocking back and forth), lying in the bath, lying on the floor (camera shot from above), lying on the floor in a crumpled position (like someone who has fallen from a height). She also looks straight into the camera, in this way establishing contact with the viewer, as if she wants to say, 'see how it feels'. As the video is shot in black and white and the sound is a non-diegetic one consisting of sombre piano music, it alludes to an artier genre than the more raw style of *HDE*. Lydia's video relies significantly on the music and the nearly static images. The differences between the styles of the videos

58 Lydiisadinosaur, *Life with Lydi: The Story from the Lens*, YouTube 2016, Viewed on 20 June 2018. https://www.youtube.com/channel/UCmQKDhwDm7rB693qlS8E3yQ/videos?sort=p&view=0&flow=grid.

59 Lydiisadinosaur. 'Description', YouTube 2016. Viewed on 31 October 2016. https://www.youtube.com/channel/UCmQKDhwDm7rB693qlS8E3yQ/about. Since 2016 has Lydia changed the text on this page and also got more subscribers.

60 Ibid.

are reflected in their names. While Stanier describes the effect of depression in an ordinary, mundane setting, Lydia, using aesthetical means, tries to mediate her inner experience.

5 Summing up and Some Final Remarks

By analysing the context in which Stanier published her video, it becomes clear that her video is part of a genre of videos with the same or a similar subject and similar ways of representing it. These media products are interwoven with each other in an intertextual meaning-making process where concepts and ideas are shared, reused and reformulated. This communal aspect of the meaning-making becomes even clearer when the comments sections are considered. Even if the structure of a YouTube page with a published video invites viewers to comment, for instance through like or dislike buttons, the communal aspect is reinforced in *HDE* by the last line of the closing remarks, 'You can make it through', that directly address the viewer.

One of the most striking results from the analysis of the different YouTube sites is how natural it was for posters to form a group by addressing viewers and readers with the pronoun 'we'. This is probably culturally coded strategy that has evolved over the years via users of YouTube and similar media. Making a group was partly achieved through communicating words of praise, acceptance and recognition. The way in which people in the videos look into the camera seems also part of a conscious strategy to establish a connection through mediation. Support for this notion is provided in the following conversation from the *HDE* site: 'number one rule of cinematography is u dont look at the camera, unless u wanna break the fourth wall'. Stanier answered: 'I am aware. I did not care. It was the point of the video.'

Important features of what constitutes this group or community are concepts of individuals who are isolated and are concealing their condition and self-destructive behaviour from the world – a world that is neglecting or mistreating them. It is a group that often alludes to female experiences of girlhood. That the protagonists in the videos presented here are girls or young women is one example of this tendency. Even if male posters sometimes appear, judging from nicknames, user icons and the content of the comments, girls and young women dominate the group. As one poster puts it, the comments section becomes a place for 'girl-to-girl' talk.

Following the notion that pathography uses a set of different myths, the myth evolving in this domain of youth and mental health could fit into what Hawkins calls the *battle* myth: we are standing together against the world. 'We' are members of a subordinated community who gather strength from each other. This strength has built up through the knowledge that we are not alone and through a distribution of reinforcing and empowering notions. It is important to remember at this point that the community alluded to as 'we' was young, powerless and without status. But the rhetoric on the sites also led to the formation of a community with a solidarity built on recognition and on the posters strengthening and empowering each other.

Personal stories are an important genre in these communities. Forming a group as described above lays the foundation for stories to be told. The importance of talk and the retrieval of buried memories is often put forward as an important aid for recovery. The analysis showed how making a community is based on having common ground and also how different utterances made a common definition of depression possible. In discourse theoretical terms, articulation was made through relating depression, as an element with a vague and uncertain meaning, to other significant notions. The articulation that dominates here is depression as a socially induced condition. In Stanier's video, depression is grounded in others' critical, and objectifying, gaze on her body. This is also put forward in BuzzFeed's version, but other types of social interaction are also emphasised here – nobody really likes or cares for you, and so forth. This is in line with Granek's findings that depression is understood as a relational phenomenon and that those suffering from the condition are characterised by 'self-criticism and self-loathing'.[61] The articulation revealed by the analysis done in this study also concurs with Issakainen's and Hänninen's informants in terms of believing that the cause of depression is life problems and 'not from biochemistry of their brain'.[62] Constructing 'they' as the hostile others ruling the world outside the group is a significant act that confirms Granek's, Issakainen's and Hänninen's results on a collective level.

In the comments sections, feelings were often indicated with emoticons. Although this could simply be an unreflecting use of internet lingua, it could be seen as an indication of a limitation regarding language's ability to mediate inner sensations.[63] This is also where *HDE* and other videos, as well as music, still images and other media, come into play. The analysis of media other than *HDE* showed how seemingly different stories, like the lyrics in 'Another Empty Bottle', could be framed by comments that are quite similar to those made in

61 Granek, 'What's Love Got': 191.

62 Issakainen and Hänninen, 'Young people's Narratives': 241.

63 Which actually is the ground for emoticons see Julianne Wyrick, 'Physics and the birth of the emoticon', *Symmetry*, 2013. Viewed on 20 June 2018. http://www.symmetrymagazine.org/article/july-2013/physics-and-the-birth-of-the-emoticon.

response to Stanier's video. This could indicate that what is recognised is something other than the specific situation that is described in the media products in question. The common ground is probably more of a feeling or an analogous situation than a situation that is recognised in more detail. Further studies might clarify what the central aspects are in these transmediations. Finding additional meaning was also made possible by analysing the media mentioned in the intertextual references or the hypertexts, for instance the manga image that illustrates Emmacore's version of 'Another Empty Bottle'. With its cracked dark sky it mediates mental distress in a more romantic and dramatic way that Stanier's video. McAllister and Lydia mediate the condition in an artier, black and white style, with voices that do not represent the outside other – instead it is the suffering subject's voice that, together with staged images and additional music, tries to capture the experience in a multimodal way. If YouTube and other kinds of multimodal social media have replaced the earlier communities for individuals struggling with mental distress, this probably affects the way the condition is articulated. This is one reason why it is important to study in what way professional commercial producers of videos with millions of followers, like BuzzFeed, might influence the communities described here. Judging from the comments section of *What It's Like Living with Depression*, it has a similar kind of audience.

Finally a reflection on the question of whether it is always positive to talk about and dwell on problematic issues. Some scholars have questioned the so-called therapeutic culture in which testimonies of the experience are crucial and where 'the narrating of experience [becomes] a way to rebuild fractured subjectivity', as Sharratt describes it.[64] Sharratt's ethnographic study of a support group for women suffering from trauma following sexual assaults showed how the opposite approach can be fruitful. Instead of narrating their trauma, members of this group favoured 'collaborative and non-vocal group-healing practices'.[65] In line with this, stories and narratives of depression could have a negative effect on the individuals involved, especially if they become part of a deviant group's activities as the constituting of 'we'. On the other hand, the practice is not as individualistic as the one questioned by the participants in Sharratt's study, and hopefully the formation of a community could lead to some improvement of the situation for the person(s) involved. In Sweden and

64 Elena Sharratt, 'Group Narratives of Trauma and Healing: Community Storytelling as a Critique of Individual "Talking Therapy" amongst Survivors of Sexual Violence' *Narrating Illness: Prospects and Constraints*, eds. Joanna Davidson and Yomna Saber (Oxford: Inter-Disciplinary Press 2016), 76. See also Sharratt, 'The Collective Production of a Shared Narrative Surrounding Sexual Violence Trauma' in this volume.

65 Ibid.

other Western countries, questions of mental health are now widely discussed and are the subject of governmental and other authorities' interventions and investigations and maybe this is due to the many voices of depression that have made themselves heard as a collective force.

Bibliography

Adler, Patricia A. and Peter Adler. 'The Cyber Worlds of Self-Injurers: Deviant Communities, Relationships, and Selves'. *Symbolic Interaction* 31.1 (2008): 33–56.

Adler, Patricia A. and Peter Adler. *The Tender Cut: Inside the Hidden World of Self-injury*. New York: New York University Press, 2011.

AZ, Katy Mcallister Lyrics. Viewed on 20 June 2018. http://www.azlyrics.com/lyrics/katymcallister/anotheremptybottle.html.

Baker, Darren and Sarah Fortune. 'Understanding Self-Harm and Suicide Websites: A Qualitative Interview Study of Young Adult Website Users'. *Crisis* 29.3 (2008): 118–122.

Brockmeier, Jens and Donal A. Carbaugh, 'Introduction'. In *Narrative and Identity: Studies in Autobiography, Self and Culture*, edited by Jens Brockmeier and Donal A. Carbaugh, 1–22. Philadelphia, PA.: Benjamin, 2001.

Busfield, Joan. 'Introduction: Rethinking the Sociology of Mental Health'. *Sociology of Health & Illness* 22.5 (2000): 543–558.

BuzzFeed. *What It's Like Living With Depression*. YouTube 2015. Viewed on 20 June 2018. https://www.youtube.com/watch?v=Ps8RcOdfHT4.

Center for Behavioral Health Statistics and Quality, Behavioral Health. *Trends in the United States: Results from the 2014 National Survey on Drug Use and Health*. HHS Publication No. SMA 15–4927, NSDUH Series H-50, 2015. Viewed on 20 June 2018. http://www.samhsa.gov/data/sites/default/files/NSDUH-FRR1-2014/NSDUH-FRR1-2014.pdf.

Chandler, Amy. 'Narrating the Self-injured Body'. *Medical Humanities* 40 (2014): 111–116.

Cresswell, Mark. 'Psychiatric "Survivors" and Testimonies of Self-harm'. *Social Science & Medicine* 61.8 (2005): 1668–1677. Viewed on 20 June 2018. http://dx.doi.org/10.1016/j.socscimed.2005.03.033.

Elleström, Lars. 'The Modalities of Media: A Model for Understanding Intermedial Relations'. In *Media Borders, Multimodality and Intermediality*, edited by Lars Elleström, 11–48. Houndmills: Palgrave Macmillan, 2010.

Elleström, Lars. *Media Transformation: The Transfer of Media Characteristics Among Media.*, Houndsmill: Palgrave Macmillan, 2014.

Emmacore. *Nightcore~ Another Empty bottle*. YouTube 2015. Viewed on 20 June 2018. https://www.youtube.com/watch?v=ClVY_X_a7HA.

Findahl, Olle and Sheila Zimic. *Unga svenskar och Internet 2008* [Young Swedes and Internet 2008]. Hudiksvall: World Internet Institute, 2008.

Foucault, Michel. *The History of Sexuality, Vol. 1: The Will to Knowledge*. Harmondsworth: Penguin, 1990.

Füredi, Frank. *Therapy Culture: Cultivating Vulnerability in an Uncertain Age*. London: Routledge, 2004.

Graneheim, Ulla Hällgren and Berit Lundman. 'Qualitative Content Analysis in Nursing Research: Concepts, Procedures and Measures to Achieve Trustworthiness'. *Nurse Education Today* 24 (2003): 105–112.

Granek, Leeat. 'What's Love Got to do With It? The Relational Nature of Depressive Experiences'. *Journal of Humanistic Psychology* 46.2 (2006): 191–208.

Gutman, Leslie Morrison, Heather Joshi, Michael Parsonage and Ingrid Schoon. *Children of the New Century: Mental Health Findings from the Millennium Cohort Study*. London: Centre for Mental Health, 2015. Viewed on 20 June 2018, http://cdn.basw.co.uk/upload/basw_120221-1.pdf.

Hawkins, Anne Hunsaker. *Reconstructing Illness: Studies in Pathography*, 2. ed. Purdue University Press, West Lafayette, Ind., 1999.

Hsieh, Hsiu-Fang and Sarah E. Shannon. 'Three Approaches to Qualitative Content Analysis'. *Qualitative Health Research* 15 (2005): 1277–1288.

Issakainen, Mervi and Vilma Hänninen. 'Young People's Narratives of Depression'. *Journal of Youth Studies* 19.2 (2016): 237–250.

Johansson, Anna. *Självskada: En etnologisk studie av mening och identitet i berättelser om skärande* [Self-injury: A ethnological study of meaning and identity in narratives about cutting] (Doctoral dissertation). Umeå: h:ström – Text & kultur, 2010.

Johansson, Anna. 'Constituting "Real" Cutters: A Discourse Theoretical Analysis of Self-harm and Identity'. In*Tracking Discourses: Politics, Identity and Social Change*, edited by Annika Egan Sjölander and Jenny Gunnarsson Payne, 197–224. Lund: Nordic Academic Press, 2011.

Johansson, Anna. 'Hybrid Embodiment: Doing Respectable Bodies on YouTube'. In *Hybrid Media Culture: Sensing Place in a World of Flows*, edited by Simon Lindgren, 34–50. London, Routledge, 2013.

Johansson, Anna and Hans T. Sternudd. 'Iconography of Suffering in Social Media: Images of Sitting Girls'. In *World Suffering and Quality of Life*, edited by Ronald E. Anderson, 341–355. Dordrecht: Springer, 2015.

Laclau, Ernesto and Chantal Mouffe. *Hegemony and Socialist Strategy: Towards a Radical Democratic Politics*. London and New York: Verso, (1985) 2001.

Lydiisadinosaur. *Life with Lydi: The Story from the Lens*. YouTube 2016. Viewed on 20 June 2018. https://www.youtube.com/channel/UCmQKDhwDm7rB693qlS8E3yQ/videos?sort=p&view=0&flow=grid.

Lydiisadinosaur. 'Description'. YouTube 2016. Viewed on 31 October 2016. https://www.youtube.com/channel/UCmQKDhwDm7rB693qlS8E3yQ/about.

Marcus. 'flame war'. *Urban Dictionary* 2004. Viewed on 20 June 2018. https://www.urbandictionary.com/define.php?term=flame%20war.

McColl, Owen. *The Voice Of Depression*. YouTube 2014. Viewed on 20 June 2018. https://www.youtube.com/watch?v=hBs6BPT50G8.

McKenna, Katelyn Y.A. and John A. Bargh. 'Plan 9 From Cyberspace: The Implications of the Internet for Personality and Social Psychology'. *Personality and Social Psychology Review* 4.1. (2000): 57–75.

nightcore_fan. 'Nightcore'. *Urban Dictionary* 2010. Viewed on 20 June 2018. http://www.urbandictionary.com/define.php?term=nightcore&defid=5043157.

Oliffe, John, L., Steve Robertson, Mary T. Kelly, Philippe Roy, and John S. Ogrodniczuk. 'Connecting Masculinity and Depression Among International Male University Students'. *Qualitative Health Research* 20.7 (2010): 987–998.

Riessman, Catherine Kohler. *Narrative Methods for the Human Sciences*. London: SAGE, 2008.

Rose, Sammy. *Katy McAllister – Another Empty Bottle – Lyrics*. YouTube 2012. Viewed on 20 June 2018, https://www.youtube.com/watch?v=Cqv9ZHveNbk.

Ross, Michael W. *Typing, Doing and Being: A Study of Men who have Sex with Men and Sexuality on the Internet*. Malmö: Faculty of Health and Society, Malmö University, 2006.

Schiano, Diane J. and Sean White. 'The First Noble Truth of CyberSpace: People are People (even when they MOO)', 352–359 Los Angeles: *Proceedings of the SIGCHI Conference on Human Factors in computing systems*, 1998.

Sharratt, Elena. 'Group Narratives of Trauma and Healing: Community Storytelling as a Critique of Individual "Talking Therapy" amongst Survivors of Sexual Violence'. In *Narrating Illness: Prospects and Constraints*, edited by Joanna Davidson and Yomna Saber, 75–82. Oxford: Inter-Disciplinary Press 2016.

Snickars, Pelle and Patrick Vonderau, eds. *The YouTube Reader*. Stockholm: National Library of Sweden, 2009.

Stanier, Saraphine. *How Depression Effects Someone's Daily Life-Short Film*. YouTube, 2015. Viewed on 20 June 2018. https://www.youtube.com/watch?v=203pnN95zHY.

Stanier, Saraphine, Status update, *Facebook* 2015. Available 1 February 2016, https://www.facebook.com/Saraphine13/timeline.

Sternudd, Hans T. 'Having the Voice of Depression: An Example of Pathographic Film Narratives on YouTube'. In *Narrating Illness: Prospects and Constraints*, edited by Joanna Davidson and Yomna Saber, 221–234. Oxford: Inter-Disciplinary Press, 2016.

Sternudd, Hans T. 'Photographs of Self-Injury: Production and Reception in a Group of Self-Injurers'. *Journal of Youth Studies* 15.4 (2012): 421–436.

Sternudd, Hans T. and Anna Johansson. 'The Girl in the Corner: Aesthetics of Suffering in a Digitalized Space'. In *Narratives of Suffering: Meaning and Experience in a Digitalized Space*, edited by Lolita Guimarães Guerra and Jose A. Nicdao, 105–115. Oxford: Inter-Disciplinary Press, 2015.

Säljö, Roger. *Lärande i praktiken: ett sociokulturellt perspektiv*, [Practice of Learning: A Sociocultural Perspective]. Studentlitteratur, Lund, 2014.

This American Life. '573: Status Update'. 2015. Viewed on 20 June 2018. https://www.thisamericanlife.org/radio-archives/episode/573/status-update.

Turkle, Sherry. 'Construction and Reconstruction of the Self in Virtual Reality: Playing in the MUDs'. *Mind, Culture, and Activity* 1.3 (1994): 158–167.

Ussher, Jane M. *The Madness of Women: Myth and Experience*. London: Routledge, 2011.

Winther Jørgensen, Marianne and Louise Phillips. *Discourse Analysis as Theory and Method*. London: Sage, 2002.

Whitlock, Janis L., Jane L. Powers and John Eckenrode. 'The Virtual Cutting Edge: The Internet and Adolescent Self-Injury'. *Developmental Psychology* 42.3 (2006): 1–11.

Wyrick, Julianne. 'Physics and the birth of the emoticon'. *Symmetry* 2014. Viewed on 20 June 2016. http://www.symmetrymagazine.org/article/july-2013/physics-and-the-birth-of-the-emoticon.

Yawata, Alex. *A Depression PSA (Short Film)*. YouTube 2014. Viewed on 30 November 2016. https://www.youtube.com/watch?v=ompcDVq_noU.

Öhman, Anneli Brännström, Maria Jönsson and Ingeborg Svensson, 'Inledning' [Introduction]. In *Att känna sig fram: Känslor i humanistisk genusforskning* [To feel ones way: Feelings in Humanistic Gender Studies] edited by Anneli Brännström Öhman, Maria Jönsson, and Ingeborg Svensson, 7–19. Umeå: Bokförlaget H:ström 2011.

PART 4

Ethical Stories: Voices in Research

CHAPTER 9

A Shared Story of Professional Practice: Therapists Make Meaning of Spirituality

Peter Bray

Abstract

This chapter presents the story of a series of nine discussions held over a twelve month period with a group of alcohol and substance addictions therapists who work with Māori clients in a residential hospital unit. Although these therapists' practices are regulated by professional bodies and a medical institution, their personal approaches to individuals in recovery are uniquely inspired by their own experiences and beliefs, and the stories they tell about their spirituality. To avoid institutional censure, they have tended to minimise their spiritual selves in the workplace and hidden these potentially controversial beliefs and experiences from their employers. Thus, as counsellors engaged with the stories and experiences of their clients, they are adept at handling the uncomfortable disjoint between the demands of their quasi-medical roles and the authentic expression of their collaborative alliances with clients. Although the group's initial goal was to identify and develop the use of spirituality as an aid to working with recovering addicts, it became clear that the group needed to examine its own spiritual experiences and pathways to meaning, particularly those experiences that replicated or closely corresponded to their clients' whose core narratives resonated at a fundamental level with their identities. While they identified spirituality as a positive factor in human health and well-being, particularly its ability to reconnect their traumatised clients with lost potentials, they were also fearful that their perspectives might not be fully understood by medical colleagues. Their stories of co-existing trauma and addiction, the hope and growth of spiritual awareness, and the struggles and rewards of working in such challenging settings, illustrates their passion for engaging with clients' spiritual resources. Their stories caution us as professionals not to disregard our clients' spiritual beliefs but to fully utilise them in support of healing and post-traumatic growth.

 | DOI:10.1163/9789004396067_011

Key Words

Addiction – counselling – co-existing problems – competence – mental health – post-traumatic growth – recovery – self-actualisation – spirituality – storytelling – therapy – trauma

*****

1 Introduction

A few years ago I was invited to present some ideas on the topic of spirituality and its role in post-traumatic growth.[1] The lecture, organised by the staff of a mental health and addictions treatment centre in New Zealand, went well and I was subsequently asked to run a special interest group to provide opportunities 'to safely articulate spirituality within the medical model'.[2] This simple invitation to work with colleagues proved a rich opportunity for therapeutic story-telling and their unique voices emerged from the recordings and their transcriptions. In a series of nine semi-structured, ninety minute group conversations the impact of spirituality on their therapeutic work and upon their relationships with clients hoping to resolve addictive behaviour were freely explored. Here group members co-constructed a common narrative which served to clearly present their group position on spirituality and enabled each to express and grow their understanding of spirituality and their professional identities.

From the beginning it became apparent that stories of spirituality, rather than experiences of religiosity were to be the main focus, and one to which we returned again and again. It was also agreed that, even in a health setting where patient-centred practices are set-up specifically to respond to unique experiences, the numinous and inexplicable are easily overlooked and discounted.

---

1 For more about Stan and Christina Grof's seminal work on psycho-spiritual transformation and the post-traumatic growth research of Richard Tedeschi and Lawrence Calhoun, please see; Peter Bray, 'A Broader Framework for Exploring the Influence of Spiritual Experience in the Wake of Stressful Life Events: Examining Connections between Posttraumatic Growth and Psycho-Spiritual Transformation', *Mental Health, Religion and Culture* 13.3 (2010): 293–308.

2 This and subsequent unreferenced quotes and comments from group members are taken from the transcripts of our meetings, made contemporaneously and with the group's permission for further dissemination.

Not uncommonly, once the formalities of clinical contracting, assessment, and the expedient assignment of authority has been dispensed with, the client and clinician are then left to negotiate the space between them to prioritise what client concerns are worthy of attention and what they are not.

Unlike the position afforded by religion, spirituality has long been regarded in Western society as a place that professional helpers enter with caution, if at all. So, it is with caution, care and respect that I bring the group's story, quite conscious that within it lies my own. In the therapeutic world of talking cures, spirituality is increasingly a factor in measuring mental wellness. Every day we are asked to demonstrate to others that we are able to function effectively in a human-sized world, and that our egos can resist the dangers of an over-expanding consciousness. Extreme behaviour in either may signal a cause for concern and a need for psychological support.

Nonetheless master narratives of human spirituality, and the conduct of therapy, permeate the literature but due to its subjectivity the former remains notoriously difficult to quantify.[3] Similarly, stories of spirituality in client work, either as it is introduced through the experiences of professional practitioners[4] or voiced by clients, require the right tools to tease out.[5] Consequently, in order to understand who the therapist is as a person, and how their world-view is inextricably linked and expressed through professional relationships, may require an ethnographic approach to research that 'acknowledges and accommodates subjectivity, emotionality, and the researcher's influence'[6] and informs the particular telling of therapists' stories. In addition, clients' use of spirituality to resource recovery also finds its expression in stories of quest and restitution,[7] as discussed by Mirjam Stuij and her colleagues in this collection.[8]

3 Peter Bray, 'Naming Spirituality in Counsellor Education: A Modest Proposal', Special Issue on Counsellor Education in Aotearoa New Zealand, *New Zealand Journal of Counselling* (2011): 76–97.

4 Arthur W. Frank, 'Why Doctors' Stories Matter', Canadian Family Physician, 56.1 (2010): 51–54, in which Frank reflects upon his own experiences with illness. This approach is also highlighted in Victorria Simpson-Gervin, 'Narrative Medicine and Storytelling: An Alternative Method for Healing', in this volume.

5 Carolyn Ellis, Tony E. Adams and Arthur P. Bochner, 'Autoethnography: An Overview', *Forum Qualitative Sozialforschung / Forum: Qualitative Social Research* 12.1 (2010): np viewed 19 June 2018, http://nbn-resolving.de/urn:nbn:de:0114-fqs1101108.

6 Ibid.

7 Arthur W. Frank, *The Wounded Storyteller* (Chicago and London, The University of Chicago Press, 1995).

8 Mirjam Stuij, Agnes Elling, Anja Tramper and Tineke Abma, 'Developing a Relational Narrative about Diabetes: Towards a Polyphonic Story', in this volume.

With these opportunities in mind, the following chapter provides something of the richness of the group's shared experiences as they reflect upon spirituality in the workplace, their professional practices and their personal lives.[9]

2 The Therapists

The discussion group comprised, in total, nine highly experienced addictions workers and registered health professionals', comprising: psychologists; social workers; psychotherapists; and, counsellors. Employed by hospital-based mental health and addictions providers, they were contracted to deliver behavioural and psycho-educational training and skill development activities designed to maintain client motivation, engagement and change. Half of the group identified as having successfully recovered from the experience of addiction and, as one group member explained, 'Some of us worked through our trauma without addiction and some of us have got addiction as a way of coping'. Guided by principles of client-centeredness, the group concurred that, if addiction can be described as 'a chronic relapsing brain disease characterized by compulsive behaviour',[10] then spirituality, used as a resource in rehabilitation, positively supports addiction management and recovery.[11]

Whilst these professionals were keen to disclose how spirituality impacted upon their counselling with clients, their initial decision to participate anonymously demonstrated how spirituality is still 'an uncomfortable fit with the medical model' and that 'medical materialism'[12] still has the power to constrain therapeutic practice even at a grass-roots level.

---

9 A companion piece to this work may be found in Peter Bray, 'Mental Health Therapists Consider the Relevance of Spirituality in their Work with Addiction and Trauma', *New Zealand Journal of Counselling* 36.1 (2016): 21–46.

10 Benita Walton-Moss, Ellen M. Ray and Kathleen Woodruff, 'Relationship of Spirituality or Religion to Recovery from Substance Abuse', *Journal of Addictions Nursing* 24.4 (2013): 224–225.

11 Harold E. Doweiko suggests that spiritual interventions have the capacity to penetrate a client's psychological defences and restore coherence and meaning in life. Harold E. Doweiko, 'Substance Use Disorders as Symptoms of Spiritual Disease', *Addiction and Spirituality a Multidisciplinary Approach*, eds. Oliver J. Morgan and Merle Jordan (St. Louis: Chalice Press, 1999), 51.

12 William James argues that psychology is unable to fully explain religious experiences. William James, *The Varieties of Religious Experience* (New York: Modern Library, 1929).

3 The Clients

> [Clients] have done things that are contrary to who they think they are and their core values. That in itself is a traumatic experience and they are traumatised by it. They will often say 'I can't believe I did that'.[13]

Members of the special interest group work principally with Māori clients who have a diagnosis of substance dependence, described by the DSM IV as 'a pattern of repeated self-administration that can result in tolerance, withdrawal, and compulsive drug-taking behaviour'[14] alongside 'PTSD and Axis II disorders'.[15] Group members described clients as adopting self-medicating lifestyles to minimise the distressing effects of their childhood traumas because they 'don't have healthy environments to grow up in, are unable to make healthy choices, or are afflicted by external traumatic events which have disempowered them'.[16] Consequently, the centre's eight week residential programme and

13 The literature confirms established connections between trauma and addiction. Center for Substance Abuse Treatment, 'Anxiety Disorders' in *Assessment and Treatment of Patients With Coexisting Mental Illness and Alcohol and Other Drug Abuse. Treatment Improvement Protocol [TIP] Series 9, DHHS Publication No. SMA 95-3061* (Rockville: Substance Abuse and Mental Health Services, 1994), viewed 19 June 2018 http://www.ncbi.nlm.nih.gov/bookshelf/br.fcgi?book=hssamhsatip&part=A30236;

Individuals who have encountered stressful life events, have histories of physical and/or sexual trauma, are more vulnerable to alcohol and substance addiction than those who have not.

Office of Applied Studies, Substance Abuse and Mental Health Services Administration (SAMHSA), 'Mental Health Screenings and Trauma-Related Counseling in Substance Abuse Treatment Facilities'. *The N-SSATS Report*, September 30, 2010; Center for Substance Abuse Treatment, *Trauma-Informed Care in Behavioral Health Service: Treatment Improvement Protocol (TIP) Series, No. 57* (Rockville: Substance Abuse and Mental Health Services Administration, 2014).

14 American Psychiatric Association, *Diagnostic and Statistical Manual of Mental Disorders*, 4th Edition (Washington: American Psychiatric Association, 2000), 192.

15 Coexisting disorders may include mood, anxiety, personality, and eating disorders, and persistent, maladaptive symptoms such as blunted emotional responses, hyper-arousal, and flashbacks related to trauma. Marian L. Logrip, Eric P. Zorrilla, and George F. Koob, 'Stress Modulation of Drug Self-Administration: Implications for Addiction Comorbidity with Post-Traumatic Stress Disorder', *Neuropharmacology* 62 (2012): 552–564.

16 In their study of childhood trauma and dissociation in patients with alcohol and drug dependence Ingo Schafer and colleagues confirmed they had been exposed to high levels of early potentially traumatic experiences. Ingo Schafer, et al., 'Childhood Trauma and Dissociation in Patients with Alcohol Dependence and Drug Dependence, or Both – A Multi-Centre Study', *Drug and Alcohol Dependence* 109 (2010); 87–88.

individualised Recovery Action Plans (RAP)[17] support the self-assessed needs of clients that, post-treatment, are later followed up to maintain long-term psychosocial functioning.

4 The Workplace

At the time of writing the centre was located in a tired and shambling colonial villa where residents have access to a number of meeting, teaching and counselling rooms, a communal kitchen and dining area. Meals are shared but otherwise there are clear professional boundaries between patients and clinical staff. In accordance with New Zealand's 'Treaty of Waitangi',[18] the centre explicitly incorporates bicultural approaches and models of practice that support the collective vision, aspirations and cultural beliefs of Māori communities and provides access to kaupapa services and kaumatua/elders. Therapists too have developed bicultural perspectives that are aligned with holistic models of Māori health such as 'Te Whare Tapa Wha'.[19] In common with other non-dominant traditional cultures, Māori carry a broader view of health and well-being, which may call upon 'spiritual connectedness, [and] access to a secure cultural identity'.[20] Elder, healer and leader Rose Pere notes that, as 'the physical realm is immersed in the spiritual realm',[21] so wairua/spirituality impacts upon relationships with the environment, the living and the dead. Thus, as clinicians who 'walk the space between'[22] and subscribe to personal change, the group questioned why spirituality is not more widely recognised as a 'fundamental pillar of the medical model in New Zealand'.

Unsurprisingly, although their programmes generally meet client needs and the organisational and clinical service requirements of the parent institution,

17 The RAP responds to five areas of need: current situation; goals and hopes; actions; sharing responsibility; and, progress.

18 Claudia Orange, *The Treaty of Waitangi* (Wellington, New Zealand: Allen & Unwin, 1987).

19 Te Whare Tapa Wha attends to taha tinana/physical health, taha whānau/family health, taha hinengaro/mental health, and makes a unique contribution to spiritual health, known as taha wairua. Mason Durie, *Whaiora: Mäori Health Development* (Auckland: Oxford University Press, 1994).

20 Fraser C. Todd, *Te Ariari o te Oranga: The Assessment and Management of People with Co-existing Mental Health and Substance Use Problems* (Ministry of Health: Wellington, 2010), 23.

21 Rose Pere, *Te Wheke: A Celebration of Infinite Wisdom* (Gisborne: Ao Ako Global Learning, New Zealand 1997), 16.

22 Melinda Webber, *Walking the Space Between: Identity and Mäori/Päkehä* (Wellington: NZCER Press, 2008).

the group felt passionately that, in order to work more effectively with the many co-existing disorders associated with substance use, they still needed to attune themselves and their service to a broader range of beliefs and experiences. Prior to our meetings, the group had accepted the received interpretation of spirituality as participation in formal religious activities. However, as we began to meet they identified the 'Spiritual and Cultural' area of their practice as one that could be significantly improved, agreeing that, of the four cornerstones of Māori health, spiritual health was the most poorly served by their institutional practices. Similarly, examining their own spiritual positions, they discovered how little they trusted their institution to honour them. 'I don't have anyone I can trust with that [spirituality] material within the medical model of practice … we don't get to talk about this stuff anywhere else'. Even conventional clinical supervisors don't always have the skill to handle this material. 'We work covertly with one eye watching our backs'.

5 Discussion and Process

The simple goal of the group was to find a place to safely articulate and deliver spirituality within the parameters of a medical institution and to understand the meaning it has for them and their clients. However, the simple became quite daunting. In this context the group had a 'unique' angle on the subject which made them uncertain about how to freely articulate it so that it might fit it into a health services model and context. Unsurprisingly, this aspiration was superseded by one closer to home – to examine personal perspectives that informed and supported them individually in their practices. This exploration depended upon three basic assumptions that: clients and counsellors bring their spirituality to therapy; spirituality is a positive resource that may be used to support clients managing the trauma of addiction; and, counsellors working in addiction recovery may be simultaneously working with their own and their clients' spiritualties.[23]

5.1 *Meeting 1*

Most journeys begin with a single step and storying spirituality resembled a group therapy session where participants have faith in the process and trust in each other. It was agreed that through increasing awareness of our own spirituality we might strengthen our capacity to work with clients. 'If we know what

23 William West, *Psychotherapy and Spirituality* (London: SAGE Publications, 2001); Bray, 'Naming Spirituality', 76–97.

spirituality means to us as practitioners we might be able to assist clients in theirs'. As a result, the creation of a 'common-sense' model of clinical spiritual practice became established as long-term goal for the group. Nevertheless, it soon became clear that, in order to discuss their work, it might be best to begin by identifying how they made meaning and defined spirituality – what it is and what it is not – and to differentiate between 'religion' and the more expansive and encompassing experience of the 'spiritual'. To come to a shared definition of spirituality it was suggested that the group consider the impact and outcomes of 'pivotal moments' or life crises.

> If spiritual understanding or belief is activated by existential concerns ... Once we have had spiritual experiences the veil is lifted and they [spiritual experiences] cannot be unseen or unlearned but they can be denied or suppressed.

It was suggested that crisis experiences block any return to the way that life used to be,[24] and that clinicians are often called upon to make judgements about whether such narrative are 'real or imaginary, growthful, or dangerous?' The group wrestled with questions of how to correctly 'interpret, diagnose, judge, or value clients' spiritual experiences', or whether all 'spiritual crises hold the potential for growth-promoting change?'[25] It was finally resolved that 'clients can have active connections with other things in their lives' but that often 'psychic phenomena may also be interpreted as psychosis', that 'inexplicable experiences are often modified by interpretation'.

As the conversation moved on to look at the work done with clients' spirituality, the group acknowledged that they might be powerfully positioned to broaden the scope of what is seen as either 'normal', 'safe', or ethically appropriate in this process. Clients, it was agreed, should be invited, given permission, to discuss their spiritual beliefs and experiences and that they might be acutely sensitive about being understood correctly, 'We need to understand the client's way of seeing the world to see what carries her through'.

This discussion took the form of a presenting of case studies, safely peppered with generalised anecdotes. The group were genuinely reluctant to

24 Ronnie Janoff-Bulman, *Shattered Assumptions: Towards a New Psychology of Trauma* (New York: Free Press, 1992).

25 Grof and Grof describe 'spiritual emergency' as a moment of crisis that loosens control of the ego and opens a doorway into the unconscious. These changes in perception are profoundly disturbing and clients require understanding and education to make sense of their new positions and grow psychologically from them. See Stanislav Grof and Christina Grof, eds., *Spiritual Emergency: When Personal Transformation Becomes a Crisis* (New York: G.P. Putnam's Sons, 1989).

reveal their own spiritualties and expressed real concern about where these discussions might be leading. Thinking that this was a natural phase in early group interaction I was surprised when it emerged that experience in the field of trauma and addiction over a number of years had made them more vigilant about becoming targets. Just as clients may be labelled or even stigmatised for disclosing their spiritual experiences, so the actions of other health professionals with their clients had made these therapists somewhat wary and vulnerable to suffering the same fate.[26] As one therapist explained,

> Even before I became a CBT therapist I've hated labels … In the therapeutic context – the language of spirituality seems loaded with value-judgements, quite a lot of which are negative, abnormal, and *unhealthy*.

The group were concerned about revealing their spiritual experiences to senior colleagues 'who may view us as mad'. Eventually, one member bravely disclosed that she was constantly aware of a parallel 'dream process that accompanies [her] day-to-day living'. She described it as a continuous and simultaneous experiencing of déjà vu, 'I am not mad but I have these experiences … so, if I am feeling like that, what must my clients be feeling?' This raised a further question about how much the group use intuition or 'clairvoyance' in their sessions with clients. It was acknowledged that some knowledge is intuitively gained but other knowledge might originate from 'elsewhere'.

> In these moments with clients, things are seamlessly unfolding – flowing – there is little or no resistance. Almost seems like we channel our responses. In these cases how can we be sure that we are being effective or do we have faith in the process? Do we accept that the [collective] unconscious may be directing our work?

Whilst the group broadly acknowledged the importance of discussing spirituality in their practices they observed that working in this area generates anxiety and tension between their personal and professional identities.

5.2 *Meeting 2*

Our previous meeting had had some beneficial effects on the group's subsequent clinical work. Up until now these practitioners had consciously withheld the spiritual parts of themselves and their experiences from colleagues and clients. Now they were feeling challenged to disclose more and to invite

26 Marc Galanter, 'Spirituality and Addiction: A Research and Clinical Perspective', *The American Journal on Addictions*, 15 (2006): 290.

others to do the same. At this point implications were explored. If 'being on the same page as the client means meeting her in her spirituality' then how does the fear of disclosing spirituality to the institution restrict therapists' relationships with clients? Here the concerns of the private person and the professional provided both an explanation and an excuse as to why 'things are getting in the way of us being fully present to ourselves and others'. One group member observed that, 'To be fully present is to have the capacity to tap into another's inner being or spirituality', which honoured the therapeutic relationship and the therapists' capacities to engage with their spiritual selves and to share their spiritual stories. Examining the many relational dichotomies it was suggested that as spirituality has its own immutable existence, its access can only be 'disengaged by a logic that defeats the ability to be fully immersed in the experience'.

Struggling with a way of defining spirituality, 'love' was suggested as a useful description of the outworking of spiritual experience. 'When special moments occur with the client could we call it a "love experience"?' This led to some consideration of spirituality as a place of sanctuary, 'in a therapeutic context [spirituality] could be a boundary ... a place where we can only go when we are feeling safe'. Another suggested that spirituality might be described in terms of energy or knowledge from the collective unconscious.

> I may use my energy to get some sense of my client. I expand my awareness to get how they are and what's going on for them – not just what they are saying – so I really get that you call it love – send your energy out and connect with someone else's energy and see how it feels. Same with spirituality, I see it as energy that permeates everything and everywhere and we can tap into that and it taps into me.

These ideas together generated further debate around professional positioning. If therapists, for example, assume that all their clients are people with lives whose pieces contribute to a greater more universal spiritual design, would this change how they engaged with their clients? It was agreed that 'Positioning with our client's consciousness should be about awareness and accommodation', so that therapy sessions are not missed opportunities to understand and enter the client's spiritual worldview. Accommodating this broader view might mean 'expanding the boundaries of our awareness in ways that more fully accommodate and appreciate the client's spiritual experiences'. This took the conversation on an imaginative journey where participants shared their own ideas on the impact of client and clinicians' beliefs concerning reincarnation and past life experiences, predestination and fate. 'When your boundaries are semi-permeable you place yourself in a much stronger position to absorb that feeling energy of excitement and anxiety that they give off' suggesting that this makes the therapist and client more vulnerable to each other. There was also some interest in sharing the client's journey and becoming a part of their story. In a truly spiritual sense it meant momentarily sharing clients' 'destinies' too.

This final comment suddenly identified the presence of an essential and profound reciprocity, not only in the group's past, present and future therapeutic relationships but in all their engagements with the world. It also signalled the importance of keeping strong personal and professional boundaries. 'Sometimes there needs to be a closing down – a detachment for our own protection so that I am not absorbing that [energy]'.

Another perspective suggested that as professional helpers

> We are exposed to experiences with some clients that will assist us with other clients further down the track. We draw upon these and take them into new contexts with new clients.
>
> If we regard all experiences as potentially useful to us and others it makes meaning of the whole of existence. We can no longer say that this is just a job.

5.3 *Meeting 3*

As we came back together one therapist noted that the group was particularly valuable as a forum to reflect upon responses to client disclosures. Another explained that the previous meeting had prompted him to undertake a spiritual inventory of his life, whilst another had been musing over what she considered to be two significant elements of spirituality, its experience and how the story of that experience is understood and explained to others. Both, it was agreed, involving a level of emotional exposure balanced by a need to be interpreted correctly and be fully understood. The point was well made in terms of the group process and in the context of clear professional communication. 'If we are experiencing reluctance or resistance to disclosing this area of our praxis, how might our clients feel in the forming stages of relationship?' As the group began to trust each other and feel safer about expressing specific spiritual beliefs and experiences, mutual sharing and a heightening of awareness enabled generous disclosures to be made and to be warmly received. As the conversation ranged on, spirituality became 'a dimension of relationship where intuition exists that can provide access to mutually satisfying ways forward'.

It was agreed that inviting clients to engage in discussions on spirituality, therapists require confidence about their use of time and space to sensitively guarantee that their interventions are comfortable, appropriate, and safe. Regarding self-care it was also suggested that 'Giving clients strength to do their work requires the practitioner to manage high levels of energy'. Knowing how to manage the draining effect on themselves of their clients' experiences and 'refilling the tanks' was very important for the group.

What followed was deeply disclosive, as individual participants told their own stories. One talked at length about his struggles with depression as a Christian that, though it severely tested his faith, had left it fragile but unbroken. He reflected upon his disequilibrium and fragmentation and observed that in his liminal position as a professional helper/observer, 'Working at the edge', he sometimes simultaneously experienced what he could only explain as supernatural excitement and fear.

Further sharing revealed personal stories of healing from addiction and trauma that had led to a greater acceptance of spirituality. One member remarked, 'Accepting it [spiritual experience] just happened – it's a huge experience ... I just allowed it to be'. Whilst another, affirming the rest, declared 'We are not insane!! We have strength that we can offer to the client, and the client carries the same responsibility'. It seemed that under their cautious professional veneer there was a broad acceptance of spiritual systems and praxis.

The group felt that the 'official' medical model dominated how spiritual experiences were being constructed, interpreted and valued in their workplaces. It seemed to them that anything even remotely considered spiritual was 'lumped together' in the same basket. Two group members, both highly experienced in working alongside Māori, shared their fears that conventional treatment packages were not appropriate in all cases. They recalled a story about how a psychologist had been deregistered by his professional body because of his beliefs about spiritual guardians. 'There needs to be an acceptance that these things exist beyond Māoridom'. In a further sharing of stories about clients from other cultures, there was a deep concern about client assessment. As one therapist remarked specifically on her multicultural practice, 'I feel like my main work since I have been in the mental health system has been to normalise peoples' experiences'.

For another the present group was cited as a way to 'to remove myself from the medical model ... to be more confident about talking about spirituality within the system we work in'. This was a challenging idea and although it was accepted that one of the group's functions was 'to support us to be agents of change – to make changes to the medical model' the question still remained, 'How do we accomplish this?'

Here the discussion turned powerfully to colonisation and the possibility that culturally specific spiritualties might be regarded as something that is owned by one culture over another. In terms of New Zealand's obligations to Māori, it was cynically suggested that institutions only pay 'lip-service' to spirituality, 'It's because of the Treaty, that it's allowed room'. Nevertheless, it was agreed that acknowledging the presence of spirituality was preferable to its being ignored and that Māori spiritual beliefs and practices had a lot to offer conventional Western approaches to client work.

At this point in the discussion the spiritual nature of the therapeutic relationship finally took centre stage. Noting the impact of her Christian beliefs, one therapist commented, 'When I am with a client I suspend my spiritual beliefs and allow space for them to bring what is valid'. Here two parallel threads: theology, 'judgement, ethics, morals, religion, rules – the cognitive and socially ordering pieces'; and, spirit 'things that we are immersed in, inform us as a human being, a faith, and being non-judgemental' emerged. A clear distinction was made between the formalising aspects of religion, and the roles of intuition and faith, described as the difference 'between the head and the body', theory and practice.

It was highlighted that the group was on a journey whose purpose was unfolding and as a result of sharing was positively influencing their everyday professional practices.

> We may now know where we are going but what is clearer is that with spirituality we can be agents of change. We are positioning ourselves relative to culture and the group helps us to find ways to safely articulate spirituality with our clients and within the medical model.

5.4 *Meeting 4*

There is a great value in awareness raising through the sharing of spiritual material from the workplace. Indeed, as a result one of the group seriously considered doing a master's thesis on spirituality and health. With limited opportunities to discuss these aspects of their lives and practices with close friends or intimate colleagues this kind of workplace forum supports its members to strengthen work with clients practically. One typical intervention described was derived from Gestalt therapy's two-chair or empty-chair work where, in this case, a deceased partner is sensitively invited to participate in a therapy session.[27] This creates a new and important memory for the client and adds to the supportive resources of the griever. As one counsellor put it, 'There are forces that we may perceive that represent less specific but nonetheless supportive entities'.

27 See also, Robert Elliott, Jeanne C. Watson, Rhonda N. Goldman, and Leslie S. Greenberg, *Learning Emotion-focused Therapy: The Process-experiential Approach to Change* (Washington, DC: American Psychological Association, 2004).

Discussing their work in addictions and trauma, the group applauded the resilience of their clients, 'how do clients retain heart, sensitivity, and optimism in the face of their past experiences?' Spirituality was regarded as a significant player in clients' recovery from addiction,[28] which has implications for the role of the therapist, 'Our work connects the lost with the living, and the living with their lives'.

The group shared that the majority of clients are often forced to become survivors from early on and, as a result they understand what makes life worth living. They identify with spirituality because they have reached rock bottom and are already on the road to recovery. They are aware that they have survived for a reason, want to trust in something beyond themselves, have a desire for something better, and can make a choice to heal. It was observed that, because of their distressing experiences, clients have 'developed spiritual muscles' that enable them to 'push the line between the natural and the supernatural – they have gone to places that have prepared their psyches to connect with the numinous'. However, it was also noted that clients want to feel special 'they need therapists who make them feel good about themselves and hold the client's hope until they are ready to pick it up again'.

It was understood that, in the same way that the experience of encouragement and mutual understanding worked in our group, so this can work for clients too. Simply, through their group process members recognised that, even though their workplace may minimise the importance of spirituality, they were comfortable accepting the fuller potential of their clients' spiritual realities and determined to work with them creatively utilising existing approaches and systems. Here the discussion returned to power and empowerment and the conceived binary between spiritual knowing and Newtonian medicine. 'It's like we believe that explaining the world will make it more controllable'. Admittedly it seems, the ineffability of spiritual experiences and concepts can feel risky to people of science but, as one brave soul observed, 'Doctors are gods with a small "g" and they don't like the competition'. Furthermore, mental health in attempting to explain and excuse human behaviour in purely scientific terms may have glossed over some important distinctions between good and evil in the modern world.

Moving on, there was so much that the group understood from their own lives that they didn't acknowledge professionally or publically,

28 An idea suggested by the work of Christina Grof, *The Thirst for Wholeness: Attachment, Addiction, and the Spiritual Path* (New York: HarperOne, 1993).

> … we identify meeting clients at many different levels but only partially discuss with them and others the deeper and more holistic nature of their experience[s] … [providing] a text-book summary of how to do things.

To avoid difficult misunderstandings with colleagues and clients, it was agreed that as professionals they needed to be more transparent in reporting their practice. Similarly, 'We cannot assume that all spirituality is the same', or that 'Some clients seem to have two dimensional lives', overlooking spirituality is 'denying them a three dimensional existence'. It was agreed that, when engaging with spirituality, previously negative experiences can make clients fearful or uncomfortable. Even in day-to-day conversations it was confirmed that 'some people are not grounded enough to manage this exposure'. A counselling session, whilst it does provide the right conditions for the intuitive sharing of spiritual perspectives can also challenge the therapist's 'groundedness' too. Similarly, 'Working with … getting in the flow of the spirit, rather than being present in body and mind, can be effective therapy [for the client] but it is also [personally] consuming'.

> You're in this intuitive flow and it's kinda only being revealed one step at a time … so you're kind of on the edge, and it's like that sensation of being pushed from behind and you take the next step, and the next step …

This approach seemed incongruent with the institution's manualised therapeutic regime for its residents. As one therapist put it, competence and accountability is measured by managers in terms of 'doing something' with clients and it is sometimes difficult to follow pre-session agenda, or map a client's therapy when it touches on areas like spirituality. For the client spontaneity often works better than a hard and fast procedure, 'you go where the energy is'. Work led by the spirit, therefore, looks different from heavily structured practice templates. They can become self-serving rather than client-serving. Experience had revealed, for this group at least, that it is judicious to 'write the reports they [medical managers] want to hear but what we do with the client is sometimes quite different … actually nobody knows what we do in the room'. One example was given that described how a report about a patient was returned to a clinician by a senior colleague who suggested that he rewrite it and remove reference to an intervention because it might be negatively misinterpreted and cast the therapist in a poor light.

The meeting closed with a discussion that further hinted at the perils of working in an institution. The group were unanimous in feeling professionally undervalued but said that it was in everyone's interests not to make waves.

To draw too much attention to their current practice, to reveal too much imagination or creativity could attract scrutiny, judgement and control over work that they considered was really benefitting their clients. When I suggested that they might be more open about their work it was explained that they had on numerous occasions attempted to describe their work to medical colleagues but without being understood. 'Management have been invited to watch what happens', but the timing hasn't worked, 'to try and explain it to people who haven't experienced it, is very difficult'. '[We] do work here that is quite hard to explain to the system that you [we] work in … when you share this with other practitioners they understand'. Another explained their dilemma. If therapeutic work

> … is hard to quantify and difficult to discuss what does that mean for spirituality? Because if that is part of your work that is not always voiced [but] it's only practiced, then how do you explain that bit when you can't explain the work that you do anyway?

5.5 *Meeting 5*

There was a degree of confusion about whether there was a meeting or not and so only half the group attended for a shorter time. After a brief recap on the group's process and changing goals it was agreed that as part of formalising work with clients' spirituality, each client's RAP might contain details that interpret the client's religious affiliations and practices in broader terms than prescribed by those safe and acceptable markers of Christianity and Māori culture. This felt challenging and activated the group, 'I don't care what you [clients] believe as long as there is no harm'. It also interested the group 'that spirituality and culture are included together' on the form. It was perceived as an unconscious Othering of minority religious and indigenous perspectives by a more dominant Western medical model. In addition, there was caution expressed that too much detail might make clients more vulnerable to adverse diagnoses, for example, 'clients who see people and hear people'. Nevertheless, it was agreed that, although naming 'spiritual' experiences could

> … change the label or diagnosis we give them, we could also be accused of being too cautious or unclear in our assessments. Does the problem originate from bio-organic sources in the individual or responses to the impact of external events? These are explainable and fit the 'this makes sense' diagnosis – this is the symptom, this is the diagnosis, and this is the drug. However, there are some experiences that don't fit the medical analysis. Spirituality is made separate from the job that we do – if you are

> unwell spirituality doesn't come into it. It's separate – from the Western perspective – DSM V.

In short, clients may be experts in their own lives but it helps if they are listened to and in turn are offered a full range of explanations, including the spiritual, for their thoughts and behaviours.

5.6 *Meeting 6*

This was also a small but again a very effective group. The integration of spirituality into counselling practice was broadly discussed and looking for 'benefit-finding' in spirituality where there is none, was considered. It was suggested that it was more about seeing the world 'with different eyes'. One member, implying that there is learning or benefit to be found in all experiences, concluded 'I can't believe that people go through things that are a waste of time'. In response to the question, 'Do professionals rationalise pain and suffering, and positively project upon client experiences spiritual explanations to justify their work or are there genuine benefits to be derived from suffering?' one suggested, 'bad stuff is bad stuff and yet there is some good that comes out of it'. Another agreed but referencing the absolute hopelessness of some cases suggested that 'what we might identify as spiritual are those moments of awareness, even in the most difficult and hopeless situations, where the client glimpses, however briefly, a moment of peace'.

Is spirituality then a moment in time when we see something good that is greater than ourselves – transcendence? A client's capacity to reach out, even in the most appalling circumstances, to connect with something that supports them to perform simple and miraculous things for themselves was appreciated. 'How or where does that energy come from that helps individuals to make it through?'[29] However, when clients with a faith find it hard to have a purpose in life, then it appears that therapists can get stuck. An example was given of a suicidal client who, before he took his life, had disclosed that he had lost connection with his soul. 'His soul had moved somewhere and his body had lost its ability to carry on'. Alternatively, there are clients who confer an awesome responsibility to the professional. They should be dead but hang by 'a thread that helps them to survive ... our job is to hold that piece ... to grow it when they can't'.

29 One of the group recalled poem 'Footprints in the Sand' (1936), a poem attributed to Mary Stevenson, that suggested that 'There's something greater at work', viewed 19 June 2018, http://www.footprints-inthe-sand.com/index.php?page=Bio.php.

There is no doubt that the group are affected by clients and their painful lives. A simple example was presented of how humour can restore balance and groundedness.

> Having worked with a particularly harrowing case, I took my student observer off for supervision. I found a box of chocolates. They were quite old but we ended up stuffing them while we talked about the case. Our conversation alternated between discussing how difficult the client was and how good the chocolates were. The student was tearful and we were laughing.

Another story shared 'The negative spiritual energy that some clients can bring'. It highlighted the subtle interplay of the therapist's mental state with the impenetrable depression of the client's. When the therapist recognised the 'dark aura' in the room where he was conducting a group session he felt that he was under attack and

> … needed to protect myself. I have definite, clear experiences of energy that is nothing to do with me but I can't do anything about it … do I need a blessing and cleansing? Does this darker energy exist within the client or is the client the conduit for it? Does it go everywhere the person goes or are we thinking it is in this particular location or group?

As he concluded, it was clear that he had become disconnecting from the discussion and from the rest of the group as he re-experienced that moment. 'Where else do I have the privilege to ask this?' It was a powerful acceptance of the group and revealed his continuing inability to discuss such things elsewhere.

5.7 *Meeting 7*

Back to its full strength the group spent time recapping and looking at the experience of working with addiction and events that might open the client to spiritual experiences. As many of the group's clients have experienced trauma, and addictions have taken them across the threshold between consensus and transpersonal realities, their trauma was addressed and carefully examined through a spiritual lens.

> Trauma with a capital 'T' and trauma with a small 't' … the latter being a number of failures or relapses that affect the psyche – I see that as a

> traumatising ... The jarring effect of addicts undertaking rehabilitation on their own without professional support, and setting themselves up with unreal expectations – almost self-sabotaging a positive outcome because it runs contrary to what they want.

It was generally accepted that addicts are caught in a self-defeating process of making meaning and finding purpose, and it was suggested that the outcome of drug use could be more meaningful than simple sedation in that it heightens experience and also allows the user to be part of a community with shared values, rituals, and recreational habits. 'Even if it's not essentially real [individuals have] a sense of connection with something, community, group or self'.

> In my experience it does open up the third eye and they can be more perceptive to certain things in life but they are not equipped to manage the fact that they have opened up something that causes more trauma in a sense because they are not strong enough ... I think it can cause more harm than good with people who are already damaged.

At this point a number of attempts were made to identify the experience of trauma in their very specific practice contexts. One offered that 'Trauma is the experience you have after the event'. Whilst another asked, 'Or is it more loss of identity, loss of self, loss of sense of safety in the world?'

> The point being that it *has* happened to you and the damage is done and that there is a realisation that this has happened and that you have arrived at a place where you can't go back. Either you have lost something or the people around you have lost you ... the next piece is when they have to come and seek out helping professionals and then make meaning without drugs, and recreate a life without that.

There was general agreement about the therapeutic role.

> You are helping clients to work through their trauma and also working with them not to re-addict – knowing that is always a danger, knowing that will take them back to a place of trauma ...
>
> Sometimes I think we do pick up aspects before the drug and alcohol came in – client developmental pieces that have been useful to the person ... What can we take with us from there? I see it as part of the client reconnecting to what they could have been had that time not happened.

> I like to feel that we hold 'hope'. We hold that potential for them that they may never see … and that's our job … if we didn't have that [passion] what would our work be like?

However, it can be difficult for clients if their therapists place too many expectations on them that they cannot share or achieve. Nevertheless,

> We have to believe it's [change] possible … that the client can achieve recovery. If we don't then what kind of message does that send to the client? I need to have faith that they can be more than they are right now. Faith in the therapeutic process, the human capacity to seek actualisation, however unconsciously.

The final part of this meeting began by attempting to define what spiritual is in the group's practice and ended up talking about their expectations and hopes. The meeting had become quite personal and reflected the therapists' widening view of their work. When the therapeutic relationship is on song then barriers to spiritual modes of communication are removed.

In summary, it was determined that trauma creates a rupture in the process, or journey, towards greater self-actualisation, 'I think that the spiritual part of them is quite depleted when they come here'. In this story addiction is the undesirable outcome of managing, or trying to understand, the affects and consequences of trauma.

> If self-actualisation is driven by the spiritual dimension and it is stopped by trauma, then we are involved in a process to reconnect the individual with the spiritual so that the journey can continue.
>
> [Clients] have to go through the process of reconnection and relearning the world a number of times. So that is the space you are working in. That's the space where informed choices are being made and actions are tentatively taken, disruptions are being challenged, and meaning and learning is happening.

As therapists who facilitate client change, they make adjustments, synchronise or attune themselves with the spiritual character of their clients, and accept their views and aspirations in the moment.

5.8 *Meeting 8*

The group goal for this meeting was to identify connections between trauma and addiction and it began with a lengthy discussion about how the controlled use of substances might develop into addiction. It was assumed that 'controlled use is likely to be a stuck place – a short-cut leading nowhere – where spiritual experience or contact is numbed-out or disconnected rather than a place of continual enlightenment'.

We reviewed our last definition of trauma to incorporate the role of addiction. There was some discussion as to whether addiction can be a result of trauma or whether the addiction creates the trauma. '[Addiction] may not be as a result of trauma but as a result of core beliefs that are formed … that then lead to the use of substance'. A case was recalled where the client's life history didn't reveal any trauma

> … but he was set-up with perfectionism, and a core-belief that he wasn't good enough and a failure … what he did to manage his inability to live up to his own expectations was to use alcohol as a way of coping with that.

Another perspective was presented that argued that through human development everyone faces major or minor disruptions to their core-beliefs but that 'addiction interrupts that continuous journey – addiction is the trauma rather than the developmental stuff which one would expect to occur for everyone'. Put simply,

> Trauma is a reaction and not the event itself. So if the reaction means that we become addicted, which is essentially the result of a coping mechanism, we have a choice as to whether we regard it as a bad thing to do or a good thing … in this context should we judge addiction as something that is wrong?

Another added,

> It is a brain disease … the primitive part of our brain tells us that if the substance feels good it is doing us good, it is keeping us alive. Whereas the pre-fontal parts of our brain tell us it is going to kill us. It's our choice as to whether we use it. … any coping mechanism indicates a dysfunction when it creates something worse than the thing you are trying to avoid.

Addiction, it seems, can be both a response to, and a cause of trauma. Grief, it was suggested, is also a fundamental part of the process of giving up addiction, 'It can create trauma when people are asked to consider not drinking again for the rest of their lives. Clients go through the grief and trauma of that realisation'.

One member disclosed that his habitual substance use led to a series of traumatic experiences, 'paranoia, low self-esteem, loss of relationships, loss of a good place in the world, hair loss, tics … a trap'.

Addiction responds to the emotional rather than the rational self.

> Addicts don't drink to feel better they drink not to feel worse … It's a 'false normal'. Keeping people on long-term methadone scripts can impact upon and numb their spirituality and connections to others. Drugs reverse our sense of reality.

Nevertheless, talking about client growth from a place of addiction, 'The addiction journey highlights [clients'] inadequacies that they can't hide from' making the road to recovery all the more challenging, an opportunity or a spiritual quest. 'Some clients can be grateful for their addiction journey because of the insights that they have provided and how they have had to learn to relate to the world'. Sadly some young addicts, it was observed, may have never had the opportunity to fully develop themselves, 'we have 12 year olds who are using and becoming addicted. They haven't a clue who they are and what they might become'.

Addiction workers, it was generally agreed, hold the tension between the negative censors of society and an obligation to honour the client's experience. Reflecting upon her own experiences of substance use one of the therapists suggested that it gave her what she needed at the time, which was an antidote to her shyness, and has helped her to become the confident person she is today. 'I wouldn't take it back …'

This group perspective was refreshing. It tended to view addiction as only one aspect of a clients' potential, a part that had lost its way but had also taught itself a lesson. 'By suggesting that the addictive part of personality is only a part of the client can be very liberating … okay so let's look at the rest of the family'. It was explained that the focus of their work is to support the client to integrate this wayward part of self – to 'love the addict'. Recognising that the client still has needs that cannot be met by the addict anymore, 'The work of the therapist is to assist in a realignment of the client on the journey'. To refill the client's depleted spiritual tanks. Clients, it seems, are so used to their trauma 'they don't actually get an insight that it was trauma'. However, removed from its context clients realise that their experiences are beyond normal.

What followed was a series of reflections on how living in a world that is not how we thought it was can, in itself, be a traumatic discovery.

> If trauma is a reaction to 'stuff' that you didn't realise was traumatic until you react to it, then the role of the therapist seems to be to reveal the trauma that is already there. There's a whole raft of stuff that then happens after that and it as that point that the client realises that these are the reasons for her behaviour and thoughts – giving them an explanation for their addictive behaviour.

As much as addiction is a response to trauma it seems that it is also a by-product of the individual's desire to make meaning. This resonated with an earlier discussion on finding meaning in existence and the search for wholeness.[30] For some even the search is impossible to understand or accomplish successfully. As one therapist realistically noted,

> I have yet to meet a person who doesn't have a reason to be addicted. Our work here is to look for what created that, why that person needs to use substance ... when they come here they are already defined as being a dependent substance user. Some accept the diagnosis and some don't but the real struggle is to accept that they will need to be abstinent for the rest of their lives. They acknowledge that they use substance in a maladaptive way but that they can never use substance again as a coping mechanism is the real struggle.

5.9 *Meeting 9*

Our final discussion began with a broad preamble from me as the facilitator that brought us back to the group's value as addictions professionals. They responded by generously expressing their appreciation of the group's process which had led to an important personal reassessment of their practices and their professional growth. 'We've come this far – we've got this document', the transcripts of our meetings, 'Something to guide [our] deliberations into the future'. They felt that they had begun to name spirituality in their practices but still had the challenge of normalising it amongst their colleagues. Nevertheless it was agreed that they had progressed from a general discussion to specifically talking about spirituality as part of a collaborative therapeutic partnership,

30 Christina Grof reminds us that human beings have a fundamental desire for wholeness that is satisfied through their attachments to each other, their environment, and with Creation through sacred and spiritual experiences. 'The only way we successfully satisfy this elemental craving for wholeness or for God is through an ongoing relationship with a vast spiritual source'. Grof, *The Thirst for Wholeness*, 1.

and that they had begun describing how the narratives of spiritual journeys could become metaphors for their clients' regenerative processes.

I reminded the group that from their original invitation to present information on post-traumatic growth and spirituality they seemed to have a clearer understanding of their stories of spirit especially when presented and heard in the context of their own beliefs and values, experiences and training. Our meetings had initiated a starting point for them to share personal stories of spirituality as useful aspects of their professional personas.

Whilst the challenge of openly recognising spirituality in their current practices remained 'an uncomfortable fit with the medical model', three members of the group shared that they had drawn comfort from a recent lecture that they had attended on neuroscience that drew attention to Jung's collective unconscious and resonated with and affirmed their work with clients. As one attendee put it, 'the human brain is uniquely responsive and does not always conform to medical model strategies or treatments – we don't know it all yet!' The lecture was timely and unsettling as it suggested that the existing medical model, in privileging medical procedures over human relationship 'just isn't working'.

Moving on to clarifying some of their centre's approaches to psychological assessment, its psycho-educational approach to recovery, post-programme support and the 'cult-like' qualities of the 12-Step Programme, there was a lively debate about the positive aspects and limitations of such programmes and also about co-existing issues of disempowerment and dependence. It was observed that even in the 12 Steps clients lack personal agency because they 'simply surrender and transfer their dependence from one force [substance addiction] to another [God]'.

A number of encouraging comments were made about the group experience and the importance of the work that individuals had decided to do for themselves.

> I realised in the course of our discussions that I have discounted the spiritual side of me and realise that it is a big part of who I am … as I unpack it it's a big component and I think I have minimised that … the writing has allowed me to reconnect with that part of myself.[31]

Although I had naively intended to assist the group to develop a theoretical model of practice, it was clear that each of the group members had come to their own model and spiritual worldview through their rich, if sometimes

31 The group were encouraged to write reflective spiritual biographies.

painful, day-to-day encounters with clients. Through their complex cases, clients had wholly presented themselves in every dimension of their disturbing experience. These powerful encounters had grown their therapists' understanding and inevitably shaped their practices. They had learned that, although this perennial wisdom could be transferred to other clients, it would be much harder to articulate to their senior managers.

> When we open ourselves up to the people we work with we are opening ourselves up to having some not-so-helpful energy with us sometimes but we are the tool of the industry and we need to look after ourselves.

Sadly this learned discretion with colleagues had resulted in disempowerment and prevented them from being fully effective in the communication of their work to others. Understanding and supporting their clients' desires to make meaning, members of the group strongly identified with their marginalised positions and had begun to make their clients' fears of judgment and stigmatisation their own. This had made our discussions more challenging but ultimately more valuable.

By our final meeting we had failed to design a model but we had begun to uncover a fundamental idea that had been present in the group's individual and collective narrative from the beginning. By examining the notoriously ephemeral qualities of spirituality they had identified their need for greater professional autonomy and understanding. Although this important idea was deeply valued and widely articulated in their work with clients it had not resonated with them as individuals in the way that it began to in our work as a group.

> The client has a central core that is comfortable and right, and if it is deviated from there is an experience of tension, dislocation, and a sense of alienation, or dissociation, from the self. At these times you are right to ask 'Who are you genuinely? Where do you want to be in the future? How do we help you to relocate your sense of self and help you to move wherever you need to be?

Acknowledgements

I would especially like to thank my colleagues whose permission, support, transparency, and enthusiastic participation in our Spirituality Special Interest Group made this chapter possible.

Bibliography

American Psychiatric Association. *Diagnostic and Statistical Manual of Mental Disorders*, 4th Edition. Washington: American Psychiatric Association, 2000.

Bray, Peter. 'A Broader Framework for Exploring the Influence of Spiritual Experience in the Wake of Stressful Life Events: Examining Connections between Posttraumatic Growth and Psycho-Spiritual Transformation'. *Mental Health, Religion and Culture* 13.3 (2010): 293–308.

Bray, Peter. 'Naming Spirituality in Counsellor Education: A Modest Proposal'. Special Issue on Counsellor Education in Aotearoa New Zealand. *New Zealand Journal of Counselling* (2011): 76–97.

Bray, Peter. 'Mental Health Therapists Consider the Relevance of Spirituality in their Work with Addiction and Trauma'. *New Zealand Journal of Counselling* 36.1 (2016): 21–46.

Center for Substance Abuse Treatment. 'Anxiety Disorders' in *Assessment and Treatment of Patients with Coexisting Mental Illness and Alcohol and Other Drug Abuse. Treatment Improvement Protocol [TIP] Series 9, DHHS Publication No. SMA 95–3061*. Rockville: Substance Abuse and Mental Health Services, 1994. Viewed 19 June 2018. http://www.ncbi.nlm.nih.gov/bookshelf/br.fcgi?book=hssamhsatip&part=A30236.

Center for Substance Abuse Treatment. *Trauma-Informed Care in Behavioral Health Service: Treatment Improvement Protocol (TIP) Series No. 57*. Rockville: Substance Abuse and Mental Health Services Administration, 2014.

Doweiko, Harold E. 'Substance Use Disorders as Symptoms of Spiritual Disease'. In *Addiction and Spirituality a Multidisciplinary Approach*, edited by Oliver J. Morgan and Merle Jordan, 33–53. St. Louis: Chalice Press, 1999.

Durie, Mason. *Whaiora: Mäori Health Development*. Auckland: Oxford University Press, 1994.

Elliott, Robert, Jeanne C. Watson, Rhonda N. Goldman, and Leslie S. Greenberg. *Learning Emotion-focused Therapy: The Process-experiential Approach to Change*. Washington, DC: American Psychological Association (2004).

Ellis, Carolyn, Tony E. Adams and Arthur P. Bochner. 'Autoethnography: An Overview', *Forum Qualitative Sozialforschung / Forum: Qualitative Social Research* 12.1 (2010): np. Viewed 19 June 2018. http://nbn-resolving.de/urn:nbn:de:0114-fqs1101108.

Frank, Arthur W. *The Wounded Storyteller*. Chicago & London: The University of Chicago Press, 1995.

Frank, Arthur W. 'Why Doctors' Stories Matter'. *Canadian Family Physician*, 56.1 (2010): 51–54.

Galanter, Marc. 'Spirituality and Addiction: A Research and Clinical Perspective'. *The American Journal on Addictions* 15 (2006).

Grof, Christina. *The Thirst for Wholeness: Attachment, Addiction, and the Spiritual Path.* New York: HarperOne, 1993.

Grof, Stanislav and Christina Grof, eds. *Spiritual Emergency: When Personal Transformation Becomes a Crisis.* New York: G.P. Putnam's Sons, 1989.

Janoff-Bulman, Ronnie. *Shattered Assumptions: Towards a New Psychology of Trauma.* New York: Free Press, 1992.

Logrip, Marian L., Eric P. Zorrilla and George F. Koob. 'Stress Modulation of Drug Self-Administration: Implications for Addiction Comorbidity with Post-Traumatic Stress Disorder'. *Neuropharmacology* 62 (2012): 552–564.

Office of Applied Studies, Substance Abuse and Mental Health Services Administration (SAMHSA). 'Mental Health Screenings and Trauma-Related Counseling in Substance Abuse Treatment Facilities'. *The N-SSATS Report,* September 30, 2010.

Orange, Claudia. *The Treaty of Waitangi.* Wellington, New Zealand: Allen & Unwin, 1987.

Pere, Rose. *Te Wheke: A Celebration of Infinite Wisdom.* Gisborne: Ao Ako Global Learning, New Zealand, 1997.

Schafer, Ingo, Willemmien Langeland, Johanna Hissbach, Christel Luedecke, Martin D. Ohlmeier, Claudia Chodzinski, Ulrich Kemper and Peter Keiper. 'Childhood Trauma and Dissociation in Patients with Alcohol Dependence and Drug Dependence, or Both – A Multi-Centre Study'. *Drug and Alcohol Dependence* 109 (2010); 84–89.

Todd, Fraser C. *Te Ariari o te Oranga: The Assessment and Management of People with Co-existing Mental Health and Substance Use Problems.* Ministry of Health: Wellington, 2010.

Walton-Moss, Benita, Ellen M. Ray and Kathleen Woodruff, 'Relationship of Spirituality or Religion to Recovery from Substance Abuse'. *Journal of Addictions Nursing* 24.4 (2013): 217–226.

Webber, Melinda. *Walking the Space Between: Identity and Mäori/Päkehä.* Wellington: NZCER Press, 2008.

West, William. *Psychotherapy and Spirituality.* London: SAGE Publications, 2001.

CHAPTER 10

Dementia Fiction: Giving Voice to an Experience beyond Language

Naomi Krüger

Abstract

Stories about dementia have ethical implications. Both cultural and fictional narratives about this disease have the potential to strengthen the fear and disgust that often surrounds it. This in turn can impact the way people living with dementia are viewed and treated. While there has been much criticism of de-humanising, biomedical approaches and much focus on the implications of language used in cultural narratives, the fact remains that dementia is a devastating degenerative disease. In light of this, how can stories and storytelling contribute towards assembling 'a new humanity in the loss,'[1] inspiring empathy and hope, without effacing the painful reality of the condition? I will attempt to answer this question by telling the story of my own creative process in writing a novel as part of my PhD thesis that is partly narrated by a character with dementia. By reflecting on the experiences that inspired my fictional narrative, and the ethical and aesthetic challenges that I faced along the way, I will argue that narrative does have an important role to play in re-visioning the lived experience of dementia and the way we approach care and support. I will draw on critics from the fields of literary disability studies and medical humanities to support my argument. Furthermore, in using creative nonfiction to express my ideas, I hope to show not only that stories can help us to re-imagine and re-characterise dementia, but also, as David Herman asserts, that 'narrative itself can work to readjust the contextual parameters in terms of which people produce and understand stories.'[2]

Key Words

Dementia – Alzheimer's – fiction – storytelling – ethics of representation

*****

1 David Shenk, *The Forgetting* (London: Flamingo, 2002), 93.
2 David Herman, *Story Logic: Problems and Possibilities of Narrative* (Lincoln: University of Nebraska Press, 2004), 23.

 DOI:10.1163/9789004396067_012

1 Beginnings

'Dementia' is an umbrella-term covering a variety of degenerative neurocognitive disorders, including but not limited to Alzheimer's, and usually associated with older adults. Diagnostic factors include the following:

> Evidence of significant cognitive decline from a previous level of performance in one or more cognitive domains (complex attention, executive function, learning and memory, language, perceptual-motor, or social cognition).[3]

My decision to write about dementia was inspired by a visit to Christine, an old family friend who had recently been diagnosed with Alzheimer's. I almost didn't go. All the most negative and reductive aspects of the disease came rushing forward. I was scared that she would no longer be herself and that she wouldn't recognise me. I was scared of blankness and violence, of seeing emptiness instead of personality. In the event, despite difficulties with short-term memory, she was cogent and lucid and reminisced about incidents from my childhood that I had forgotten. I was struck with the complexity of memory, and ashamed that my fear and ignorance had almost stopped me from connecting with her.

I began to read various books – both fact and fiction – about Alzheimer's and memory, misfiring neurons and the accumulation of plaques and tangles. The research took me to the Lake District to attend a conference on ageing and creativity. It was in a panel session, among therapists and doctors, carers and social scientists, listening to a discussion about how people deal with dementia in the absence of God, in the absence of belief in a soul that I started to feel overwhelmed. Our attitude to death can shape our life for good or bad, they said. Moments of transcendence are possible, but there will also be anger, rage and impotence. The psychic retreat from reality is unsustainable and damaging, but that kind of stasis is often more attractive than the risks of life and intimacy. Or, as Freud puts it: 'Our unconscious has as little use now as it ever had for the idea of its own mortality.'[4]

Later, at an evening reading I listened to a poem about dementia and the difficulty of connecting with or coming to know a close relation who, in living memory has always been 'elsewhere.' I started crying. It came from nowhere.

3 American Psychiatric Association, *Diagnostic and Statistical Manual of Mental Disorders*, 3rd ed. (Arlington, VA: American Psychiatric Publishing, 2013), 602.

4 Freud quoted by, Julia Kristeva, *Strangers to Ourselves*, trans. Leon S. Roudicz (New York: Columbia U.P., 1991), 185.

The sudden recollection of my grandfather's final year – shaking hands, hallucinations, memories that were not so much lost as mutilated, distorted, transformed into new and living truths it was useless to contradict. And the mortification of crying in public, the fear that someone might notice, the necessity of concealing all the traces. What surprised me most was my own ability to forget. I had been researching dementia and memory for months, writing about it, thinking about it. I had printed out journal articles on semantic restriction, consciousness and confabulation. And yet, until that moment I had not once connected my research to my immediate family.

Looking back, this seems hard to believe. But that's how it was. It's possible that these memories were not simply repressed. Perhaps it was also the pathology that allowed me to keep things so separate. I was researching Alzheimer's. My grandfather had Parkinson's. The hallucinations, confusion and memory loss were part of his condition but I never used the term 'dementia' in connection with his experience.

I was sixteen when he died. It was January. I don't remember crying. Not once. He had lived with us for my whole life. A constant presence. Walks to the park, mud pies in the garden, the wonky Wendy house he built and the play pit filled with damp builder's sand because the proper stuff was too expensive. Telling me stories in his room as the sun went down across the fields, the pastel stripes filtering through the leaves of the copper beech tree. The endless, ugly rose bushes and sour grapes in the greenhouse and feeding the tomatoes with so much fertilizer they smelt like chemicals. My mother would send me upstairs with his food on a tray because 'we were too bloody noisy,' and I remember the thrill of him asking me to pour some 'Adam's Ale' from the crystal jug on his windowsill. I remember him one Sunday after church whistling 'How Great Thou Art' and mumbling 'If all those silly buggers are going to heaven then please Lord, send me somewhere else.'

Years later he would search for missing keys that he had hidden from 'all the people' who came to his room and wouldn't leave him alone. I would find countless ways to avoid taking the tray to his room. His whiskery goodnight kisses would become alien and unsettling. He would tell my mother that she ran a grand hotel, fall out of bed more than once and eventually end up in a home where she would visit him every day without fail to the amazement of the care staff. I would visit him much less often. The day before he died he would grip her hand. 'I don't know who you are,' he'd say, 'but I know that I love you.' Seeing the words written down now, it seems a little sentimental. I would hesitate before putting it into a story, but it happened all the same.

Perhaps this – my own bewilderment and failure to deal with his loss is the real reason I began to write about dementia. To try to make sense of it and replace fear with some kind of hope. But it's really impossible to be sure. 'Writers,' David Lodge argues, 'discover what it is they want to say in the process of saying it, and their explanations of why they wrote something in a particular way are therefore always retrospective extrapolations, working back from effect to cause – wisdom after the event.'[5]

2 The Ethics of Story

A diagnosis of Alzheimer's has become a terrifying prospect. People living with the condition are often referred to as zombies or 'the living dead' and the disease itself is increasingly personified as a merciless thief, a brutal enemy or an impending natural disaster.[6] As critics point out, Alzheimer's is regularly framed in terms of warfare and 'understood as an antagonist that "attacks" or "strikes" the brains of "victims."'[7] Hannah, Zeilig asserts that language and representations like these, result in a popular perception of dementia that is shot through both with images of natural disaster and mass destruction on one hand, and the idea that the condition hunts down, attacks and destroys individuals in a cruel and targeted way on the other. 'In both cases,' she argues, 'the effect is to make us feel both terrified and powerless.'[8]

When I began writing the novel it was with these damaging metaphors in mind. I wanted to write against reductive, biomedical representations that were so prevalent in the western media. I wanted to narrate dementia from 'the inside,' to write from the perspective of a character struggling with memory and perception in a rich and empathetic way, to reduce the distance between reader and character, to complicate the neat division of self/other. I posted an early draft chapter onto an online conference for peer review and was startled when a fellow student – not actually in my group, and therefore not obliged or expected to offer feedback – put forward a passionate critique of the work.

5 David Lodge, *Consciousness and the Novel* (London: Penguin, 2002), 110.

6 Susan M. Behuniak, 'The Living Dead? The Construction of People with Alzheimer's Disease as Zombies,' *Ageing & Society* 31 (2011): 70–92.David Cameron, 'UK Calls on World to Tackle Global Crisis of Dementia,' Department of Health Press Release, 30 August 2018, https://www.gov.uk/government/news/uk-calls-on-world-to-tackle-global-crisis-of-dementia. Caroline David, 'Martin Amis in New Row over Dementia Booths' *The Guardian*, 30 August 2018, http://www.theguardian.com/books/2010/jan/24/martin-amis-euthanasia-booths-alzheimers.

7 Daniel R. George, and Peter J Whitehouse, 'The War (on Terror) on Alzheimer's,' *Dementia* 13 (2014): 122.

8 Hannah Zeilig, 'Dementia as a Cultural Metaphor,' *The Gerontologist* 54.2 (2013): 261.

Parts of it were nicely written, she said, but as a story about dementia it just didn't ring true. She questioned the clarity of the character's thoughts, the neat flow of the writing. Then she told me about the reality: 'My mother-in-law,' she said, 'appears to me to be pretty much on a daily acid-trip, replete with hallucinations and some occasional moments of lucidity. So I had difficulty believing your protagonist was really suffering from dementia, even the early stages of it, as her memories were far too coherent.'

I was bruised by the truth of her criticism. And, not for the first time, I wondered if I was, in fact, just wasting my time trying to narrate something fundamentally un-narratable, trying to humanise something that was unremittingly bleak and hopeless. In replacing those totalising narratives with something more layered and positive, was I actually just effacing the real pain and distress that dementia brings? As Joe Moran argues, dementia 'can never be narrated adequately – part of it will always slip through the discursive sphere into raw experience, being a depressing, terrifying experience for both sufferers and those close to them.'[9]

I began to see this tension – the need for positivity and challenge pitted against the harsh lived reality of dementia – played out on online forums and in the comments sections of articles about the effects of the disease. One particularly telling exchange was a Daily Mail article about Dr David Hilfiker, in which he describes some of the positive aspects of living with Alzheimer's:

> We tend to be scared of Alzheimer's or embarrassed by it.... We see it as the end of life rather than a phase of life with all its attendant opportunities for growth, learning, and relationships. We see only the suffering and miss the joy. We experience only the disappearing cognitive abilities and ignore the beautiful things that can appear.[10]

In the comments that followed, among the many people who admired his positivity and courage there were also suspicious dissenters. One particularly emphatic response by a subscriber writing under the name 'usednurse' read as follows:

---

9 Joe Moran, 'Aging and Identity in Dementia Narratives,' *Cultural Values* 5.2 (2001): 258.

10 David Hilfiker quoted by, Hayley Peterson, 'Doctor with Alzheimer's writes About "watching the lights go out" – and says he's never felt happier,' *The Daily Mail*, 2 April 2013 <http://www.dailymail.co.uk/news/article-2302625/Doctor-David-Hilfiker-Alzheimers-writes-watching-lights-out.html>.

> In a short while he won't remember or recognise his wife, what about that 'renewed love' then? He must have had a **** life before if he finds dementia a cause of happiness.[11]

Of course, it is possible for both these viewpoints to be valid. No two people who are diagnosed with a form of dementia have the same experience.[12] Symptoms are likely to be alleviated or exacerbated by life history, existing health problems, environmental factors and the kind of treatment and care that is received.[13] Furthermore, as the disease progresses and the lived experience inevitably slips through the 'discursive sphere' it could be argued that trying to represent this experience using only language is a hopelessly misguided endeavour.

Despite these moments of doubt, I began to experiment. I started to write a polyphonic novel called *May*, partly narrated by the eponymous character, a Lancashire postmistress, housewife, mother and grandmother in the later stages of dementia. Her fragmented account of one particular day in the care home is filled with her longing for the truth about Ned – a mysterious red-haired boy who haunts her with his need to be remembered.[14]

I wanted to plunge readers into May's disordered consciousness so that they were – if only momentarily – forced to imagine what it might be like to be in that situation, forced to search for meaning and connection. May's voice, consciousness, or, more accurately 'mentalese' – to borrow from Oliver Sacks – is necessarily fragmented, fractured, full of gaps, song lyrics, idioms, confabulations and brief, intense flashes of memory.[15] She feels as though people are lying to her. She's not entirely sure where she is or why:

> 9:42 am
> They only think about themselves. I could tell them a thing or two.
> I could –

11 Ibid (from the online comments).

12 Margaret Lock, *The Alzheimer Conundrum: Entanglements of Dementia and Aging* (Princeton: Princeton University Press, 2013), 63.

13 Tom Kitwood, *Dementia Reconsidered: The Person Comes First* (Maidenhead: Open University Press, 2012).

14 Naomi Krüger, 'The "terrifying question mark": Dementia, Fiction and the Possibilities of Narrative,' *Popularizing Dementia: Public Expressions And Representations of Forgetfulness* (*Aging Studies Volume 6*) ed. Aagje Swinnen, Mark Schweda (Transcript, 2015), 109–133.

15 Oliver Sacks, 'The Mind's Eye: What the Blind See,' *New Yorker*, July 28 2003, Viewed 04 July 2018. https://www.newyorker.com/magazine/2003/07/28/the-minds-eye.

> if they stopped putting these whatsits all over the place, don't need the things
> on my knees don't need them everywhere. I like a straight back. I like to be able to see in the corners in the dark places behind
> trees and feathers and bird's eggs he brought
> messages
> I see the stars, I hear the rolling thunder I want to hear the music but there are people talking on the watching thingy
> talking and clapping and shouting their uncouth ways. Why
> would anyone want to see this when there is so much
> more
> the boy, the boy, the boy. The sun in his hair as he runs to the trees there are
> more things in heaven and earth[16]

If dementia destroys the ability to makes connections between past, present and future – and by implication to tell coherent, linear stories or even imagine yourself as part of one – then it seemed appropriate that this disruption would find its way into the texture and structure of the novel.[17] Many stories about dementia, including true accounts, make use of traditional linear narrative techniques. And while this could be seen in some ways as an act of defiance or a way to make some sense out of chaos, there are also more complex ethical implications:

> Although such a perpetuation of traditional concepts of authorship may appease the fears of readers who suffer from early symptoms of dementia themselves, it impedes more flexible, encompassing, and indulgent concepts of vulnerable narrative selves and excludes all sufferers who have no 'success stories' to tell.[18]

Throughout the writing process I struggled to find a balance between ethical and aesthetic concerns. There was a constant tension produced by the desire

16 Naomi Krüger, *May* (Brigend: Seren, 2018), 47–48.

17 Lars Christer-Hyden, Linda Orulv, 'Interaction and Narrative Structure in Dementia,' *Telling Stories: Language, Narrative, and Social Life*, ed. Deborah Schriffin, Anna DeFina, and Anastasia Nylund (Washington, D.C.: 2010), 149–160.

18 Irmela Marei Krüger-Fürhoff, 'Narrating the Limits of Narration: Alzheimer's Disease in Contemporary Literary Texts,' *Popularizing Dementia: Public Expressions And Representations of Forgetfulness* (*Aging Studies Volume 6*) ed. Aagje Swinnen, and Mark Schweda (Transcript, 2015), 95.

to provide coherence, connection and accessibility for readers but also to write in a way that would not misrepresent or oversimplify the condition. I wanted to produce a text that would be challenging, flexible and encompassing. I tried to move towards this with experiments in stream of consciousness, the inclusion of multiple voices, deliberate gaps and jumps in time.

One chapter in the novel, loosely inspired by my time volunteering in a dementia day centre, is narrated by Afsana, a new care-worker on her first day in the job. Gill, the more experienced staff member prompts the residents to share their life histories one-by-one in a therapeutic storytelling session:

> He looks at me.
> 'What's your name again, hen?'
> 'Afsana.'
> 'Afsana. Af. Sana. Well, that's a new one.' He angles his chair away from Gill and leans across the table. 'What is it we're doing here Afsana? What are we waiting for? What's expected?'
> I sit down next to May who mutters something under her breath. Before I can answer him Gill steps in. 'Life stories, Malcolm,' she doesn't look up, 'we're sharing memories.'
> 'Well in that case let's start at the beginning. Picture it: The Glasgow slums, nineteen.... nineteen...,' he waves his hands around and almost hits Tony in the head, 'oh, sod it. A bloody long time ago. One cold morning when the rain is shitting down, a baby slips out of its mother a month too early. Slips out of her like a mackerel from the Clyde.'
> Gill sighs. 'It's Tony's turn now, Malcolm, we're listening to Tony's memories.' She reaches out and touches Tony's sleeve. He jumps a little and looks up, adjusts his glasses, tries to focus. 'That's right, isn't it, love. You remember? We were talking about where you met you wife, Jean.'[19]

Here, Malcolm's fragmented but imaginative storytelling fails to be acknowledged by the session leader both because of the 'improper' language he uses and because it transgresses the order of the group, violating the requirement for linearity and coherence. As Afsana settles into the job she finds it increasingly difficult to ignore these strange and intriguing fragments, often wondering about the real experiences behind them. In a wider sense I am interested in the way narrative is valued and often seen as essential to meaningful existence,[20]

19 Krüger, *May*, 66–67.

20 Alasdair MacIntyre, *After Virtue: A Study in Moral Theory* (London: Gerald Duckworth, 1985), 218–219.

and, by extension, what this could possibly mean for people who are unable to produce it. Although the nature of dementia means that this question is particularly charged – dementia is not the only condition that prompts us to consider the value and production of narrative. This can be seen in discussions elsewhere in this collection that consider the problematic nature of restitution narratives and the importance of considering the way meaning is 'socially and collectively produced.'[21]

Stephen Post argues that in a hyper-cognitive society that situates memory as the source of humanity and personhood, people living with dementia are easily written off.[22] It is possible that at a certain point in the progression of the disease, trying to restore a coherent account of life history, however well-meaning, could be a continual, distressing reminder of everything that has been lost, everything that has now become impossible.[23]

Anne Davis Basting outlines an alternative: a pioneering project called Time*Slips*, which involves 'free-form storytelling' facilitated by trained staff who use varied visual prompts to generate collaborative stories in dementia care homes.[24] By leaving behind 'preconceived notions of what constitutes a "story,"'[25] facilitators regard all responses to the open questions as valid and incorporate them into inevitably meandering but often creative and entertaining storylines. As Basting states, this kind of storytelling 'runs counter to theories of narrative healing' and can seem much closer to what Arthur Frank describes as a 'chaos narrative,'[26] but this deliberate rejection of beginning, middle and end also has the potential to be valuable and therapeutic:

> People with dementia, silenced by confusion and the social pressure to say the right thing, learn to experiment with language and form social bonds with staff and participants in the process.[27]

---

21 Mirjam Stuij, Agnes Elling, Anja Tramper and Tineke Abma, 'Developing a Relational Narrative about Diabetes: Towards a Polyphonic Story,' in this volume. Hans T. Sternudd, 'Voices of Depression: An Analysis of a Collective Narrative,' in this volume.

22 Stephen G. Post, 'The Concept of Alzheimer Disease in a Hypercognitive Society,' *Concepts of Alzheimer Disease: Biological, Clinical and Cultural Perspectives*, ed. Peter Whitehouse, Konrad Maurer, Jesse F. Ballenger (Baltimore: Johns Hopkins University Press, 2003), 245–256.

23 Helen Small, *The Long Life* (Oxford: Oxford University Press, 2007), 204–205.

24 Time*Slips* Organisation: https://www.timeslips.org, Viewed 04 July 2018.

25 Anne Davis Basting, 'Creative Storytelling and Self-Expression among People with Dementia,' *Thinking About Dementia: Culture, Loss, and the Anthropology of Senility*, eds. Annette Leibing, Lawrence Cohen (New Brunswick: Rutgers University Press, 2006), 181.

26 Ibid., 182.

27 Ibid., 181.

3 Finding Connection

Just as the Time*Slips* project seeks to restore voice to people who have 'few meaningful social roles available to them,'[28] the decision to allow May to 'speak' for herself in the novel was ethically charged. More than this, though, by situating her in a community of voices, I wanted to echo the ideas prominently advocated by Tom Kitwood and other proponents of 'person-centred care,'[29] that her identity – while fragile and disintegrating – is inter-subjective. She is not just her diagnosis. She is also part of a family, community and wider society. Thus, her sections of the novel are interspersed with the voices of other characters speaking from shifting moments in time: her husband, daughter, grandson and the only care assistant she trusts or connects with. In this excerpt, May is trying to make sense of her present surroundings, to put herself in context:

> because nobody will tell me what it is I'm expected to do. There'll be a backlog at the Post Office before long. They'll know something's up because I'm never
> and I can't think how to get a message through. No one will give me any stamps.
>
> The ink runs and the letters get mixed up. All the
> words words words
> they never stay put.
>
> The birds try to get in.
> Not the right kind for carrying messages. No one has given me the code. One for sorrow, two for sorrow
> all that peck, peck pecking on the glass.[30]

Although in this extract it seems likely that the birds are imaginary and May is hallucinating, this interpretation is actually complicated earlier in the novel in another chapter narrated by Afsana, a character who is herself, struggling to find a secure sense of identity and belonging:

> I pour May's tea but she doesn't want to talk. She's watching a bird at the window. The first time I've seen one using the feeder Alison put up. It's

28 Ibid., 180.

29 Kitwood, Tom, *Dementia Reconsidered: The Person Comes First* (Maidenhead: Open University Press, 1997), 7–19.

30 Krüger, *May*, 93.

> perching there on the clear plastic, attached to the window with transparent suction cups. Almost like it's trying to get in. A brown bird pecking away. I wish I knew its name.[31]

Afsana's narrative sheds light on the fact that May is not always as unreliable as she seems. Although her lucidity and ability to evaluate reality are in decline, May's perception is also influenced by her environment and her embodied experience of the moment. In this way the novel is a challenge to the individualistic tragedy narratives often present in contemporary dementia fiction.[32] May's confusion and distress is, of course, a source of sadness, but she is not simply a lone figure descending into darkness. She still has moments of awareness and her opportunities for communication and connection are not limited simply to her ability to speak.

And this in turn reflects the idea that it may be more useful to think about dementia and its associated symptoms as one point on a continuum rather than as a dark, terrifying experience impossibly removed from 'normal' consciousness. Our lives may have more in common with this fragmented, momentary experience than we like to think. While some critics cite an obsession with memory and cognition as a harmful framework from which to view dementia, Joe Moran has pointed out that the idea of the postmodern condition as 'an image-obsessed, technologized world' that has excluded memory from our experience and produced a 'perpetual present,' could easily be mistaken for a description of dementia.[33] Indeed, Fredric Jameson characterises this diffuseness and discontent as 'our utter forgetfulness of the past exhausted [...] in the vacant but mesmerized contemplation of a schizophrenic present,' or, in other words, the 'narrative of the end of narratives.'[34]

This way of being in the world has been described as a lack of certainty; the experience of selfhood 'not as an ordered narrative but as a multiple identification amongst the babble of discourses.'[35] Indeed, Mark Currie argues that this produces a kind of space–time compression. Technology allows us to be more connected and unified than ever, while at the same time highlighting our disconnection and distance both physical and otherwise.[36]

31 Ibid., 13.

32 Anne Davis Basting, *Forget Memory: Creating Better Lives for People with Dementia* (Baltimore: John Hopkins University Press, 2009), 40.

33 Joe Moran, 'Aging and Identity,' 251.

34 Fredric Jameson, *Postmodernism or the Cultural Logic of Late Capitalism* (Durham: Duke University Press, 1991), xii.

35 Mark Currie, *Postmodern Narrative Theory* (Basingstoke: Palgrave Macmillan, 2011), 107.

36 Ibid., 107.

It is arguable that our increased ability to record, narrate and 'share' our lives through social and digital media influences the way we experience the present. The developing symptoms of this 'archive fever' mean that the present is never simply present, but is also constantly and exhaustingly imagined in terms of its potential significance for posterity. In other words, it 'anticipates its own pastness in its very form, and is experienced, like everything else in the contemporary world as the object of a future memory.'[37]

Highlighting the way these complex and disorienting cultural shifts affect characters other than May allowed me to draw further attention to these connections. In one telling scene in the novel May's grandson Alex, who is depressed and struggling with a lack of certainty about his future, sits in bed staring at the screen of his laptop 'with the cursor blinking. The whole world at [his] fingertips' unable to 'think of a single thing to type.'[38]

Fredric Jameson suggests, even the idea of the end of narrative is, in itself, another kind of narrative.[39] And while 'grand narratives are the object of critique [...],' it has been argued, 'for little narratives it is business as never before.'[40] There are meta-fictions, almost-stories, counter-narratives and quiet little flash-fictions. Dementia reminds us that some of us may find it more useful, more humane, to consider life in in terms of more fragmentary, episodic structures.

Furthermore, there are also aspects of selfhood which lie outside cognition, outside the realms of language. In her ethnographic study of 'embodied selfhood' in a Jewish care home, Pia Kontos recounts incidents in which patients with severely reduced cognitive function and linguistic ability enact physical processes, sing songs and complete religious rituals independently from reflective cognition. She goes on to suggest that 'selfhood resists the ravages of Alzheimer's disease precisely because it resides in corporeality.'[41] If many of us are encompassed by narrative, then perhaps it is only narrative that can hope to draw our attention to these ideas, these important possibilities that lie beyond the discursive sphere. It could be argued that the need to move our focus from memory to imagination has never been so urgent.

---

37 Mark Currie, *About Time: Narrative, Fiction and the Philosophy of Time* (Edinburgh: Edinburgh University Press, 2007), 9.

38 Krüger, *May*, 162.

39 Jameson, *Postmodernism*, p. xii.

40 Currie, *Postmodern Narrative Theory*, 110.

41 Pia C. Kontos, 'Embodied Selfhood: An Ethnographic Exploration of Alzheimer's Disease,' *Thinking About Dementia: Culture, Loss, and the Anthropology of Senility*, ed. Annette Leibing, Lawrence Cohen (New Brunswick: Rutgers University Press, 2006), 203.

4 Open Endings

On Christmas Eve 2013 I went with a group of relations and friends to sing Christmas carols at a specialist dementia home, the place where Christine was now resident, after her care needs had become too severe for her to continue living alone. It was warm and stuffy inside. No time to take our coats off and nowhere safe to leave them. A member of staff in uniform escorted us inside. Security, it seemed, was important. There were special locks and key codes.

We walked through a corridor decorated with tinsel and paper chains. Notice boards covered with photographs, posters and collages of past events. A legendary local football player from the 1950s, a 1940s wedding, a family of girls standing on a promenade – probably Blackpool – in their printed dresses, circle-skirts puffed out with net petticoats, tight sweaters, handbags and carefully rolled hair.

In the public lounge we almost outnumbered the residents. We were a disruption, a talking point. We arranged ourselves into a messy group in one corner. One man got up immediately to move away. A woman demanded to know who we were and what we wanted.

> 'We're going to sing you some carols,' my sister said.
> 'What's that, Betty?'
> 'They're going to sing us some carols.'
> 'Who said we wanted any?' And then to us: 'we don't want any carols.'
> One of the workers said 'Hush now.' There was some nervous laughter.

We were about to start 'Joy to the World' when my father pointed out where Christine was sitting. She was in the far corner and none of us had noticed because she looked so small and slumped and different. We had almost forgotten she was the reason we were there in the first place. Her hair was entirely white. Her eyes were closed and I couldn't tell whether she was asleep or not. Her teeth must have been somewhere else because her mouth was slack and puckered. He walked across the room to sit with her. She'd remember him because he still visited so often, but the rest of us would just have to wait and see.

The final couple of bars were played as an introduction and we launched into the first verse of the song, finding our parts a few notes in, settling into the melody. My daughter wound her way through the squashed mass of the choir to find my hand and lean against me. She wanted reassurance; she wanted to know that things would be ok. I put my arm around her and carried on singing the harmony. *Let every heart prepare him room, and saints and angels sing*. I've never had any major problems with the high notes but I like alto better. I don't like to do the obvious. I like to complicate things.

The songs went on and at the back of the room two women sat shoulder to shoulder, swaying and smiling and singing along. Word perfect. We didn't sound too bad. Even the protesters didn't look outraged. Christine woke up – was woken up – and my father said something to her. He pointed to us and she looked up and back to him. He was explaining who we were. She didn't look particularly interested.

And then, during the refreshments we mingled and spoke to people. We had to be careful; the usual small talk wasn't going to cut it. *So what are you doing for Christmas?* sounded even more hollow than normal. It was bordering on mockery. Asking about the future was dangerous and there just wasn't enough time to inquire seriously into the past. I sat next to Christine for a minute but she was already surrounded.

> 'What did you think of our singing?' someone asked her, 'did you enjoy it?' 'More or less,' she said.

She was never easily impressed. Always exacting and slow to give praise. Always a dry sense of humour and a keen awareness of human frailty. Some things don't change. I heard my name from across the room. My dad was beckoning me over. My daughter had attracted attention. Young children were probably a rarity.

One woman was standing up, beckoning her forward. 'Come here,' she said, and then 'Oh! You're lovely.' She took my daughter's hand and turned it over.

'Let me give you something, just a little something.'

The woman opened her handbag and pulled out a couple of white paper tissues. She pressed them into her hand.

'There you go,' she said, 'just a little something. You can treat yourself.' She turned to me. 'Can you use it?' she said, 'to get her something nice?'

'Yes,' I said, 'thank you, that's really kind of you.'

'Wait,' she said, 'take these, have some more, you're a lovely little thing.'

She drew out another wedge of them, and I wondered if she had a whole box of the things stashed at the bottom of the bag. I wondered what else she had hidden in there. I thought of Mary Poppins pulling a cheval mirror and wooden hat stand out of her magical tapestry carpetbag. My daughter looked at the tissues and then at me and then back to the woman. She smiled and whispered a thank you and passed them to me behind her back so I could slip them straight into my pocket. We backed away. It was time to get going.

'She thought she was giving you money,' I said as we walked back towards the corridor.

'I know. She was nice.'

That was it. She was off, running ahead of me to catch up with her cousins. We said our goodbyes and walked back past the bedrooms with name plaques on every door and photographs of the people the residents used to be. I reached into my pocket to get my gloves ready and felt the thick wad of tissues and wondered about the ethics of playing along. If the money had been real it would've been too much by far. I would've had to refuse. But sometimes pretending – I won't say lying – seems to be the humane thing to do. It was a harmless enough fiction after all. And it's not hard for things to get mixed up, for an untenable gap, a jarring absence to be filled in or neutralized or occupied by a mind that is constantly searching for sense and coherence. Linda Orulv argues that in dementia, confabulations are more than simply false statements with no connection to the immediate context:

> Rather they should be regarded as meaning – or sense-making processes for the persons telling, listening to and acting upon them, and closely linked to the local context as well as the life-history context.[42]

Out in the cold again, walking over to the car, it didn't take a minute for my mind to turn to home. There were things to be done. The stove to restock with wood, presents to wrap, the food and drink to lay ready on the table. I checked my phone to see if my husband was home from work, whether he had managed to get out early.

Tomorrow there would be games to play. Lego to assemble, films to watch, more books to fit on the shelf. And in a couple of weeks, when she was bored of all the new stuff, I would probably be co-opted into my daughter's favourite fantasy again. She'd put a tea-towel over the footstool in the living room, set up her pretend cooker, write out a comprehensive lunch menu and demand that I order a strange variety of dishes: ham soup and a fried egg followed by yoghurt and Battenberg cake. A slice of lemon on the side. She'd serve me wooden food on plastic plates and order me to pay for it, to leave her a generous tip with banknotes she'd shaped and drawn and authenticated herself out of little scraps of paper rescued from the recycling pile.

42 Linda Orulv, and Lars-Christer Hyden, 'Confabulation, sense-making, self-making and world-making in dementia,' *Discourse Studies* 8 (2006): 653.

5 Conclusion

Telling stories about dementia has ethical implications. I am not the first or last writer to attempt to write against reductive perspectives by trying to represent the disease from 'the inside.' The challenge of this process has been managing the continual tension between the ethical implications of aesthetic decisions and the need to tell a story coherent enough that it would remain 'readable.' This is a tricky balance, but the process of textual experiment has enabled me to become more aware of my own narrative expectations and how much I rely on memory to imagine my place in the world and narrate my hopes for the future. David Shenk argues that the challenge of dementia is to 'escape the medical confines of *disease* and to assemble a new humanity in the loss.'[43] I believe that fictional representations of this condition can have value as they seek to complicate the idea of a single story about dementia. As the novelist Chimamanda Ngozi Adichie argues so eloquently, 'the problem with stereotypes is not that they are untrue, but that they are incomplete.'[44] In a cultural atmosphere that is dominated both by reductive master-narratives and the idea that complex cognition and individual success is the ultimate achievement, stories that draw attention to the need for connection, the need to think beyond traditional narrative structures, are vital. There is still work to be done. I hope that my novel can contribute towards this new humanity, a more expansive, hopeful and informed response to a disease that inspires such terror and disgust. I hope that telling stories about a condition that seems to be unarratable, about people who are increasingly unable to tell their own stories in a coherent way – and reflecting on the challenges of the process – can be part of a more imaginative approach to care and connection.

Bibliography

Adichie, Chimamanda Ngozi. 'The Danger of a Single Story' Viewed 04 July 2018. https://www.ted.com/talks/chimamanda_adichie_the_danger_of_a_single_story/transcript?language=en.

American Psychiatric Association. *Diagnostic and Statistical Manual of Mental Disorders*, 3rd ed. Arlington, VA: American Psychiatric Publishing, 2013.

43 Shenk, *The Forgetting*, 93.

44 Chimamanda Ngozi Adichie, 'The Danger of a Single Story' Viewed 04 July 2018, https://www.ted.com/talks/chimamanda_adichie_the_danger_of_a_single_story/transcript?language=en.

Basting, Anne Davis. 'Creative Storytelling and Self-Expression among People with Dementia,' in *Thinking about Dementia: Culture, Loss, and the Anthropology of Senility*. Edited by Annette Leibing and Lawrence Cohen. New Brunswick: Rutgers University Press 2006, 180–194.

Basting, Anne Davis. *Forget Memory: Creating Better Lives for People with Dementia*. Baltimore: Johns Hopkins University Press, 2009.

Behuniak, Susan M. 'The Living Dead? The Construction of People with Alzheimer's Disease as Zombies.' *Ageing & Society* 31 (2011): 70–92.

Cameron, David. 'UK Calls on World to Tackle Global Crisis of Dememtia,' Department of Health Press Release, 11 December 2013. Accessed 30 August 2018. https://www.gov.uk/government/news/uk-calls-on-world-to-tackle-global-crisis-of-dementia.

Currie, Mark. *Postmodern Narrative Theory*. Basingstoke: Palgrave Macmillan, 2011.

David, Caroline. 'Martin Amis in New Row over Dementia Booths' *The Guardian*, 24 January 2010. Accessed 30 August 2018. http://www.theguardian.com/books/2010/jan/24/martin-amis-euthanasia-booths-alzheimers.

George, Daniel R. and Peter J Whitehouse. 'The War (on Terror) on Alzheimer's.' *Dementia* 13 (2014): 120–130.

Herman, David. *Story Logic: Problems and Possibilities of Narrative*. Lincoln: University of Nebraska Press, 2004.

Hyden, Lars-Christer and Linda Orulv. 'Interaction and Narrative Structure in Dementia.' *Telling Stories: Language, Narrative, and Social Life*. Edited by Deborah Schriffin, Anna DeFina and Anastasia Nylund, 149–160. Washington, D.C.: 2010.

Jameson, Fredric. *Postmodernism or the Cultural Logic of Late Capitalism*. Durham: Duke University Press, 1991.

Kitwood, Tom. *Dementia Reconsidered: the Person Comes First.* Maidenhead: Open University Press, 2012.

Kontos, Pia C. 'Embodied Selfhood: An Ethnographic Exploration of Alzheimer's Disease.' *Thinking about Dementia: Culture, Loss, and the Anthropology of Senility*. Edited by Annette Leibing and Lawrence Cohen, 195–217. New Brunswick: Rutgers University Press, 2006.

Kristeva, Julia. *Strangers to Ourselves*. Translated by Leon S. Roudiez. New York: Columbia, 1991.

Krüger, Naomi. *May*. Brigend: Seren, 2018.

Krüger, Naomi. 'The "terrifying question mark": Dementia, Fiction and the Possibilities of Narrative.' *Popularizing Dementia: Public Expressions and Representations of Forgetfulness* (*Aging Studies Volume 6*). Edited by Aagje Swinnen and Mark Schweda, 109–133.Transcript, 2015.

Krüger-Fürhoff and Irmela Marei. 'Narrating the Limits of Narration: Alzheimer's Disease in Contemporary Literary Texts.' *Popularizing Dementia: Public Expressions and*

Representations of Forgetfulness (*Aging Studies Volume 6*). Edited by Aagje Swinnen, Mark Schweda, 89–108. Transcript, 2015.

Lock, Margaret. *The Alzheimer Conundrum: Entanglements of Dementia and Aging*. Princeton: Princeton University Press, 2013.

Lodge, David. *Consciousness and the Novel*. London: Penguin, 2002.

MacIntyre, Alasdair. *After Virtue: A Study in Moral Theory*. London: Gerald Duckworth, 1985.

Moran, Joe, 'Aging and Identity in Dementia Narratives.' *Cultural Values* 5.2 (2001): 245–260.

Orulv, Linda and Lars-Christer Hyden. 'Confabulation, sense-making, self-making and world-making in dementia.' *Discourse Studies* 8 (2006): 647–673.

Peterson, Hayley. 'Doctor with Alzheimer's Writes About "watching the lights go out" – and Says he's Never Felt Happier,' *The Daily Mail*, 2 April 2013. Viewed 04 July 2018. http://www.dailymail.co.uk/news/article-2302625/Doctor-David-Hilfiker-Alzheimers-writes-watching-lights-out.html.

Post, Stephen G. 'The Concept of Alzheimer Disease in a Hypercognitive Society.' *Concepts of Alzheimer Disease: Biological, Clinical and Cultural Perspectives*. Edited by Peter Whitehouse, Konrad Maurer and Jesse F. Ballenger. 245–256. Baltimore: Johns Hopkins University Press, 2003.

Sacks, Oliver. 'The Mind's Eye: What the Blind See.' *New Yorker*, July 28 2003. Viewed 04 July 2018. https://www.newyorker.com/magazine/2003/07/28/the-minds-eye.

Shenk, David. *The Forgetting*. London: Flamingo, 2002.

Small, Helen. *The Long Life*. Oxford: Oxford University Press, 2007.

Time*Slips* Organisation: https://www.timeslips.org, Viewed 04 July 2018.

Zeilig, Hannah. 'Dementia as a Cultural Metaphor.' *The Gerontologist* 54.2 (2013): 258–267.

CHAPTER 11

Developing a Relational Narrative about Diabetes: Towards a Polyphonic Story

Mirjam Stuij, Agnes Elling, Anja Tramper and Tineke Abma

Abstract

The restitution story, the type of illness story about living a healthy life again, is the most prominent type in Western society. Patients who are unable to realise a restitution story might need an alternative 'corpus of stories' to draw on, for example narratives that more explicitly incorporate quest and/or loss. In this chapter, we present the narrative of Anja, a woman with diabetes who wanted, but was unable to live the restitution story. Although she seemed to have all characteristics in favour of 'restitution', such as willingness, capacities, and a higher socioeconomic background, she encountered losses and was not able to go back to her 'normal life'. Through a sociological lens, her narrative habitus was influenced by her privileged position and expressed in her emphasis on 'starting all over again', departing from dominant health discourses that emphasise restitution and individual responsibility. The encounters with the voice of the researcher(s) made her aware of the dominant storyline and, as an incidental outcome of the research process, enabled her to reconstruct her story. Along the way, Anja's story became more polyphonic, as she began to incorporate the voices of the researcher(s) and others. A detailed elaboration of this specific case shows the relational dynamics of narrative development and interpretation, and offers important implications for health care. It points towards the importance of attentiveness, responsibility, and responsiveness as well as solidarity with a broader group of patients suffering from diabetes, including those in less privileged positions.

Key Words

Voices – relational narratives – narrative habitus – care ethics – sociological lens – health care practices

*****

 | DOI:10.1163/9789004396067_013

1 Introduction[1]

An illness, or first signs of an illness, may signify a biographical disruption or a moment of re-orientation as well as a confrontation with formerly taken-for-granted life and bodily ability.[2] In such times, when expectations for continuity are disrupted, (re-)constructing a story can help someone to make sense of events and find new destinations.[3] This construction is not only a personal issue, but also a social one: stories are told to someone, either directly or indirectly, and created in a certain social context that defines what is appropriate to tell and what is not.[4] Furthermore, stories can be (co-)constructed in interaction,[5] for instance in interaction with a health care professional.

Today, the most prominent and culturally recognised type of illness story is the restitution story, with the underlying storyline emphasising recovery from illness and living a healthy life again: 'Anyone who is sick wants to be healthy again. Moreover, contemporary culture treats health as the normal condition that people ought to have restored'.[6] Interestingly, this aim is also underlined by the expression of 'health'-care.

Although restitution might seem incompatible with a chronic condition like diabetes, diabetes treatment generally is directed at maintaining the blood sugar level within the 'normal' range in order to minimise symptoms and future complications. Therefore, certain treatment strategies – like insulin, medication, following a healthy diet and/or being sufficiently physically active – are prerequisite. Implementation of these strategies is aimed to result in a kind of restitution: in feeling healthy and being able to live a nearly 'normal life' again.

In order for this implementation to be successful, these treatment strategies must be incorporated in daily life. Therefore, part of diabetes treatment is aimed at 'behavioural change', or, more precisely, changes regarding smoking,

---

1 This work is part of the research programme Sport: Participation, which is financed by the Netherlands Organisation for Scientific Research (NWO).

2 Michael Bury, 'Chronic Illness as Biographical Disruption', *Sociology of Health and Illness* 4.2 (1982): 167–182; Juliet C. Corbin, 'The Body in Health and Illness', *Qualitative Health Research* 13.2 (2003): 256–267.

3 Arthur W. Frank, *The Wounded Storyteller: Body, Illness, and Ethics* (Chicago: University Press, 1995), 1; Elliot G. Mishler, *Storylines: Craftartists' Narratives of Identity* (Cambridge, MA: Harvard University Press, 1999), 15; Catherine K. Riessman, *Narrative Methods for the Human Sciences* (London: Sage, 2008), 10.

4 Frank, *Wounded Storyteller,* 3.

5 Mishler, *Storylines,* 15.

6 Frank, *Wounded Storyteller,* 77.

exercise and eating behaviour, respectively.[7] To achieve restitution – to get and keep control over one's blood sugar level and feel healthy again – the individual with diabetes needs to become active and make these treatment strategies part of 'normal life'. This fits within a larger neoliberal political and social discourse that strongly emphasises individual autonomy and places the responsibility for health, and illness, with the individual.[8]

Although advice regarding diet and physical activity behaviours are embedded in treatment protocols for people with type 1 and type 2 diabetes, it is especially emphasised in the protocols for the latter, as both the origin of and 'medicine' for type 2 diabetes are to a large extent considered to be related to lifestyle behaviour.[9] The prevalence of type 2 diabetes is much higher among people from lower social classes and ethnic minorities.[10] Moreover, in high-income countries in general, people from the higher social strata tend to be more active and attach more importance to individual responsibility and healthy living.[11] Therefore, many elements in this study are related to intersecting social status positions.

7 Guy E.H.M. Rutten, et al., 'NHG-Standard Diabetes mellitus type 2' [Standard of the Dutch College of General Practitioners on Diabetes mellitus type 2], 3rd ed., *Huisarts en Wetenschappen* 56.10 (2013): 516.

8 Julianne Cheek, 'Healthism: A New Conservatism?' *Qualitative Health Research* 18 (2008): 974–982; Robert Crawford, 'Health as a Meaningful Social Practice', *health: An Interdisciplinary Journal for the Social Study of Health, Illness and Medicine* 10.4 (2006): 401–420; Elizabeth E. Wheatley, 'Disciplining Bodies at Risk: Cardiac Rehabilitation and the Medicalization of Fitness', *Journal of Sport & Social Issues* 29.2 (2005): 198–221.

9 There are several types of diabetes, with type 1 and type 2 being the most commonly known. Type 2 results from an ineffective use of insulin by the body and is the most common form. Type 1 diabetes is characterised by an absolute deficiency in insulin production and insulin needs to be injected daily. Not all individuals easily fit into a single category. Sources: American Diabetes Association, '2. Classification and Diagnosis of Diabetes', *Diabetes Care* 38 Suppl. 1 (2015): S8–S16; World Health Organisation, Diabetes: Fact sheet N°312, Updated March 2013', viewed on 21 June 2018, https://web.archive.org/web/20130826174444/http://www.who.int/mediacentre/factsheets/fs312/en/.

10 Jetty A.A. Dalstra, et al., 'Socioeconomic Differences in the Prevalence of Common Chronic Diseases: An Overview of Eight European Countries', *International Journal of Epidemiology* 34.2 (2005): 316–326; Joanne K. Ujcic-Voortman, Miranda T. Schram, Monique A. Jacobs-van der Bruggen, Arnoud P. Verhoeff and Caroline A. Baan, 'Diabetes Prevalence and Risk Factors among Ethnic Minorities', *European Journal of Public Health* 19.5 (2009): 511–515.

11 Jane Wardle and Andrew Steptoe, 'Socioeconomic Differences in Attitudes and Beliefs about Healthy Lifestyles', *Journal of Epidemiology & Community Health* 57.6 (2003): 440–443.

Elements of the restitution story are recognized by many people with a chronic condition like diabetes.[12] A downside of the dominance of this type of story is the potential limited availability of other storylines when restitution does not work, or is not working anymore.[13] In this chapter, we present the story of Anja, a woman with diabetes who wanted and tried to, but was unable to live the restitution story. Her story illustrates the necessity, but scarcity, of other storylines to fall back on and to remain or regain a sense of self. Furthermore, it shows the importance of relational narrative autonomy, the bringing of actions in line with a sense of self and life story, using the support of others.[14] As Anja's story further developed in interaction with the researcher(s), the aim of this chapter is to give an interpretation of this relational process of narrative development, and to offer implications for the improvement of health care.

2 Storytelling and Narrative Habitus

According to Arthur Frank, people use commonly available narrative ideal types, like the restitution story, as resources to create their own individual story.[15] These are part of what he calls the 'narrative habitus', based on Pierre Bourdieu's concept of habitus. Bourdieu defined this as a durable internalisation of all sorts of habits, a 'second nature' that serves as an unconscious basis for behaviour, thoughts and emotions.[16] Frank identified the following core elements of the narrative habitus:

> knowing a corpus of stories; feeling comfortable telling and hearing certain stories (and not others); and sharing with others a sense of where events in a story are likely to lead. This issue is not only expectations for how plots develop in stories, but also expectations for how people ought to emplot their lives.[17]

12 Mirjam Stuij, Agnes Elling and Tineke Abma, *Mensen met diabetes over sport, bewegen en ziekte. Resultaten kwantitatieve studie* [*People with Diabetes about Sport, Physical Activity and Illness. Results of the Quantitative Study.*] (Utrecht: Mulier Instituut, 2014).

13 Frank, *Wounded Storyteller*, 94. See also Naomi Krüger, 'Dementia Fiction: Giving Voice to an Experience beyong Language', in this volume.

14 Kathryn Abrams, 'Redefining Women's Agency: A Response to Professor Williams'. *Indiana Law Journal* 72 (1997): 459.

15 Frank, *Wounded Storyteller*, 77; Arthur W. Frank, *Letting Stories Breathe: A Socio-Narratology* (Chicago: University Press, 2010), 14.

16 Pierre Bourdieu, *The Logic of Practice* (Cambridge: Polity Press, 1990).

17 Frank, *Letting Stories Breathe*, 195.

In other words, these habitual dispositions lead to a sort of continuity in the stories a person tells.[18] Furthermore, related to health care, it points towards the importance of a shared repertoire, as this offers a certain familiar basis to build on together. Moreover, Frank adds the concept of the 'inner library' as the organization of the narrative habitus: 'people make sense of a story by placing it among similar stories (…) stories they know, including stories they might have heard, or that are resonant in stories they once heard'.[19] Therefore, people are predisposed to pay attention to some stories and not to others.

This predisposition is related to and reflects social status, as people with similar intersecting social positions – like class, ethnicity and gender – partly 'know' one another's experiences and face similar (im)possibilities and living conditions.[20] Furthermore, the narrative habitus is also influenced by political hegemonic stories, like those emphasising health and individual responsibility as important values. According to Marjo Buitelaar, in order for a personal story to be convincing, the narrator needs to make use of the 'collective voice' of the group he or she belongs to, by 'using the rules, conventions and world views that dominate in that group'.[21] These are established in the narrative habitus, and expressed through a 'voice' that has appropriated the collective story.

Despite its durability, someone's habitus is neither unchangeable nor all-decisive.[22] This means that in spite of a certain tendency to fall back on familiar storylines, there is room for development outside this known repertoire, for instance when a story is not sufficient anymore. Therefore, the concept of narrative habitus might offer us a focus to search for underlying plots in a story that are well-known, powerful and persistent, as well as possibilities for changes or resistance to these or other plots that could help us to see openings for narrative development.

---

18 Stephanie Taylor, 'Narrative as Construction and Discursive Resource', *Narrative – State of the Art*, ed. Michael Bamberg (Amsterdam: John Benjamins Publishing Company, 2007), 114; Brett Smith, 'The State of the Art in Narrative Inquiry. Some Reflections'. *Narrative Inquiry* 17.2 (2007): 395.

19 Frank, *Letting Stories Breathe*, 55.

20 Bourdieu, *Logic of Practice;* Diane Reay, '"They employ cleaners to do that": Habitus in the Primary Classroom'. *British Journal of Sociology of Education* 16 (1995): 353–371; Anne Townsend, 'Applying Bourdieu's Theory to Accounts of Living with Multimorbidity'. *Chronic Illness* 8.2 (2011): 3.

21 Marjo Buitelaar, 'De Stemmen van Tahara. De Orkestratie van Verschillende Zelf-Representaties in het Levensverhaal van een Nederlandse Moslimvrouw van Marokkaanse Afkomst'. [The Voices of Tahara. The Orchestration of Different Self-Representations in the Life Story of a Dutch Muslim Woman of Moroccan Background.] *Amsterdams Sociologisch Tijdschrift* 29.1 (2002): 73–77.

22 Bourdieu, *Logic of Practice.*

3 A Case Study on Multiple Voices

The story of Anja was collected as part of a larger research project on meanings of sport and physical activity for people with a chronic illness, called Sport in Times of Illness.[23] We selected this particular story because it presented an 'opportunity to learn';[24] it is not a story representative of all the stories collected, but one with specific tensions and complexities, and a story that further developed as a result of an ongoing interaction between the storyteller and the researcher(s). It is precisely the detailed interpretation of this interaction, including attentiveness towards the wider social context in which this interaction took place, that provided us with 'a concrete demonstration'[25] of opportunities for narrative development.

During the first meeting between Anja and Mirjam, the first author of this chapter, Mirjam asked Anja the 'grand tour question'[26] 'you have diabetes, can you tell me what happened?'. She introduced some follow-up topics during the course of the conversation, however, Anja was strongly encouraged to tell her own story and to take her time in doing so, and prepared not to expect many questions.[27] The session took two hours, was audio taped and transcribed ad verbum. Then Mirjam wrote down the story, mainly in the words and order of Anja, and concluded it by a first interpretation based on Frank's work and some other literature. She discussed the transcript and the account with the other researchers, Agnes and Tineke, and sent it back to Anja as a 'member check'. This was followed by a short email conversation, a second meeting a year later, and another email conversation.

To illuminate the narrative habitus, we look at different voices – informed by different intersecting social status positions – present in this process of narrative development.[28] First, there is the voice of Anja. To present this voice,

---

23 The research proposal was approved by the Medical Ethical Committee of the Free University (VU) Medical Centre. See for more information about the project: www.stzverhalen.nl.

24 Robert E. Stake, 'Qualitative Case Studies', *The SAGE Handbook of Qualitative Research*, ed. Norman K. Denzin and Yvonna S. Lincoln (Thousand Oaks: Sage Publications, 2005), 451.

25 Elliot G. Mishler, *The Discourse of Medicine: Dialectics of Medical Interviews* (Norwood, NJ: Ablex Publishing Corporation, 1984), 182.

26 James P. Spradley, *The Ethnographic Interview* (New York: Holt, Rinehart and Winston, 1979), 86.

27 Gerhard Nijhof, *Levensverhalen: Over de Methode van Autobiografisch Onderzoek in de Sociologie* [*Life Stories: On the Method of Autobiographical Research in Sociology*] (Amsterdam: Uitgeverij Boom, 2000), 86–91.

28 Actually, the voice of the editor of this volume directed us towards this focus and we noticed that it got our thinking moving in a helpful direction.

we used the account of her story and several 'narrative summaries'[29] that we wrote based on a close analysis of her words. The email conversations also provided us with fragments of her voice. Moreover, Anja was actively involved in writing this chapter, as she provided valuable feedback on several versions.[30] Second, the voice of the researchers, who, by accident, became part of this process of narrative development, is of importance. They are also the tellers of this process. Finally, the third voice in this chapter comes from the perspective of several care ethicists. We need this to place the other voices in a broader context and offer recommendations for health care.

4 A Short Introduction to the Voice of the Researchers

Although Anja is the main character in this chapter, her story, necessarily, is told through the voice of the research team. We – Mirjam, Agnes and Tineke – are three white, higher-educated women, from middle-class backgrounds, and without any chronic conditions. This voice consists of different levels which are interdependent.[31] There is 'my' voice, the voice of Mirjam (33). I graduated in medical anthropology and sociology and then started to work as a sports researcher focussing on social class differences – related to habitus – and dominant discourses concerning health, body weight and self-control.[32] With Agnes

29 Michael Murray and Anneke Sools, 'Narrative Research', *Qualitative Research in Clinical and Health Psychology*, ed. Poul Rohleder and Antonia C. Lyons (London: Palgrave Macmillan, 2015), 138–150. We did not use this storyline analysis during the member check procedure as the story we sent back to Anja was written in the third person. But we decided to use it in this chapter because it offered us a guideline to write a very dense I-person fragment that presents the core of a storyline. Following Murray and Sools (pp. 140–143), we composed these 'narrative summaries' based on a combination of content and structural analysis, following these three steps: (1) the formulation of a storyline title to capture the essence of the storyline, (2) the identification and characterization of five storyline elements, namely agent/character, acts/events, means and/or helpers, setting/scene, purpose/intention/desired or feared goal, and the breach, which refers to an imbalance between two storyline elements and makes clear how these elements are connected into a meaningful whole, and (3) the writing of a storyline summary in which the narrative causal connections between the parts are explicated.

30 This is the reason Anja is included as an author of this chapter. It emphasizes the co-construction and co-authoring of this relational narrative, a process involving several voices. These voices each made their own contribution as we carefully described in this chapter.

31 These levels are based on the work of Peter Reason and William R. Torbert, 'The Action Turn: Toward a Transformational Social Science', *Concepts and Transformations*, 6 (2001): 18–28.

32 Mirjam Stuij, 'Explaining Trends in Body Weight: Offer's Rational and Myopic Choice vs Elias' Theory of Civilizing Processes', *Social History of Medicine* 24.3 (2011): 796–812;

and Tineke, I was involved in the set-up of the research project *Sport in Times of Illness* and currently I am one of the executing researchers in this project. I practised sports – gymnastics and badminton – until ten years ago, when I decided to quit because of the strain on my hypermobile joints.

My voice is influenced by the combined voice of the research team. Agnes (47) is a critical sport scholar with a long career in competitive sports. Tineke (52) identifies herself as an engaged and interdisciplinary scholar in the fields of social sciences, humanities and medical sciences. As a research team, we discussed the transcripts of the conversations with Anja, the account of her story and this chapter several times. Our combined reflections influenced my – Mirjam's – voice during the conversations and correspondence with Anja, and while writing this chapter.

Our voice as a research team, in its turn, is influenced by the broader theoretical and empirical research framework we are familiar with: it is the literature we refer to in this chapter but it is also the literature we are influenced by, but not explicitly aware of. As Annemarie Mol states,

> there are so many [links to the literature], so many more. They are *embedded,* indeed, in the questions asked, the topics raised, the words used throughout [a] study. Is it possible to make all the partial connections between a text and its relevant others explicit? I don't think so.[33]

These links are part of our 'researcher habitus', with its specific inner libraries.

5 Anja's Voice – Mediated by the Voice of Mirjam

After reading an online call to participate in the project, Anja emailed me that she wanted to tell her story because she recently had to quit horse-riding due to physical discomfort and this decision caused her pain. At that time, she was 54 years old and diagnosed with type 2 diabetes twelve years earlier. She had lived with the same man for 25 years and had two daughters of 17 and 20 years old. They are a white, middle-class family. Anja completed her higher education and worked several years as a manager, but resigned when her second

---

Mirjam Stuij, 'Habitus and Social Class: A Case Study on Socialisation into Sports and Exercise', *Sport, Education and Society* 20:6 (2015): 780–798; Mirjam Stuij and Ruud Stokvis, 'Sport, Health and the Genesis of a Physical Activity Policy in the Netherlands', *International Journal of Sport Policy and Politics* 7.2 (2015): 217–232.

33 Annemarie Mol, *The Body Multiple: Ontology in Medical Practice* (Durham and London: Duke University Press, 2002), 16.

daughter was born, stayed at home, and started to do voluntary work a few years later.

Sitting in her backyard, she told me about her life with diabetes, her experiences with health care and the meaning of physical activity in her life. She described herself as 'always busy, I always look for something to do'. She enjoys activities 'that may not be called sport, but are active, just during the pleasure of everyday life'. This has always been part of her life; she did gymnastics in her youth, regularly went (roller-)skating since she was young, and emphasised that she had never had a sedentary job because she was always 'on the road, walking stairs at peoples homes'. Lately, along with her continuing enjoyment of roller-skating, she especially liked cycling and horse-riding with her daughters.

Her story consisted of four general storylines, namely with respect to the period of her first complaints and diagnosis, diabetes related health care experiences, current complaints relating to menopause, and her decision to quit horse-riding. These all fit under the theme 'pick up the pieces and start all over again'. She mentioned this several times. Responding to her diagnosis she said:

> At the moment you hear that you have diabetes you have tears in your eyes and think: 'It really is true'. You have this for life and you don't know where it ends. But well, then I started to collect all information available and thought: 'What next?' So, then you go for it. That is my attitude: if it doesn't work out, I go and look for what I can do. Picking up the pieces and starting all over again, literally.

This fragments shows some elements that return more often in her story. It illustrates a certain attitude that is oriented towards the future and aimed at doing something to solve a 'problem'. Furthermore, it shows her need to collect and have information to make decisions, as is also illustrated by this narrative summary:

> *So then I determined my own programme about what I wanted and how I wanted this*
> That I would have such a type of diabetes wasn't expected. I was really young, not overweight and I didn't have any other symptoms. There was little experience with this in the countryside where I lived. I got a lot of medication right away, tablets, but with this, I couldn't influence anything. I couldn't decide to go cycling very fast after dinner, because then my sugar would decrease too soon. That's why I collected information myself and told my general practitioner that I wanted to use insulin.

> They didn't think it was wise, because you can't go back, but I did do it. It has been difficult for a while, but it did give me much more freedom. So I was very happy I did it, but it was without any support. Overall, I find the support minimal, and actually, when you are young like me, it is limited and short-sighted.

This summary illustrates an important experience for Anja: the feeling that her health care practitioners didn't respond well enough to her needs. She told me that 'you needed to be lucky to have a good health care professional'. She elaborated on this a bit more and said that, after having experienced resistance several times, she didn't ask for a referral to a professional specialised in exercise this time, 'because care is always very person-dependent, so you're very dependent on your care taker'. By 'short-sighted' support, she referred to some 'strict regimes' she was told to follow by a dietician, that didn't bring her enough relief. With 'limited' support, Anja found that she experienced limited possibilities for help, especially when she didn't know what to do. This was the case at the moment she applied for participation in this research project. The essence of that moment is captured by the following narrative summary:

> *The fun has gone out of it*
> I started horse-riding when I was 46. It was a wish come true, from my childhood onwards. My children started horse-riding and they told me: "We'll give you a sample lesson for your birthday". I started and then, in fact, it started wrong right away. After an hour, I totally did not feel my lower legs anymore. They did an examination of my blood vessels, that was all fine. That's about seven years ago, it went fairly well for quite some time then. I did it with so much pleasure, we had so much fun. My daughters and I, we [rode] at a riding school, for the fun and doing something together. I also experienced that my blood sugar levels decreased because of this, that's just an extra. However, I had so much trouble with my legs during the past year, I just can't anymore. So, then the fun has gone out of it. I held on until the summer. I told myself: 'This is not going to work, you have to quit, you have to prepare yourself for this'. I truly did. I cried a lot about it, still, I really find it awful, but yes, that's how it is. It was picking up the pieces and starting all over again.

She added to this that she recently 'started over again' by doing yoga, not because she liked it – actually, she didn't – but because she hoped this would strengthen her body and make it more flexible and enable her to do more intensive activities again. Here, again, her daughters were of importance, because one of them practiced yoga already, albeit 'a very intensive' kind, that Anja felt she would 'never' be able to practice because of the troubles with her legs. Instead, she did a 'simplistic' form of yoga, together with 'people aged 70 and older'.

Some elements in the story of Anja returned in all four storylines, albeit with slightly different details and emphasises. Firstly, they all concerned living a 'good life' which, for her, was being able to be active 'in everyday life', experience pleasure, and have sufficient freedom to do what she wants. Secondly, taking responsibility for her own health, mainly by strictly controlling her blood sugar level, was an important element. This was revealed by sifting through and considering all information available, measuring her blood sugar level every morning and accurately keeping track of all measurements from the beginning, not only to set her insulin level for the day, but also in order to follow the trend. Finally, there was an element of loss that clearly emerged throughout her story. Not only because of what she told me – such as the loss of fun and doing things together, physical abilities, activities, feelings of youth – but also because she was sometimes emotional during the conversation. Together with her email, I felt a kind of urgency for Anja to tell her story. She also made an appeal to me, when I asked her at the end of the interview what she thought about it. She seemed to search for a means of making sense of the things that had happened in her life, as she said:

> I'm always curious to find out how someone else looks at it. (…) I do see that this doesn't happen as it is not how it should be in an interview like this, but I would have liked to get some reply. (…) Because you're always in your own circle and there are really few people who can offer you that reply, knowledge-wise.

I told her that I would send her an account of our conversation and that I would keep this request in mind.

6 Where Voices Meet: Polyphonic Voices

As stated before, our 'member check procedure' included a reflection from us as researchers on the individual story and this offered me the opportunity to give a reply. I found it quite difficult to write the story, so I sent an email to one of the other researchers:

> Attached you find the story of Anja (…). I would like you to read it (…) because I find it quite a 'heavy' story and reflection. (But this is probably also because of my tendency to prefer restitution terminology and, at least in part, a positive story to send back, as, in the end, I am part of society as well.) Besides this, I would like to offer her something more concrete in the reflection, because of her explicit request for help/a reply. But I don't know what, exactly. And of course, this is not the aim of the member check, but maybe you have some suggestions?

We decided to aim for recognition: maybe for Anja it was helpful to read her story herself and to see the reflection from an outsider perspective. In this reflection, which consisted of more than four sides, I mentioned the elements stated in the former section as well as:

> Anja mainly departs from the dominant storyline (…): the restitution story.[34] (…) This is dominant because it is the type of illness story most told and the one people prefer to hear. Her departure is displayed in a lot of different elements, but mainly in the strict control and regulation of her blood glucose level and by taking responsibility for this herself. She clearly strives towards restitution, for instance by starting to practice yoga in the hope that she regains control. Furthermore, her story mainly is a linear story, in which she keeps harping on 'picking up the pieces and starting all over again' after several events. Therefore, it is a future-oriented story: Anja doesn't seem to be thinking about the "what" and "when", but mainly about a solution, the "what next". However, as Frank argues, a major limitation of the restitution story is that if it doesn't work anymore, there is no other story to fall back on. This seems to be the case for Anja right now, indicated by the many aspects of loss in her story and her explicit request for help. (…)

I emailed my account to Anja and she quickly replied:

> What a story. I needed to sit down to read it. (…) My first impression is that it is useful for me. It clearly displays how you see this moment in my life. If I also see it that way, I might be able to do things differently. Make it easier for myself. (…) At that part about the restitution story and finding another form, maybe Eastern wisdom can help. I do have a passionate

34 Frank, *Wounded Storyteller.*

> yoga teacher, which is inspiring. I need to reread your piece and think about it carefully. (…) Thank you very much.

A year later, out of curiosity, I asked her how she was and whether she would like to meet again. She answered:

> I would like to meet again. (…) The last year, several "small" things have changed in my life. Even the diagnosis of my chronic illness. Funnily, the only thing left is sport. I still practice yoga.

We met again and she told me about these changes, amongst others concerning her diagnosis. Based on an article she read, she 'felt' that something was wrong and strongly insisted on a referral to the internist, who immediately changed her diagnosis into type 1 diabetes.[35] Furthermore, because of several major events concerning both herself and people close to her, she noticed that 'at the moment, physical activity and diabetes are relatively small in my life, just because the other things take up a great deal of time'. However, during this conversation she did imply a sort of change in attitude. An example is her decision to quit her voluntary work and do nothing:

> Everyone immediately asked: "What are you going to do next?" (…) And I told them: "I'm just going to do nothing, I'm just going to leave it at that". (…) That's very hard, because everyone looks at you like, that is also what you mentioned in your account, what is expected from you, that's what you're going to fulfil. (…) Of course you have the tendency to do so [but I didn't this time].

Moreover, she added that although she still did not like yoga, she experienced her yoga teacher as someone helpful:

> [She helps me] to gain insight into what particular outlook you have on life, how you handle things and how you should handle things. I cannot explain it precisely, but this made that I'm looking at things more easily now, how difficult they might be. (…) It is here and it is now, and it is not yesterday and not tomorrow. And of course, you anticipate what happens in the future, you cannot live by the day, but it is very important to look

35 This was later further specified as 'LADA', Latent Autoimmune Diabetes in Adults, a slow form of type 1 diabetes which is often mistakenly diagnosed as type 2.

> at *this* day and to keep close to yourself and not always place oneself in someone else's position. (…) That really was very helpful to me.

When we said goodbye, she mentioned that she would like to stay involved in the research project. A few months later, I wrote a conference paper about her story and our interaction and I sent it to her, being curious about what she would think of it.[36] In her reaction, she acknowledged that 'the essence of the paper was put into words very well'. And we, again, had a short email conversation in which I told her about the aim of the conference and she answered:

> [It is] nice to know what you're working on. Now, I am able to place it better. I also find it good for myself, because then I also look at myself more critical.

This reaction indicates an ongoing process of narrative development.

Over time in the course of our interaction, both of our voices became more 'polyphonic', because they became 'characterised by overlaid, interwoven and (…) contradictory'[37] voices and values, influenced by other voices.[38] To put it in black-and-white, I started as an 'observing' sociologist, interviewing people in order to analyse their story with a certain theoretical framework and making recommendations for health care. An interview setting is quite a fixed setting in which one person asks questions and another answers. This was also recognised by Anja, when she realised that asking for a reply 'is not as it should be' in such a setting. However, Anja told me a very personal story that moved me. It touched on other facets of me as a person.[39] Therefore, I felt a moral responsibility to do something with this story and give her something in reply. My voice further developed during the discussions with the other researchers, in which I became more aware of the importance of an elaboration on narrative development for the aims of the research project.

Anja, at first, presented herself as someone feeling the need to know, decide and do everything concerning her diabetes herself. Individual autonomy and

36 Mirjam Stuij, Agnes Elling and Tineke Abma, '"Starting All Over Again". Living with Diabetes and the Quest for Restitution' (paper presented at the Storytelling, Illness and Medicine 11th Global Meeting of the Health project, Budapest, Hungary, March 14–16, 2016).

37 Douglas Ezzy, 'Illness Narratives: Time, Hope and HIV', *Social Science & Medicine* 50 (2000) 613.

38 Among these other voices is the voice of the Anja's yoga teacher, a voice that I only know through Anja's telling.

39 Tineke A. Abma, 'Struggling with the Fragility of Life: A Relational-narrative Approach to Ethics in Palliative Nursing', *Nursing Ethics* 12.4 (2005): 345.

informed decision making were important to her. This was probably partly because of her experiences with health care: she didn't experience the care and expertise she felt she needed, and the regimes she was told to follow didn't fit with her notions about living a good life. But over time, when her attitude seemed to have changed, her voice also became more polyphonic; to a certain extent, she seemed to accept some uncertainty about what the future might bring.[40] Furthermore, she was aware that she needed to take care of herself as well.

7 Implications for Health Care Practices: Voices of Care Ethicists

Although both Mirjam's and Anja's voice became more polyphonic over time, for the purpose of health care practices especially, the changes in Anja's voice are of importance. Departing from dominant health discourses, which emphasize restitution and one's own responsibility, in her story, told during the first conversation, Anja repeatedly emphasised to 'start all over again'. Based on her reactions to the account of this conversation, she was not explicitly aware of this. It seemed to be a familiar storyline to fall back on, as part of her taken-for-granted narrative habitus. However, at the moment of the interview, this storyline did not seem to work for her anymore and she asked for help, even if the interview setting was not an appropriate one. In a sense, she changed the context into a therapeutic one. In this section, we draw from the voices of care ethics to understand what happened next and discuss some implications for health care.

The essence of what happened seemed to be the development of a 'relational narrative'[41] that we composed together. This type of narrative 'yields ethical knowledge that is co-authored, contingent and contextual'.[42] Firstly, the co-authoring refers to 'the joint and collaborative development of ways to handle [this particular] situation'.[43] This was started by Anja's request for a reply, which changed, to some extent, the purpose of our interaction. This co-authoring is intertwined in the extracts included above and it is explicitly visible in Anja's comment: 'that is also what you mentioned in your

40 Ezzy, 'Illness Narratives', 615; Abma, 'Struggling with Fragility', 345.

41 Sally Gadow, 'Relational Narrative: The Postmodern Turn in Nursing Ethics'. *Scholarly Inquiry for Nursing Practice* 13.1 (1999): 3–16 in Robin Lindsay and Helen Graham, 'Relational Narratives: Solving an Ethical Dilemma Concerning an Individual's Insurance Policy'. *Nursing Ethics* 7.2 (2000): 152.

42 Lindsay and Graham, 'Relational Narratives', 152.

43 Abma, 'Struggling with Fragility', 345.

account'. Secondly, contingency emphasises that a narrative can always change; it doesn't have a final answer.[44] This was shown by the ongoing interaction between us, in which we both continue to develop our voices, influenced by a broader chorus of voices. Thirdly, it was contextual as it depended on certain particularities.[45] What these particularities were is not easy to pin down precisely, however, some elements might be considered.

Most importantly, although Anja and Mirjam did not know each other before the first meeting, there was an environment in which Anja felt safe enough to tell a personal story, to be vulnerable. This might be because Mirjam travelled more than two hours to visit Anja at home and emphasised that she didn't have any other appointments to go to. In other words, she wanted to hear the story and had the time to do so. Or, because Anja knew about the topic of our research project, and she therefore knew Mirjam was interested in her story. Or, because Mirjam asked open-ended questions, didn't interrupt Anja and mainly let her decide the course of the conversation. Or, because there was an interpersonal 'fit', partly fostered by having several social characteristics in common – level of education, social class, gender, ethnic background – as a 'familiar' basis for interaction. Or, perhaps, all or some of these factors combined together.

Furthermore, some of Mirjam's personal experiences, that Anja wasn't aware of, might have influenced her interest in this particular story. Although it wasn't her first interview with someone with diabetes, it was the first 'difficult' story; a story that didn't have a foreseeably 'good end' and a narrator that was at times emotional. Moreover, Mirjam had experienced a loss related to sports herself. While it already was some years ago and she wasn't regretful about it anymore, Mirjam could recognise Anja's pain, and it was easy for her to show a genuine interest and to build a rapport with Anja.[46]

As said before, we don't know what it was exactly that created this process of narrative development. Most importantly, Mirjam was there at that moment and listened. However, as Elliot Mishler states, although listening is an important and necessary condition for care giving, it is not sufficient: 'someone [also] must be heard'.[47] Mishler stressed the importance of recognition 'of the distinctive humanity of patients and respect for the contextual groundings of their problems in their life worlds'[48] as the essential ingredient for humane

44 Ibid.

45 Ibid.

46 See also Peter Bray, 'A Shared Story of Professional Practice: Therapists Make Meaning of Spirituality', in this volume.

47 Mishler, *Discourse of Medicine*, 181. See also Miranda Quinney, Alison Ward and Jane Youell, 'Life Story Sharing: A Therapeutic Intervention in Palliative Care', in this volume.

48 Mishler, *Discourse of Medicine*, 192.

care. The feeling of recognition and being heard, probably was given to Anja by the carefully phrased outsider reflection on her story through the member check account. Here Mirjam and the other researchers acknowledged her request by being both understanding and critical towards her independent and responsible attitudes by pointing out to her that her story, sense of self and actions seemed incongruent.[49]

According to Annemarie Mol, 'good care' is about improving someone's life, however, the question of how to do this is multifaceted and complicated; it needs 'tinkering',[50] a process in which a patient and a health care professional try and explore what is suitable and what not. Part of this is a local fine-tuning of health care standards that entails an adjustment to daily life.[51] Therefore, health care professionals need to pay attention to life circumstances and their effects, but, 'these are not [always] acceptable topics in health care settings'.[52]

Joan Tronto emphasises that care should be considered as a 'relational practice',[53] which means that attention must be paid to purpose, power and particularity. The 'purpose' of care, in general terms, is related to activities that repair and maintain a good life. 'Power' refers to good care being democratic, and not protective or paternalistic; care is an activity where decision-making power should be shared. 'Particularity' means that care needs to be adjusted to the personal needs of a unique person, at a particular moment in time and place. 'Good care' requires the moral virtues of being attentive, accepting moral responsibility, actually doing the caring work and being responsive, to evaluate whether caring activities meet needs.[54] This is exactly what Mirjam did in her engagement with Anja. She was attentive to the needs of Anja, felt a responsibility, and acted and checked to see if Anja's needs were met. This enabled Anja to develop a polyphonic story and broaden her narrative habitus. Her narrative autonomy was engendered by the support she received from other people.

But, as political scientist Tronto alerts us, there is more to care than covering the intimate relations, because the institutional context in which care is provided is also of importance. It is in this context that approaches to purpose,

49 Abrams, 'Redefining Women's Agency', 459.

50 Annemarie Mol, *The Logic of Care: Health and the Problem of Patient Choice* (London and New York: Routledge, 2008), 88.

51 Ibid., 85.

52 Elliot Mishler, 'Patient Stories, Narratives of Resistance and the Ethics of Humane Care: A la recherche du temps perdu'. *Health: An Interdisciplinary Journal for the Social Study of Health, Illness and Medicine* 9.4 (2005): 438.

53 Joan Tronto, 'Creating Caring Institutions: Politics, Plurality, and Purpose'. *Ethics and Social Welfare* 4.2 (2010): 161.

54 Ibid.

power and particularity may be conflicting.[55] Tronto especially mentioned the danger of parochialism, which means that we preferably take care of those close to us.[56] In a way, this is illustrated by the story we told in this chapter, because we privileged the story of Anja, a woman with a comparable social status position, more than others.[57] But at the same time, by making this explicitly visible, we aimed to raise consciousness about these processes and underlying sociological concepts, like status positions and habitus. Ideally, in the context of health care, both the ill person and the health care professional are able to reflect on and if necessary adapt their 'narrative preferences'[58] as part of a relational process. This requires moral virtues like attentiveness, responsibility, doing care and responsiveness as well as trust and solidarity.[59]

8 Concluding Remarks

The story of Anja shows that life sometimes is much more complex than the restitution story presupposes. Although she seemed to have all of the characteristics that favour 'restitution', Anja was not able to continue horse riding, which was an important part of her 'normal life' and also a means to keep control over her blood sugar level. This elaboration of a personal story reveals the necessity of other storylines besides the restitution story, or, in the case of a chronic illness, dominant storylines emphasizing control and normality.[60] People who are unable to live this type of story need an alternative 'corpus of stories'[61] to draw on, for example storylines which more explicitly incorporate quest and/or loss. Furthermore, it shows that changing a narrative habitus requires consciousness about the storylines someone applies and a (joint) search for alternatives.

When people need to reconstruct their story because of an illness, they benefit from being part of a relational process of co-construction or 'tinkering'.[62]

55 Tronto compared this to care in the context of the family, were the purpose, lines of power and particularities are unquestioned. Ibid., 161.

56 Ibid.

57 Although we definitely will tell other stories (forthcoming).

58 Frank, *Wounded Storyteller*, 77.

59 Tronto, 'Creating Caring Institutions'.

60 Fadhila Mazanderani and Sara Paparini, 'The Stories we Tell: Qualitative Research Interviews, Talking Technologies and the 'Normalisation' of Life with HIV'. *Social Science & Medicine* 131 (2015): 66–73.

61 Frank, *Letting Stories Breathe*, 195.

62 Annemarie Mol, 'Living with Diabetes: Care Beyond Choice and Control'. *The Lancet* 337 (2009): 1757.

In the story of Anja, health care professionals were conspicuous by their absence, however, others – a researcher passing by, her yoga teacher – seemed to have offered help in this direction. Our case study illustrated how relational storytelling is important for narrative development, feelings of recognition and coping with, or managing, a chronic condition like diabetes in daily life. We argue that health care professionals can and should play a role in such relational, patient-centred processes to be able to provide better care for privileged people and even more for people belonging to underprivileged social groups.

Bibliography

Abma, Tineke A. 'Struggling with the Fragility of Life: A Relational-narrative Approach to Ethics in Palliative Nursing'. *Nursing Ethics* 12.4 (2005): 337–348.

Abrams, Kathryn. 'Redefining Women's Agency: A Response to Professor Williams'. *Indiana Law Journal* 72 (1997): 459–462.

American Diabetes Association. '2. Classification and Diagnosis of Diabetes'. *Diabetes Care* 38 Suppl. 1 (2015): S8–S16.

Bourdieu, Pierre. *The Logic of Practice.* Cambridge, MA: Polity Press, 1990.

Buitelaar, Marjo. 'De stemmen van Tahara. De Orkestratie van Verschillende Zelf-Representaties in het Levensverhaal van een Nederlandse Moslimvrouw van Marokkaanse Afkomst' [The Voices of Tahara. The Orchestration of Different Self-Representation in the Life Story of a Dutch Muslim Woman of Moroccan Background]. *Amsterdams Sociologisch Tijdschrift* 29.1 (2002): 73–98.

Bury, Michael. 'Chronic Illness as Biographical Disruption'. *Sociology of Health and Illness* 4.2 (1982): 167–182.

Cheek, Julianne. 'Healthism: A New Conservatism?'. *Qualitative Health Research* 18 (2008): 974–982.

Corbin, Juliet M. 'The Body in Health and Illness'. *Qualitative Health Research* 13.2 (2003): 256–267.

Crawford, Robert. 'Health as a Meaningful Social Practice'. *health: An Interdisciplinary Journal for the Social Study of Health, Illness and Medicine* 10.4 (2006): 401–420.

Dalstra, Jetty A.A., Anton E. Kunst, Carme Borrell, Elizabeth Breeze, Emanuelle Cambois, Guiseppe Costa, José J.M. Geurts, Eero Lahelma, Herman Van Oyen, Niels K. Rasmussen, Enrique Regidor, Teresa Spadea and Johan P. Mackenbach. 'Socioeconomic Differences in the Prevalence of Common Chronic Diseases: an Overview of Eight European Countries', *International Journal of Epidemiology* 34.2 (2005): 316–326.

Ezzy, Douglas. 'Illness Narratives: Time, Hope and HIV'. *Social Science & Medicine* 50 (2000): 605–617.

Frank, Arthur W. *The Wounded Storyteller: Body, Illness, and Ethics.* Chicago: University Press, 1995.

Frank, Arthur W. *Letting Stories Breathe: A Socio-Narratology.* Chicago: University Press, 2010.

Gadow, Sally. 'Relational Narrative: The Postmodern Turn in Nursing Ethics'. *Scholarly Inquiry for Nursing Practice* 13.1 (1999): 3–16.

Lindsay, Robin and Helen Graham. 'Relational Narratives: Solving an Ethical Dilemma Concerning an Individual's Insurance Policy'. *Nursing Ethics* 7.2 (2000): 148–157.

Mazanderani, Fadhila and Sara Paparini. 'The stories we tell: Qualitative research interviews, talking technologies and the 'normalisation' of life with HIV'. *Social Science & Medicine* 131 (2015): 66–73.

Mishler, Elliot G. *The Discourse of Medicine: Dialectics of Medical Interviews.* Norwood, NJ: Ablex Publishing Corporation, 1984.

Mishler, Elliot G. *Storylines: Craftartists' Narratives of Identity.* Cambridge, MA: Harvard University Press, 1999.

Mishler, Elliot G 'Patient Stories, Narratives of Resistance and the Ethics of Humane Care: A la recherche du temps perdu'. *health: An Interdisciplinary Journal for the Social Study of Health, Illness and Medicine* 9.4 (2005): 431–451.

Mol, Annemarie. *The Body Multiple: Ontology in Medical Practice.* Durham and London: Duke University Press, 2002.

Mol, Annemarie. *The Logic of Care: Health and the Problem of Patient Choice.* London and New York: Routledge, 2008.

Mol, Annemarie. 'Living with Diabetes: Care beyond Choice and Control'. *The Lancet* 337 (2009): 1756–1766.

Murray, Michael and Anneke Sools. 'Narrative Research'. *Qualitative Research in Clinical and Health Psychology*, edited by Poul Rohleder and Antonia C. Lyons, 133–154. London: Palgrave Macmillan, 2015.

Nijhof, Gerhard. *Levensverhalen: Over de Methode van Autobiografisch Onderzoek in de Sociologie.* [*Life Stories: On the Method of Autobiographical Research in Sociology.*] Amsterdam: Uitgeverij Boom, 2000.

Reason, Peter and William R. Torbert. 'The Action Turn: Toward a Transformational Social Science'. *Concepts and Transformations* 6 (2001): 1–37.

Reay, Diane. '"They employ cleaners to do that": Habitus in the Primary Classroom'. *British Journal of Sociology of Education* 16 (1995): 353–371.

Riessman, Catherine K. *Narrative Methods for the Human Sciences.* London: Sage, 2008.

Rutten, Guy E.H.M., Wim J.C. de Grauw, Giel Nijpels, Bas T. Houweling, Floris A. van de Laar, Henk J. Bilo, Frits Holleman and Jako Burgers. 'NHG-Standaard Diabetes mellitus type 2 (3rd edition)' [Standard of the Dutch College of General Practitioners on Diabetes mellitus type 2]. *Huisarts en Wetenschappen* 56.10 (2013): 512–525.

Smith, Brett. 'The State of the Art in Narrative Inquiry. Some Reflections'. *Narrative Inquiry* 17.2 (2007): 391–398.

Spradley, James P. *The Ethnographic Interview*. New York: Holt, Rinehart and Winston, 1979.

Stake, Robert E. 'Qualitative Case Studies'. *The SAGE Handbook of Qualitative Research*, edited by Norman K. Denzin and Yvonna S. Lincoln, 443–466. Thousand Oaks: Sage Publications, 2005.

Stuij, Mirjam. 'Explaining Trends in Body Weight: Offer's Rational and Myopic Choice vs Elias' Theory of Civilizing Processes'. *Social History of Medicine* 24.3 (2011): 796–812.

Stuij, Mirjam. 'Habitus and Social Class: A Case Study on Socialisation into Sports and Exercise'. *Sport, Education and Society* 20:6 (2015): 780–798.

Stuij, Mirjam, Agnes Elling and Tineke Abma, *Mensen met diabetes over sport, bewegen en ziekte. Resultaten kwantitatieve studie.* [*People with Diabetes about Sport, Physical Activity and Illness. Results of the Quantitative Study.*] Utrecht: Mulier Instituut, 2014.

Stuij, Mirjam, Agnes Elling and Tineke Abma. '"Starting All Over Again". Living with Diabetes and the Quest for Restitution'. Paper presented at the Storytelling, Illness and Medicine 11th Global Meeting of the Health project, Budapest, Hungary, March 14–16, 2016.

Stuij, Mirjam and Ruud Stokvis. 'Sport, Health and the Genesis of a Physical Activity Policy in the Netherlands'. *International Journal of Sport Policy and Politics* 7.2 (2015): 217–232.

Taylor, Stephanie. 'Narrative as Construction and Discursive Resource'. *Narrative – State of the Art*, edited by Michael Bamberg, 113–122. Amsterdam: John Benjamins Publishing Company, 2007.

Townsend, Anne. 'Applying Bourdieu's Theory to Accounts of Living with Multimorbidity'. *Chronic Illness* 0.0 (2011): 1–13.

Tronto, Joan. 'Creating Caring Institutions: Politics, Plurality, and Purpose'. *Ethics and Social Welfare* 4.2 (2010): 158–171.

Ujcic-Voortman, Joanne K., Miranda T. Schram, Monique A. Jacobs-van der Bruggen, Arnoud P. Verhoeff and Caroline A. Baan. 'Diabetes Prevalence and Risk Factors among Ethnic Minorities'. *European Journal of Public Health* 19.5 (2009): 511–515.

Wardle, Jane and Andrew Steptoe. 'Socioeconomic Differences in Attitudes and Beliefs about Healthy Lifestyles'. *Journal of Epidemiology & Community Health* 57.6 (2003): 440–443.

Wheatley, Elizabeth E. 'Disciplining Bodies at Risk: Cardiac Rehabilitation and the Medicalization of Fitness'. *Journal of Sport & Social Issues* 29.2 (2005): 198–221.

World Health Organisation. 'Diabetes: Fact Sheet N°312, Updated March 2013'. Viewed on 21 June 2018. https://web.archive.org/web/20130826174444/http://www.who.int/mediacentre/factsheets/fs312/en/.

PART 5

Challenges to the Institutional Illness Discourse

CHAPTER 12

Self-Reflexivity in Oral History Research: The Role of Positionality and Emotions

Verusca Calabria

Abstract

In this chapter I explore the notion of self-reflexivity in qualitative research that engages both oral history and participatory action research methodologies. I focus on the interplay between the researcher's voice and the subject of research, weaving in auto-ethnographic reflections by taking account of these processes within my own research into the oral history of the now closed psychiatric hospitals in Nottinghamshire, United Kingdom (UK). This chapter presents the value of thinking in psychoanalytic terms as a resource for interpretation of the oral history material, the implications of my social position and ideology, and moving from the position of being an outsider to an insider during the process of the research. Self-reflexivity in research enhances the analytical process and interpretation, it can become a political act, and it can bring about psychoanalytical and critical awareness that enhances the research project. I draw insights from my own research to provide a lens on how prior knowledge, experience and new forms of knowledge interact in the process of making meanings and shaping the outcome of research projects.

Key Words

Reflexivity – self – oral history – participatory action research – feminist methodology – inter-subjectivity – positionality – emotions – transference – insider – liminality – mental health – loss.

*****

 | DOI:10.1163/9789004396067_014

1 Introduction

'Every qualitative thesis has a story attached to it, an impetus for engaging in the research'.[1]

My research project aims to record the voices of mental health service users who received care in a specific geographic cluster of United Kingdom (UK) mental hospitals in the latter part of the 20th century, along with those of the staff who provided care at those same hospitals; the objective is to shed light on the impact of closing the large-scale mental hospitals and the move to care in the community on service users and staff. The methodologies I employ are oral history and participatory action research. The fieldwork focuses on what has been lost through the modernisation of mental health services, where the relationships between staff and patients are typically short-term and veer towards crisis management. The interviews center around peer-to-peer and staff-to-service user relationships and on the experiences of care provided within the hospital environment.

In the first part of this chapter I introduce how I came to research the memories of people who have been inpatients and former workers in the now closed psychiatric hospitals of Nottinghamshire, including my motivations for doing the research, my social and ideological positions, and my prior assumptions in relation to the research topic and methods. In the second part of this chapter I provide a reflexive account of the role of emotions in the oral history encounter for both the interviewer and the informant, and I consider how the psychological impact of a narrative can be utilized as an analytical tool in research. In the final part of the chapter I present the conceptual shift that I have made, moving from the position of an outsider to the position of an insider during the process of carrying out the research, by recognizing that I share some of the 'knowledge by experience'[2] with research participants who have been mental health service users. I outline the effects of participation in the research project on me, as the researcher in the context of engaging in dialogue with former patients of the psychiatric hospitals, and the impact the engagement has had on the research project. I re-evaluate my review of the narratives

1 Katherine Janzen, 'Into the Depths of Reflexivity and Back Again—When Research Mirrors Personal Experience: A Personal Journey into the Spaces of Liminality', *The Qualitative Report* 21.8 (2016): 1495.

2 Julie Repper and Rachel Perkins, *Social Inclusion and Recovery: A Model for Mental Health Practice* (Edinburgh: Baillière Tindall, 2003), 14.

of life in the mental asylum in light of the conceptual shift that has occurred during the process of the fieldwork.[3]

2 The Story behind the Story

In this section I introduce the key aspects of reflexivity in the research process, namely how my motivations, social position, assumptions, values, gender, cultural background, personal experiences, biases, and political and ideological stances affect the process of interpretation of qualitative research.[4]

When I applied for the fully funded PhD position at Nottingham Trent University in the summer of 2015, I could not have predicted the influence and the impact the research would have on me. The scope of the project – the geographic focus on mental hospitals in Nottinghamshire and the focus on staff-patient relations – were all pre-established. I sought this opportunity to critically reflect on my experience of working in the field of oral history in the medium of academic publications, while also retaining the community engagement aspects that are central to my vision of oral history. Oral history is the recording, preservation and interpretation of first-hand accounts of the past, based on the personal experiences and opinions of the speaker; it is a qualitative method of interview where the interviewer and the interviewee spend extended time together engaged in a process of storytelling and listening.[5] A major drive to conduct the research was the chance to bring about progressive change in the field of mental health provision, coupled with a desire to counteract the vilification of asylum care.

A key aspect that bears on my identity is my involvement in the oral history movement in the UK; I have been volunteering as a regional networker and trustee for the Oral History Society for the last ten years, a not-for-profit membership organisation set up by historian Paul Thompson some 40 years ago to encourage the collection and preservation of oral histories.[6] I have enjoyed a

3 Verusca Calabria, 'Insider Stories from the Asylum: Peer and Staff-Patient Relationships' in *Narrating Illness: Prospects and Constraints*, eds. Joanna Davidson and Yomna Saber (Oxford: Inter-Disciplinary Press, 2016), 3–12.

4 Mats Alvesson and Kaj Sköldberg, *Reflexive Methodology: New Vistas for Qualitative Research* (London: Sage, 2009), 321–340.

5 Sharlene Nagy Hesse-Biber and Patricia Leavy, 'Focus Group Interviews', *The Practice of Qualitative Research* (California and London: Sage, 2011), 163–192.

6 The Oral History Society, viewed 10 June 2018, http://www.ohs.org.uk.

prolific career in the field of community oral history, scoping and delivering participatory-based oral history projects for the last ten years.

My passion for oral history began in the late 1990s when I emigrated from Italy to England and undertook a degree in Historical and Cultural Studies at the University of Brighton. I felt disillusioned with the project of gaining knowledge through the regurgitation of other people's work and, to remedy this, I sought a way of creating new knowledge that challenged the traditional concepts and traditional orthodoxy of knowledge. The method of oral history appealed greatly to me, not only for its potential to democratise history – changing both the content and purpose of history-making – but also for the specificity of oral history as a window into the realm of subjectivity.[7] Oral history draws on memory and testimony to gain a more complete or different understanding of the past, experienced both individually and collectively. The method has often been linked to grassroots and progressive politics, the democratic impulse to give voice to the marginalized and the oppressed and those forgotten by traditional documentary history.[8] At that time I undertook an independent research project to record the oral histories of refugees in Britain. Subsequently I worked for a decade as a community oral historian, seeing myself as someone who helps foster memory work in communities whose stories have not yet become part of the mainstream historical record.

Reflecting on the assumptions and values I hold in relation to the study and use of oral history as a method of research, my practice as a community-based oral historian has been influenced by the main paradigms in oral history.[9] Firstly, I have been influenced by Paul Thompson's socialist approach to oral history, which gives both legitimacy and value to histories from below.[10] The impetus behind my career in oral history has come from my unflinching passion to give a voice to people who are usually excluded from public discourse, and to preserve their histories for future generations. Secondly, I have embraced the feminist methodological stance of listening 'in stereo' by learning to subjugate my own agendas to the process of listening in order to encourage narrators to speak in their own terms.[11] Feminist methodology recognises

---

7 Paul Thompson, *The Voice of the Past: Oral History* (Oxford: Oxford University Press, 2017); Alessandro Portelli, 'What Makes Oral History Different', in *Oral History, Oral Culture, and Italian Americans,* ed. L.D. Giudice (New York: Palgrave Macmillan, 2009), 21–30.

8 Ibid.

9 Alistair Thomson, 'Four Paradigm Transformations in Oral History', *The Oral History Review* 34.1 (2007): 49–70.

10 Thompson, *The Voice of the Past.*

11 See Jack, Dana C., and Kathryn Anderson. 'Learning to listen: Interview techniques and analyses', in *The Oral History Reader*, eds. Robert Perks and Alistair Thomson (Abingdon,

the political importance of oral history for women, who are often silenced in public discourse, and considers ways of addressing the power imbalance in the interview setting.[12] Feminist oral history literature calls for the interviewing and interpretative practices to encourage empathy with the interviewee in order to investigate the questions of subjectivity, memory, and emotion in the interview. It fosters a more collaborative and interactive process, which becomes key in unfolding the subjective elements that shape individuals' perceptions of the past.[13]

My research shares the same epistemological assumptions as the research into the collective narrative of depression by Hans T Sternudd, namely that meaning is socially produced and is a product of multivocality.[14] My overall research project is informed by participatory action research (PAR). PAR invites participants into all aspects of the research through the iterative cycles of planning, acting, observing and critical reflection.[15] It is an applied research that searches for practical outcomes with the aim of bringing about positive change by engaging participants to co-produce action towards change; at the heart of PAR is the commitment to challenge the traditional location of power within research.[16] It is particularly important to involve participants in the decision making process throughout each stage of the research from the beginning to the end in order to ensure power is shared as equally as possible between the researcher and the participants.[17] I established a collaborative plan of action that has been iterative and reflective to allow for modifications in the research process. The collection and analysis of data has evolved through the active participation of former staff and patients in shaping the research as much as possible through the planning, action and reflection stages. I adopted

---

Oxon: Routledge, 2016), 179–192; Luisa Passerini, *Fascism in Popular Memory: The Cultural Experience of the Turin Working Class* (Cambridge: Cambridge University Press, 1987), 1–10.

12 Susan Armitage and Sherna Berger Gluck, 'Reflections on Women's Oral History: An Exchange' *Frontiers: Journal of Women's Studies,* 19.3 (1998): 1–11.

13 Sherna Berger Gluck, and Daphne Patai, *Women's Words: The Feminist Practice of Oral History* (Abingdon, Oxon: Routledge, 2013), 35–43.

14 Hans T Sternudd, 'Voices of Depression: an Analysis of a Collective Narrative', in this volume.

15 James Ward, Di Bailey, and Sian Boyd, 'Participatory Action Research in the development and Delivery of Self-Harm Awareness Sessions in Prison: Involving Service Users in Staff Development', *Prison Service Journal,* 202 (2012): 20–25.

16 Yvonna S. Lincoln, 'Engaging Sympathies: Relationships between Action Research and Social Constructivism', in *Handbook of Action Research: Participative Inquiry and Practice,* eds. Peter Reason and Hilary Bradbury-Huang (London: Sage, 2001), 124–132.

17 Robin McTaggart et al., 'Introducing Critical Participatory Action Research', in *The Action Research Planner,* eds. Robin McTaggart, Stephen Kemmis and Rhonda Nixon (New York: Springer, 2014), 1–31.

Michael Frisch's notion of 'shared authority', which embodies the principles of PAR within the oral history interview encounter and in the interpretation and the presentation of the data.[18] The initial iterative phase of PAR took place in meetings prior to gathering participants' memories of their experiences in the hospital. These 'off the tape' encounters served to negotiate what individuals wanted to talk about; explored their motivations for taking part, and enabled them to contribute to the research question. I gathered individuals' perspectives on key themes and topics that formed their experiences in the hospital. Participants were given the option of using different methods to participate, such as one-to-one oral history interviews, group reminiscence events, or life writing. I set out to build trust, rapport and common ground in order to establish equal relationships with participants and to facilitate the co-production of research findings.[19] Moreover, preparation is key to producing rich data in any research context.[20] I consciously made an effort to spend extensive time with participants prior to recording the interviews, not only for rapport building and establishing good working relationships but also to get basic information and understand their experiences in the context of their own lives. I negotiated the themes of my interview schedule with participants, who chose to speak about whatever theme was most relevant to them. I shared transcripts and audio recordings of the interviews with participants in regular individual and/or group events, including my findings, and gathered feedback. Participants' perspectives that emerged as a result of 'shared authority' will inform the interpretation and final writing of my thesis. Most of the participants opted for a one-to-one oral history interview. Some participants chose to recite poetry and songs inspired by their time at the hospital; some wrote their life stories.

Another story I seldom told before I started this research project is that I have first-hand experience of mental illness in my immediate family, which has a direct bearing on the topic of my research. Following the birth of my younger brother, my mother suffered from post-natal psychosis that became chronic, largely I believe through the lack of support and understanding at the time of her breakdown. However, when I began my research into the memories of people who received and provided care in the Nottinghamshire psychiatric

---

18 Michael Frisch, *A Shared Authority: Essays on the Craft and Meaning of Oral and Public History* (Albany: State University of New York, 1990).

19 Mary, Brydon-Miller, 'Education, Research, and Action Theory and Methods of Participatory', in *From Subjects to Subjectivities: A Handbook of Interpretive and Participatory Methods,* eds. Deborah L. Tolman and Mary Brydon-Miller (New York: New York University Press, 2001), 76–89.

20 Lee Ann Fujii, *Interviewing in Social Science Research: A Relational Approach.* (Abingdon, Oxon: Routledge, 2017), 12–24.

hospitals, I saw myself as an outsider; I have no personal experience of being a mental health service user and have never worked in the field of mental health in the UK.

In terms of my ideological position and how it bears on researching the lives of mental health service users and staff and the value of relationships in mental health service provision, I have been a social justice activist for some years supporting local and national campaigns. I have also been a carer and an advocate for my mother by helping to amplify her voice in relation to the care she has been receiving from the mental health services in Italy.

There are three major ways in which the researcher's positionality may affect the research: firstly, by helping to gain access to participants, as they may be more willing to share their life experience with someone who is sympathetic towards their life circumstances; secondly, the nature of the research and the researched is affected by the researcher's position; thirdly, the researcher's worldview and background shapes the lens of the research.[21] I believe my identity as a community-based oral historian has enabled me to gain a certain degree of credibility with both mental health service users and staff who had been either receiving or giving care in local mental hospitals. The main motivation for participants to take part has been a strong desire to preserve the legacy of the local mental hospitals for future generations. Before starting the fieldwork I set up a partnership with the local archive so that I could give participants the option to deposit their oral history interviews. To date, all participants have opted in. I found that most of the mental health service users who were interested in the research asked about whether I have experience of the mental health services. Talking about my experiences of my mother's mental illness has helped to build trust and common ground with research participants, a crucial aspect of the oral history encounter.[22]

I address the aspect of how the nature of the research itself and the person who is the subject of the research is affected by the researcher's position and the researcher's worldview and background, including my own biases, in part three of this chapter.

I now turn to the importance of identifying the emotional states of both parties in an oral history interview and detecting its effects on the narration, which are often rendered invisible. Emotions are usually left out of the

21 Roni Berger, 'Now I See it, Now I Don't: Researcher's Position and Reflexivity in Qualitative Research', *Qualitative Research* 15.2 (2015): 220.

22 Valerie Yow, *Recording Oral History: A Guide for the Humanities and Social Sciences* (Lanham, Maryland: Rowman and Littlefield, 2014), 96 101.

interview when it is turned into a transcript, with the exception of optional notes that may be added by the interviewer.

3 The Role of Emotions in the Oral History Encounter

In this section, I reflect on the role of emotions as an interpretative tool; that is, how the unconscious processes that play out in an oral history interview and its interpretation can be recognised, examined and evaluated. I will examine the role of unconscious emotions in the interpretation of one of the in-depth interviews I conducted as part of my research into the legacy of the psychiatric hospitals in Nottinghamshire, UK.

The paradigm shift towards reflexivity in the social sciences has been prompted in part by feminist methodology. It acknowledges that the knowledge produced in an interview is always situational, the product of the interaction between two people.[23] However, Michael Roper and others have pointed out that reflexivity in interviewing tends to focus on 'too-conscious' notions of the self, with the subjectivities at play in the encounter being seen as the product of the social structures and the agenda of the interviewer. The role of unconscious emotions, 'elements of desire, memory and primitive conflicts, the realm of the psyche, seem curiously absent'.[24] The oral history interview must be viewed not only as a relationship between the subjectivities of both the interviewer and the narrator; the encounter is also informed by unconscious dynamics. Roper offers useful insights into taking into account the role of psychodynamics in the interview encounter – not only to help interviewers deal with difficult situations during the interview, but also to enhance the process of interpretation.[25]

Quoting Karl Figlio, Roper explains how transference is always present during the process of an interview, the unconscious material from past relationships that both parties bring to the encounter, which in turn affects the level of empathy that is reached between interviewer and narrator.[26] A strong analogy exists between the role of the analyst and that of the oral historian. Oral history interviewing encourages the participants to actively develop their

---

23 Rosanna Hertz, 'Reflexivity and Voice', in *Feminist Methodology: Challenges and Choices*, eds. Caroline Ramazanoglu, and Janet Holland (London: Sage, 1997), 1–17.

24 Michael Roper, 'Analysing the Analysed: Transference and Counter-transference in the Oral History Encounter', *The Journal of the Oral History Society* 31.2 (2003): 12.

25 Ibid., 20–32.

26 Karl Figlio, 'Oral History and the Unconscious', *History Workshop Journal*, 26.1 (1988): 120–132.

narration in whatever way they like; as oral historians, 'we encourage people to allow us to feel, with them, something of what they have been through'.[27] Aspects of this emotional context are inevitably brought to life in the interview process, since narrators have a tendency to respond in ways that approximate relationships with significant people in their lives. This is where transference occurs – as interviewers, we need to deal with the counter-transference, 'a triggering of anxieties and conflicts from our own pasts, brought alive by the material of the interview'.[28] In other words, by asking our informants to recall their past, we must be prepared to hold any difficult emotions. I recognised the possibility of participants experiencing psychological and emotional distress as recounting past events can bring up painful emotions.[29] I addressed this potential risk by informing participants that they would be provided with information about support offered by appropriate organisations, however the situation did not arise.

I have often witnessed narrators revealing far more than they had anticipated in an oral history interview, and remembering aspects of their experiences they had forgotten, a rather similar process to that of free association in a therapeutic setting. Conducting an oral history interview is a balancing act of holding on to the process of active listening and being present to the needs of the interviewee – all the while also keeping track of what is being said and formulating the follow-up questions to ask as part of the researcher's agenda. As oral history interviewers we must be prepared to subjugate our own agendas to the process of listening, to balance the unequal power we hold in the encounter and to encourage new areas of inquiry and new understandings to emerge.[30] Roper suggests examining 'moments of difficulty, when the counter-transference makes itself felt', through an analysis of how interviewees make us feel, focusing on what happens in the encounter by capturing the non-verbal behaviour of an interview, what he calls our sense of 'the mood' of the interview.[31]

Taking Roper's account of the psychodynamics at play in interviewing, I critically evaluated the role of unconscious emotions in the first oral history interview I conducted as part of my research with a former patient of a psychiatric

27 Michael Roper, 'Analysing the Analysed': 22.

28 Ibid.

29 Valerie Yow, 'Ethics and Interpersonal Relationships in Oral History Research', *The Oral History Review* 22.1 (1995): 51–66.

30 Dana C. Jack, and Kathryn Anderson, *Learning to Listen: Interview Techniques and Analyses* (New York: Routledge, 1992), 180.

31 Michael Roper, 'Analysing the Analysed': 22.

hospital in Mapperley, Nottinghamshire.[32] Kay is an active member of a local community centre that is currently run by mental health service users; she has been actively involved in the promotion of service user involvement in mental health research and services design. I met Kay fairly frequently as a result of her involvement with the centre where I conducted most of the oral history interviews with service users who received in-patient care in the Nottinghamshire mental hospitals before their closure. During one of my early visits to the centre, I organised one-to-one meetings with four service users, including Kay, to discuss the purpose and uses of the research and to build trust, rapport and common ground with potential participants. Before I left the centre on that occasion, I found them all sitting together, spontaneously reminiscing about their time in the psychiatric hospital. They said to me that it felt good to remember and that most of them did not get the opportunity to talk about their time in the psychiatric hospital with their families, who tend to find it painful to look back at that time of their lives. The oral history interviews I have conducted tend to be in-depth accounts of their life stories, often recorded over an average of two to three sittings. Kay helped by introducing me to other service users who had received care in the local psychiatric hospitals; I felt that the connection I had built with Kay coupled with her understanding and support for my research made her an ideal candidate for my first interview.

I interviewed Kay in her home over the course of a day. Before I started the recording, I explained to Kay about the areas of inquiry I planned to ask her about with the proviso that she should choose where to start with the story of her life and that I would guide her through the process by asking open-ended questions and following up on 'clues' in relation to her experiences of mental illness and the mental health services in the UK. The total length of the recording was three and a half hours. The duration and frequency of the interviews were negotiated with each participant; the interview was informed by a life history approach to explore how participants give meanings to their lives and how meaning is interpreted in narrative forms.[33] I adopted a life history approach in order to enable participants to reflect on their own lives over time and to make comparisons between their time at the hospital and their experiences of care in the community. The approach has produced fairly lengthy interviews. I created three tracks during the course of the interview that I have fully transcribed into a 35-page verbatim transcript. During the course of the

32 For the purpose of this paper, I have changed the names of the participants and the name of places to ensure I respect the confidentiality of all research participants.

33 Kenneth Plummer, *Documents of Life 2: an Introduction to a Critical Humanism*, (London: Sage, 2001), 27.

lengthy interview I asked Kay only a handful of questions, and Kay spoke eloquently in great detail about her life experiences. The interview was emotionally intense. She spoke candidly about her experiences of abject depression and suicide attempts throughout her life. In her own words: 'I had a very unsettled early life… I was alienated from my family for most of my adult life due to my mental health condition'.[34] Kay wove her life story from memories of school and the first incident of thinking she was 'different', to her first attempt to commit suicide as a young adult, her experiences of moving abroad, and of returning to England, including experiencing a major breakdown that led to the loss of her business, home and all of her possessions. I found her life story highly emotive and felt a high degree of empathy when Kay recounted her troubled teenage years, the difficult relationship with her family and the lack of support she endured throughout her life.

I came to realise that I experienced counter-transference during the course of the interview after I left her home and began to jot down my reflections in my fieldnote diary. The content of Kay's narrative had triggered painful emotions about my past. I was able to identify the exact moment the unconscious emotions were triggered while preparing the verbatim transcript. Towards the end of the first interview track, Kay began to recount her attempt to commit suicide while visiting her sister in Nottingham, which led to her hospitalisation at Mapperley psychiatric hospital. Kay gave a highly descriptive account of the event. When recounting her exchanges with mental health staff, she put particular emphasis on the way in which staff at the hospital had not taken her seriously because of the unusual behaviour she was displaying:

> I was quite high, as the tablets were being metabolised in my body, so I was laughing all the time, I remember, so it was very strange because the psychiatrists were saying: "Oh you just tried to kill yourself and you are laughing"; and people misunderstand and misinterpret things like that. They think "That was stupid, that was just a cry for help, but does she think she was joking?"; and they get very angry about those things, but I believe it was just the metabolites, the drugs in my body that were doing it to me.[35]

At this point in the interview, I found myself being transported back to the memory of my mother's distinctive laughter during her breakdown. Through the process of listening back to the audio recording, I realised that from that

34 Verusca Calabria, verbatim transcript, (unpublished, 2016), 1.
35 Ibid., 10.

point on in the interview I had subconsciously been piecing together what might have happened to my mother during the worst moments of her illness. Looking back, in that moment Kay had become my mother, I was reliving some of the grief from the loss I experienced from my past when my mother became severely ill. As a child, I had not been able to properly grieve about my mother's breakdown as I was denied access to my mother's own narrative of events until my mid-twenties.

I met Kay a few weeks later for a debriefing on the interview and asked about how she felt about the interview after reading the transcript. Kay had found reading back the transcript painful, but she was pleased to have provided a record of her life experiences for research purposes in the hope that it may bring about change in mental health policy. More recently, at a mental health recovery event, Kay has made use of this interview material to talk about what Mapperley hospital had provided for her as a place of safety during her mental health crisis.

Consequently, as oral historians, we may be witnessing not only our informants' unresolved grief but also the triggering of our own unresolved emotions about past events, which may affect our responses. Barbara Erskine has reflected on the meaning of grief and loss in her work on collecting oral histories of people who have experienced the Second World War. During an oral history interview with a former war pilot, the interviewee became emotional when recounting the loss of his friends. Erskine found herself reliving the grief of losing her own father when she was a child, which she had not processed.[36] Like Erskine, I found myself experiencing the grief of losing my mother to severe mental illness; I also experienced the cathartic effects of bringing to light repressed emotions, which has helped me to heal. Through the active dialogue with service users about the effects of mental illness on their lives, during the interviews and in the debriefing sessions, I have found a voice from my own experiences. As I have progressed into the fieldwork, the inevitability of dealing with painful emotions and the past resurfacing has become apparent. When I hear the life stories of mental health service users that are too often punctuated by grief and loss, I have been acutely reminded of the suffering my mother experienced, not only as a result of her illness but also due to the devastating effects of the stigma she experienced that led to the loss of her status in the community. The act of sharing my personal story with the research stakeholders has helped me heal; the articulation of my own story has helped me to reclaim a certain degree of empathy for myself. The healing effect of storytelling

36 Barbara Erskine, 'Loss and Grief in Oral History', *Oral History Association of Australia Journal* 18 (1996): 1.

within doctor-patient relationships as a form of narrative medicine is examined in Victorria Simpson-Gervin's study.[37]

I now move my focus onto the conceptual shift I have experienced as researcher moving from the position of an outsider to the position of an insider during the course of the fieldwork, and onto the effect this has had on the research data and its interpretation.

4 From Outsider to Insider: Liminal Spaces

Dealing with difficult emotions that arose in my fieldwork has forced me to re-examine my position not only as a researcher and a person interested in improving care for individuals with long-term mental ill health, and to take into account the things I had not seen or heard previously. In this section of the paper I explore the challenges and opportunities offered by the transition from the position of outsider to that of an insider during the course of the research project, including the liminal spaces researchers can occupy when engaging in research into sensitive topics.

Roni Berger experienced moving from being an outsider to an insider during the process of her research studying the struggles faced by couples that remarried to create stepfamilies.[38] She was forced to re-evaluate some biases and commonly held assumptions that influenced her research in the light of her new experience of remarrying someone who already had a child from a previous marriage. Her way of understanding marriage and parenting changed to include her experience of becoming a stepmother. She was able to critically evaluate the experiences of her participants in light of her new awareness that tension and strife are not the only dominant characteristics in relationships between stepparents and stepchildren; her perspectives included new dimensions of these roles and relationships. This conceptual shift brought her to re-analyse her interviews and to arrive at a more nuanced understanding of what these new relationships provide in the context of the formation of new stepfamilies.[39] Berger argues that researchers ought to lay bare the intimate involvement of the role of personhood in both process and product of the research enterprise. Quoting Horsburgh, researchers must 'evaluate the extent to which an author identifies and explicates their involvement and its potential

37 Victorria Simpson-Gervin, 'Narrative Medicine and Storytelling: An Alternative Method for Healing,' in this volume.

38 Roni Berger, 'Now I See it, Now I Don't,' 220.

39 Ibid., 226.

or actual effect upon the findings'.[40] In doing so, the researcher can enhance the quality of the research by considering the ways in which the nature of who they are and what they bring to the encounter can both assist and hinder the process of the co-construction of meanings.

Berger asks us to critically evaluate how 'different perspectives that we bring as researchers hold possibilities for seeing some meanings embedded in the data and for obscuring such meanings'.[41] In this light, I will here re-examine the literature review of the counter-narratives of life in the asylum that I presented in my earlier conference paper to take into account my shifting sense of self.[42] The awareness that most published stories of life in the mental hospital focus on abuse and resistance led me on a search to unravel the tensions and contradictions in the narratives of care in the psychiatric hospitals in Britain.[43] I wanted to explore the apparent contradiction of mental hospitals as institutional settings within which some aspects of care could be beneficial for patients' recovery; I found that Goffman's concept of 'total institution' was inadequate to describe what most people felt about living and working in psychiatric hospitals from the middle of the 20th century onwards.[44] For some in the UK, psychiatric hospitals were a place of belonging, where a sense of community and kinship operated amongst staff and patients, and where having access to a place of safety, a sanctuary in time of severe mental distress, was of paramount importance.

Like Berger, the recognition that I share some common experiences with my research participants has led me to face up to my own blind spots, and to become familiar with my own biases. In my literature review I presented instances of patients and staff liking some aspects of life in the psychiatric hospitals; I consciously left out an analysis of the motif of nostalgia, commonly found in narratives of lost communities.[45] The specificity of oral history rests on memory, viewed as an active process of creation of meanings. Alessandro Portelli suggests that the constructed nature of meaning is to be understood both in

40 Dorothy Horsburgh, 'Evaluation of Qualitative Research', *Journal of Clinical Nursing* 12 (2003): 307–312.

41 Berger, 'Now I See it, Now I Don't', 222.

42 Calabria, 'Insider Stories from the Asylum'.

43 Sheena Rolph and Jan Walmsley, 'Oral History and New Orthodoxies: Narrative Accounts in the History of Learning Disabilities', *Oral History* 34.1 (2006): 42.

44 Erving Goffman, *Asylums: Essays on the Social Situation of Mental Patients and other Inmates* (New York: Anchor Books, 1961), 18–22.

45 Mike Savage, 'History, Belonging, Communities', *International Journal of Social Research Methodology* 11.2 (2008): 151–162.

terms of the interplay between public, and the private spheres and the form and content of those that the life narratives can reveal.[46] As recent scholarship claims, narratives steeped in nostalgia must be understood in the context of conflicting moral claims to place and belonging. A good example is Mike Savage's notion of nostalgia as a key narrative tool for defining a sense of belonging by local rootedness through kinship connections or long residence.[47] I felt uncomfortable about invoking nostalgia, for fear of delegitimising the testimonies of service users and staff. However, I have come to recognise the value of thinking about nostalgia as a way of making sense of the importance that psychiatric hospitals held for some service users and staff. Stefan Ramsden has argued that narratives of community decline can serve as a means of registering and understanding dramatic change, helping to preserve a sense of place at a time when collective memories are threatened by the destruction and remaking of urban environments.[48] In the context of the history of psychiatric hospitals in the UK, almost all of the old county asylums have either been razed to the ground or turned into luxury flats, thus materially effacing the memories of place held by those who lived and worked in them. I have come to the conclusion that the presence of nostalgia in asylum narratives may serve as a testament to former residents' sense of place and their need to belong. These memories may act to simultaneously preserve a hidden and forgotten past for those who considered the institution their homes and to create an alternative site of memory to validate alternative, and often contradictory, meanings of the hospital; on the one hand the hospital was seen as governed by totalizing institutional practices designed to induce passivity and loss of autonomy on the patients,[49] on the other a place of safety and refuge where many former patients expressed a sense of receiving good care. These new meanings may challenge the official history, and those negative myths that surround the dominant narrative of psychiatric hospitals as total institutions.

I now turn to examine the implications of moving from the position of outsider to insider during the course of the research project, by making reference to the liminal space, a state of in-betweenness that a researcher may occupy

---

46 Alessandro Portelli, *The Battle of Giulia: Oral History and the Art of Dialogue* (Madison: University of Wisconsin Press, 1997).

47 Mike Savage, *History, Belonging, Communities*, 151–162.

48 Stefan Ramsden, 'The Community Spirit was a Wonderful Thing: On Nostalgia and the Politics of Belonging', *Oral History* 44.1 (2016): 89–97.

49 Erving Goffman, *Asylums: Essays on the Social Situation of Mental Patients and other Inmates, 10–15.*

when engaging in sensitive topic research. Katherine Janzen has written about reflexivity on the part of the researcher when the research mirrors the personal experiences of the researcher. Drawing from her research with mothers who experienced the loss of custody of their children, Janzen discusses the dilemmas that come about in working with sensitive topics in research. She is particularly interested in the emotional responses that can arise in both the researcher and/or the participants when engaging in research with groups of people considered vulnerable, such as people experiencing mental, or physical, health issues.[50] The end result of engaging in research in the field of sensitive topics may generate researcher distress as a consequence of being exposed to the suffering experienced by research participants.[51] Janzen considers the place of liminality that researchers can enter when engaged in sensitive topic research. Quoting Beech, Janzen sees liminality as 'a state of in-betweenness and ambiguity', a significant disruption in a person's sense of self within the social structure.[52] Janzen experienced liminality during the process of the research in the form of fear and anxiety emerging from her experience of losing custody of her own children.

I found Janzen's notion of liminality and her frank exposition of her own doubt and painful emotions useful in clarifying my own sense of shifting self in the context of this research. Through the process of listening to the life stories of people who have received or given care in psychiatric hospitals, my own repressed memories of the social stigma I was exposed to as the child of a woman with mental health problems began to emerge. My mother has been a service user of the mental health services in Italy for the past 25 years. I find myself in a temporary liminal space, occupying a third position in the research. I am no longer an outsider by virtue of the knowledge by experience that I possess – I feel closer to being an insider.

My shifting sense of positionality has certain implications for my research. First, sharing similar experiences with research participants has diminished the distance between the research participants and myself. It has paved the way for me to open up in a way I had not anticipated; I had been struggling to find a way to write myself back into my research writing; I felt anxious about

50 Janzen, 'Into the Depths of Reflexivity and Back Again', 1496–1497.

51 Jacqueline L. Crowther and Mari Lloyd-Williams, 'Researching Sensitive and Emotive Topics: the Participants' Voice', *Research Ethics* 8.4 (2012): 200–211; Lesa L. Woodby, Beverly Rosa Williams, Angelina R. Wittich, and Kathryn L. Burgio, 'Expanding the Notion of Researcher Distress: The Cumulative Effects of Coding', *Qualitative Health Research* (2011): 1–9.

52 Nic Beech, 'Liminality and the Practices of Identity Reconstruction', *Human Relations* (2010): 285.

disclosing deeply personal experiences concerning not only myself but also my mother in my academic writing. My mother has agreed that I can discuss her history and I have translated the parts used in this paper and read them back to her to ensure she is in agreement. In retrospect I see that this struggle was caused by the fear of revisiting difficult emotions and the lack of clarity about the value of writing myself back in. I now see that writing myself back into the research project has given me the ability to gain in-depth knowledge and perspectives that I would otherwise not have had access to. Secondly, because of the rediscovery of the part of myself that experienced stigma due to my mother's mental illness, I find myself experiencing doubt regarding my newly found position. I wonder whether, by entering the realm of the 'other', I could be silenced as a result of speaking up about my experiences, or whether my newly discovered position of being a researcher with knowledge by experience becomes a conscious political act. I developed a intense feeling of solidarity with participants who not only have to the difficult task of managing long term mental health problems in their every day lives but also the social exclusion they face due to their diagnosis, issues that mirror my mother's experiences. Being mindful of the influence of my positionality on the research process and being forthright in communicating it to participants is an ethical imperative. Writing myself into the research by positioning myself intentionally and transparently has now become central to my research efforts. Incorporating my own reflexive practice in the write up demonstrates that what we bring to the research encounter can be used to help give voice not only to those typically silenced within research but to recover my own. As Margaretta Jolly has asserted, the practice of speaking personally, academically 'can be a way to get the particular to speak to the general and just as crucially the general to speak back'.[53] In this sense, autobiographical writing has helped restore my own agency in the process of re-inserting myself back into the research writing.

Second, becoming aware of my closeness to the subject of the research has thrown up some questions about how I go about representing research participants' experiences of loss, stigma, discrimination and the instances of institutional control while honouring their appreciation for the valuable aspects of life in psychiatric hospitals, such as the quality and availability of care, the calm and safe environment and access to social networks within the hospital. I have been asking myself what kind of responsibility I hold by having the position of authority as researcher. I have embraced collaboration as a key aspect of the research. However as researcher there are certain constraints I face in the context of participatory action research. I illustrate some of these constraints

53 Margaretta Jolly, 'Speaking Personally, Academically', *Feminist Theory* 6.2 (2005): 216.

through a request to co-present at an academic conference I received from one of my research participants, who has a lived experience of mental illness. Stan is an artist, and he wanted to express his memories of his time as a psychiatric hospital in-patient by performing poetry. I welcomed his request and felt pleased that he took an active interest in the research. However, I did not hear back from conference organisers for some time and Stan and I decided it was no longer viable to co-present. Stan asked me to let him know the reasons for the silence when I could. I started to feel what Cassell and Symon refer to as the 'disruption, the doubting, unsettling element of reflexive research'.[54] I began to share his anxieties, fearing the consequences of the rejection; I considered that it may have had to do with the stigma associated with mental patients, triggering my own memories of the societal attitudes towards my mother. I felt that perhaps I had been naïve and had not been prepared for a rejection. I eventually understood the significance – Stan had likely experienced the rejection to attend the conference as form of social exclusion commonly experienced by people with long-term mental health problems.

The scenario presented above highlights the tensions at play within oral history and participatory action research. My overall aim is to give a voice and share my authority as researcher with participants through collaborative approaches, however I still remain an academic researcher with a need to exercise a certain level of detachment and objectivity within the context of collaboration with participants. This tension problematises the notion of seeing myself as an insider; I am no longer an outsider by virtue of the knowledge by experience that I possess, so the distance between participants and myself has been reduced. However, I have not directly experienced the often devastating consequences of mental illness or the kinds of exclusions and social discrimination that people with a psychiatric label have often had to face. It brings to light the realisation that I occupy a third position in the research, a liminal space of in-betweenness – but that I have the privilege of entering and leaving this third space at my own choosing. As a result, I now see myself as insider with outsider agency.

As a result of my involvement with research participants, with whom I share some common experiences, I have experienced a shift in my political consciousness with reference to my own knowledge and by the experiences that I bring to this research project. I recognised the impact of the stigma I experienced as a child as a result of my mother's mental health diagnosis in

54 Catherine Cassell and Gillian Symon. 2004. *Essential Guide to Qualitative Methods in Organizational Research* (London: Sage, 2004), 75.

suppressing my own understanding of social exclusion experienced by people with mental ill health. I have had to readjust my view of mental health stigma and discrimination and I feel I am better equipped to represent the marginalisation that people with the lived experience of mental health problems face – experiences that are too often muted in the public discourse.

The research has unexpectedly given me a voice to talk about the experiences of mental health in my family in the context of oral history and participatory action research, therefore sharing my own interpretative authority with participants. Not only have my basic assumptions and values been challenged, but I have been forced to confront my pre-existing value judgments, my own kind of resistance – and to examine the impact of the privileged position I occupy as researcher when engaging in sensitive topic fieldwork. Through the process of self-reflexivity, I have found a greater awareness and capacity to include the multitude and contradictory stances within the research.

5 Conclusion

The multiple forms of reflexivity discussed here acknowledge the need for researchers working with research participants in the oral history encounter and participatory action research to be open to the notion of self-scrutiny with the aid of both the conscious and unconscious dynamics that are at play in their fieldwork. Researchers ought to allow for the process of change and to adapt to multiple levels of reflexivity in the process of scrutinising the connections between the self in relation to the object of the research, the methodology and the inter-subjectivities at play. I found the use of a fieldnote journal a useful reflexive tool to capture the difficult emotions that arise in my research. Moreover, I found a way of making sense of my thoughts and feelings in dialogue with participants through regular debriefs. The research data may trigger memories from our own lived experiences that can become tools to unravel the rich and complex web of meanings, which in turn can bring about new understandings and allow us to get closer to the experiences of those we research. Recognising the stages of the grieving process both on the part of the interviewer and the interviewee by recalling loss will not only sharpen our practice as oral historians and help to heal our own internal wounds, but in doing so enable us to get closer to the experiences and needs of our informants. Thinking reflexively about the voice of the researcher within qualitative research offers an additional interpretative lens to research practice by engaging with the notion of liminality. Reflexivity can enhance research rigor by monitoring the tension between involvement and detachment of the researcher.

The continuous process of reflexivity can help to go beyond questioning the truth of others and our own; it is not just a tool but also a moral and ethical project. It has forced me to re-evaluate my own past, and has brought about new kinds of conversations and ways of interpreting the research at hand; in so doing it has given me the opportunity to not only to reclaim some agency but also the possibility of personal healing.

Bibliography

Armitage, Susan, and Sherna Berger Gluck. 'Reflections on Women's Oral History: An Exchange'. *Frontiers: Journal of Women's Studies* 19.3 (1998): 1–11.

Beech, Nic. 'Liminality and the Practices of Identity Reconstruction'. *Human Relations* (2011). Viewed 16 June 2018. http://hum.sagepub.com/content/64/2/285.full.pdf+html.

Berger, Roni. 'Now I see it, Now I don't: Researcher's Position and Reflexivity in Qualitative Research'. *Qualitative Research* 15.2 (2013): 219–234.

Berger Gluck, Sherna and Daphne Patai. *Women's Words: the Feminist Practice of Oral History*. Abingdon, Oxon: Routledge, 2013.

Brydon-Miller, Mary. 'Education, Research, and Action Theory and Methods of Participatory'. *From Subjects to Subjectivities: A Handbook of Interpretive and Participatory Methods*, edited by Deborah L. Tolman & Mary Brydon-Miller. New York: New York University Press, 2001, 76–89.

Calabria, Verusca. 'Insider Stories from the Asylum: Peer and Staff-Patient Relationships'. *Narrating Illness: Prospects and Constraints,* edited by Joanna Davidson and Yomna Saber. Oxford: Inter-Disciplinary Press, 2016, 3–12.

Cassel, Catherine, and Gillian Symon. *Essential Guide to Qualitative Methods in Organisational Research*. London: Sage, 2004.

Crowther, Jacqueline L., and Mari. Lloyd-Williams. 'Researching Sensitive and Emotive Topics: The Participants Voice'. *Research Ethics* 8.4 (2012): 200–211.

Erskine, Barbara. 'Loss and Grief in Oral History'. *Oral History Association of Australia Journal* 18.1 (1996): 1–6.

Figlio, Karl. 'Oral History and the Unconscious'. *History Workshop Journal* 26.1 (1988): 120–132.

Frisch, Michael. *A Shared Authority: Essays on the Craft and Meaning of Oral and Public History*. Albany: State University of New York, 1990.

Fujii, Lee Ann. *Interviewing in Social Science Research: A Relational Approach*. Abingdon, Oxon: Routledge, 2017.

Goffman, Erving. *Asylums: Essays on the Social Situation of Mental Patients and other Inmates*. New York: Anchor Books, 1961.

Hamilton, Carrie. 'On Being a 'Good' Interviewer: Empathy, Ethics and the Politics of Oral History'. *Oral History* (2008): 35–43.

Hesse-Biber, Sharlene Nagy and Leavy Patricia. 'Focus Group Interviews'. *The Practice of Qualitative Research.* London: Sage, 2011.

Hertz, Rosanna. *Reflexivity and Voice*. London: Sage, 1997.

Horsburgh, Dorothy. 'Evaluation of Qualitative Research'. *Journal of Clinical Nursing* 12. 2 (2003): 307–312.

Janzen, Katherine. 'Into the Depths of Reflexivity and Back Again—When Research Mirrors Personal Experience: A Personal Journey into the Spaces of Liminality'. *The Qualitative Report* 21.8 (2016): 1495–1512.

Jolly, Margaretta. 'Speaking Personally, Academically'. *Feminist Theory* 6.2 (2005): 213–220.

Lincoln, Yvonna S. 'Engaging Sympathies: Relationships between Action Research and Social Constructivism'. *Handbook of Action Research: Participative Inquiry and Practice*, edited by Peter Reason and Hilary Bradbury-Huang. London: Sage, 2001, 124–132.

McTaggart, Robin, Kemmis Stephen and Nixon Rhonda. 'Introducing Critical Participatory Action Research'. *The Action Research Planner*, edited by Robin McTaggart, Stephen Kemmis and Rhonda Nixon, 1–31. New York: Springer, 2014.

Plummer, Kenneth. *Documents of Life 2: An Invitation to a Critical Humanism*. London: Sage, 2001.

Portelli, Alessandro. 'What Makes Oral History Different?' *Oral History, Oral Culture, and Italian Americans*, edited by L.D. Giudice. New York: Palgrave Macmillan, 2009, 21–30.

Portelli, Alessandro. *The Battle of Valle Giulia: Oral History and the Art of Dialogue*. Madison: University of Wisconsin Press, 1997.

Ramazanoglu, Caroline, and Janet Holland. *Feminist Methodology: Challenges and Choices*. London: Sage, 2002.

Ramsden, Stefan. "The Community Spirit was a Wonderful Thing': on Nostalgia and the Politics of Belonging'. *Oral History* 44.1 (2016): 89–97.

Repper, Julie, and Rachel Perkins. *Social Inclusion and Recovery: A Model for Mental Health Practice*. Edinburgh: Baillière Tindall, 2003.

Ritchie, Donald A. *The Oxford Handbook of Oral History*. Oxford: Oxford University Press, 2011.

Roper, Michael. 'Analysing the Analysed: Transference and Counter-Transference in the Oral History Encounter'. *The Journal of the Oral History Society* 31.2 (2003): 20–32.

Savage, Mike. 'Histories, Belongings, Communities'. *International Journal of Social Research Methodology* 11.2 (2008): 151–162.

Taylor, Barbara. *The Last Asylum: A Memoir of Madness in Our Times*. Chicago: University of Chicago Press, 2015.

Thompson, Paul. *Voice of the Past: Oral History*. Oxford: Oxford University Press, 2000.

Thomson, Alistair. 'Four Paradigm Transformations in Oral History'. *Oral History Review* 34.1 (2007): 49–70.

Ward, James, Di Bailey, and Sian Boyd. 'Participatory Action Research in the Development and Delivery of Self-Harm Awareness Sessions in Prison: Involving Service Users in Staff Development'. *Prison Service Journal* 202 (2012): 20–26.

Woodby, Lesa L., Beverly Rosa Williams, Angelina R. Wittich, and Kathryn L. Burgio. Expanding the Notion of Researcher Distress: The Cumulative Effects of Coding'. *Qualitative Health Research* (2011): 1–9.

Yow, Valerie. 'Ethics and Interpersonal Relationships in Oral History Research'. *The Oral History Review,* 22.1 (1995): 51–66.

Yow, Valerie. *Recording Oral History: A Guide for the Humanities and Social Sciences.* Lanham, Maryland: Rowman and Littlefield, 2014.

CHAPTER 13

The Voiceless and the Vocal: Infection Literature and *The Sign of the Four*

Justyna Jajszczok

Abstract

The final decades of the nineteenth century and the beginning of the twentieth century are remarkable in that they witnessed an unprecedented interconnectedness of literature, natural sciences and medicine. Between the 1870s and the 1910s the literary phenomenon of so-called invasion literature occurred. Regarded today as an inferior genre and an expression of political propaganda, its themes included two kinds of invasions: from without, i.e. by military attacks by enemy states, or from within, in the process of reverse colonisation in which the conquered nations of the Empire rebelled against the Crown. The same decades also saw the rise of tropical medicine, which focused on identification and the elimination of the causes of exotic diseases. The heyday of invasion literature and tropical medicine coincided not only with British imperial expansionism but also with significant advances in biomedicine. The years between 1875 and 1910 are considered the golden age of microbiology during which the majority of disease-causing agents, such as bacteria, viruses and parasites, were discovered. The predominant aim of this chapter is to show how these three sources of influence – invasion literature, bacteriology and tropical medicine – inspired the emergence of the time-specific literary genre: infection literature. Different from invasion literature, which is predominantly informed by military propaganda, infection literature relies mostly on medical and scientific rhetoric, and combines the science-derived ideas of virulence and immunology with the literature-inspired themes of invasion and the exotic Other. Secondly, this chapter includes an analysis of Arthur Conan Doyle's novel *The Sign of the Four*[1] which is identified as an example of infection literature. Particular attention is paid to the issues of voice; namely, which of the characters interpreted here as pathogenic are vocal and able to tell their stories directly and which are kept in silence – and for what reasons.

1 Arthur Conan Doyle, *A Study in Scarlet* and *The Sign of the Four* (Ware: Wordsworth, 2004).

 | DOI:10.1163/9789004396067_015

Key Words

Bacteriology – infection – infection literature – invasion – invasion literature – Sherlock Holmes – tropical medicine – the vocal – the voiceless

*****

1 Introduction

In September 2016, many people – myself included – were introduced to the tragic story of Helen Titchener, a woman who was charged with attempted murder of her husband, Rob. After years of enduring emotional and physical abuse, Helen had decided to leave her husband. However, when she finally confronted him, a fight ensued, and Helen stabbed Rob, apparently in self-defence. The following trial and verdict were heavily publicised with many articles dissecting the causes and consequences of this case, or concerning the broader issue of domestic violence were published. A number of British celebrities posted photos of themselves drinking cups of 'solidari-tea' to support Helen and other victims of domestic abuse, while the hashtag #FreeHelen was trending on Twitter.[2] For a brief moment in time, it seemed that almost everyone was rooting for Helen.

Except, of course, that Helen Titchener is a fictional character from the long-running BBC Radio 4 soap *The Archers*.[3] Nonetheless, the impact her storyline had not just on regular listeners of the show but on English language media consumers in general was immense, to such an extent that journalists Paul Kerley and Claire Bates tentatively referred to it as 'the Rob and Helen effect'.[4] The Helen Titchener Rescue Fund was set-up by one of the listeners affected by the storyline, and its rationale was expressed in one simple sentence: 'We're raising money for Refuge because for every fictional Helen, there are

2 Haroon Siddique and Kevin Rawlinson, 'The Archers: Call to Help Domestic Abuse Victims as Titchener Trial Starts', *The Guardian*, 4 September 2016, viewed 16 June 2018, https://www.theguardian.com/tv-and-radio/2016/sep/04/the-archers-call-to-help-domestic-abuse-victims-as-titchener-trial-starts.

3 In fact, *The Archers* has been the longest running radio soap in the world, with more than 18,000 episodes released since 1950. 'The Archers', *BBC Radio Four*, viewed 16 June 2018, http://www.bbc.co.uk/programmes/articles/5xGwGj4NgfGRJ1B2mFqg6QM/frequently-asked-questions.

4 Paul Kerley and Claire Bates, 'The Archers: What Effect Has the Rob and Helen Story Had?', *BBC News Magazine*, 5 April 2016, viewed 16 June 2018, http://www.bbc.com/news/magazine-35961057.

real ones'.[5] As of June 2018, the fund has raised over £170,000. In a sense, Helen went beyond the limitations of her fictional character and became the voice of the hitherto voiceless: the unrepresented or misrepresented survivors of domestic abuse, victims of controlling or coercive behaviour of their partners. This case also proved an interesting social commentary: among countless examples of actual survivors telling their stories, it was the voice of the fictional Helen that was heard and then amplified to reach as many people as possible. As journalist Yvonne Roberts observes, '[f]ar more powerfully than polemics and statistics, fictional characters in popular culture can open the mind and surprisingly speedily'.[6] Helen and Rob may be fictional characters but their storyline resonated with people affected by these issues in real life.

Fictional stories that deeply affect audience, perhaps contrary to popular belief, are not a new phenomenon. When Arthur Conan Doyle introduced Sherlock Holmes to the world, he could not have anticipated the impact the great detective would have on his readers. However, quite soon he realised that his creation surpassed its fictional status. This is what he wrote in his autobiography:

> That Sherlock Holmes was anything but mythical to many is shown by the fact that I have had many letters addressed to him with requests that I forward them. Watson has also had a number of letters in which he has been asked for the address or for the autograph of his more brilliant confrère. A press-cutting agency wrote to Watson asking whether Holmes would not wish to subscribe. When Holmes retired several elderly ladies were ready to keep house for him and one sought to ingratiate herself by assuring me that she knew all about bee-keeping and could "segregate the queen". I had considerable offers also for Holmes if he would examine and solve various family mysteries.[7]

After Doyle, fed up with what he regarded 'a lower stratum of literary achievement',[8] had Sherlock Holmes fall to his death in 'The Final Problem',[9]

5 Paul Trueman, 'The Helen Titchener (nee Archer) Rescue Fund', *JustGiving*, viewed 16 June 2018, https://www.justgiving.com/fundraising/helentitchener.

6 Yvonne Roberts, 'The Real-World Bonus of The Archers Abuse Drama', *The Guardian*, 4 September 2016, viewed 16 June 2018, https://www.theguardian.com/commentisfree/2016/sep/03/archers-shines-light-on-rarely-discussed-issues-domestic-abuse.

7 Arthur Conan Doyle, *Memories and Adventures* (Ware: Wordsworth, 2007), 84.

8 Ibid.

9 Arthur Conan Doyle, 'The Final Problem', in: *The Adventures and Memoirs of Sherlock Holmes* (Ware: Wordsworth, 1996).

he received many unpleasant letters from his readers outraged by what they considered a blatant murder of their favourite detective. He recalls how one lady addressed a letter to him with 'You Brute', on which he remarked: 'I expect she spoke for others beside herself'.[10] The public was disappointed and upset with such a development and continued to pressure Doyle into resurrecting the detective, which he eventually did,[11] first in *The Hound of the Baskervilles*[12] and then in 'The Adventure of the Empty House'.[13]

The stories of Helen Titchener and Sherlock Holmes share a number of similarities: they show the extent to which the attachment of the fan base can grow; they introduce their audience to new subjects and new angles from which common stories can be read. They also suggest the existence of a certain level of overlap between fiction and real life, caused either by the audience's wilful suspension of disbelief in the fictional, or their downright inability to tell the truth and fiction apart. As a result, stories such as these have the power to influence and shape public opinion on the issues they present. The case of Helen Titchener demonstrates that this power can be employed to support a great cause. But it can also be used to propagate stereotypes and misconceptions, and to assert, rather than to challenge, the *status quo*. In addition, the perceived overlap between fiction and real life can ultimately undermine the most basic assumption of creative texts of culture: fiction – precisely because it is not real – is governed by rules which are inapplicable to real situations. Stendhal famously said of the novel that it is a mirror which is carried along a main road,[14] noting its ability to reflect life as it appears. Yet, a mirror reflecting the world is limited by its frame; it reflects only what is present directly in front of it – or, what the person holding the mirror wants to be reflected. Stendhal's analogy thus accounts for the possibility of manipulation inscribed within the properties of fiction. Once any text becomes the voice or the expression of something particular, it reflects a certain fragment of reality, omitting or excluding other, perhaps equally or more important than the ones given prominence to.

Infection literature is a prime example of such a manipulation in which political and medical stereotypes are accentuated while other possible points of

---

10 Doyle, *Memories and Adventures*, 84.

11 Richard Lancelyn Green, Introduction to *The Return of Sherlock Holmes* by Arthur Conan Doyle (Oxford: Oxford University Press, 1994), xii.

12 Arthur Conan Doyle, *The Hound of the Baskervilles* (London: Penguin Books, 2009).

13 Arthur Conan Doyle, *The Return of Sherlock Holmes* (Oxford: Oxford University Press, 1994).

14 Stendhal, *The Red and the Black: A Chronicle of the Nineteenth Century*, trans. Catherine Slater (Oxford: Oxford University Press, 1998), 371.

view are either ridiculed and undermined or omitted altogether. In this respect, Arthur Conan Doyle's novel *The Sign of the Four* can be read as a narrative of infection which employs imperial propaganda to support the power structure existing during the time of its publication. To this end, the present chapter is divided into two parts of unequal emphasis: the first one briefly explains the concept and origin of infection literature, and the reasons why I choose to read *The Sign of the Four* as an example of this genre. The second, larger part focuses on a particular reading of this novel, in which the issue of voice is being examined on two planes: the voices of the medical propaganda of the time, that is Sherlock Holmes's, Dr Watson's – but also Conan Doyle's – and these particular characters which I read as 'pathogenic', who are either vocal, and able to narrate their stories, or who remain voiceless.

2 Infection Literature

The forty years between the 1870s and the beginning of the First World War witnessed a number of developments in three distinct fields: bacteriology, tropical medicine and literature. At the time when European colonial expansion reached its peak, specialists in biomedicine discovered many disease-causing pathogens, from *Tubercle bacillus* to malarial *Plasmodium*. These discoveries directly influenced the newly established science of tropical medicine which combined imperialist prejudices with bacteriological and parasitological methodology. Within the same time-frame, a politically-inspired genre of popular literature emerged, i.e. invasion literature. Distinct as all these fields were, they appear closely connected through their emphasis on a number of similar social and political issues. For instance, the purpose of invasion literature, as defined by literary critic A. Michael Matin,[15] was to shake the reading public – and, by extension, the entire nation – into alertness and vigilance, and prepare them for the inevitable attack, either by foreign military forces or by revengeful colonised peoples. To this end the British were portrayed in those narratives as inert and apathetic when faced with impending invasion, a reaction as inadequate as it was despicable. The clear message of invasion literature was not

15 Matin defines invasion literature as 'pre-Great War invasion narrative, a once immensely popular although now little studied Tory-Conservative genre whose chief polemical aim was to stimulate public and Parliamentary support for increased military expenditure by depicting French, Russian, and German attempts on Great Britain and on the territories of the British Empire'. A. Michael Matin, '"We Aren't German Slaves Here, Thank God": Conrad's Transposed Nationalism and British Literature of Espionage and Invasion', *Journal of Modern Literature*, 21.2 (1997–98): 252.

only that such passivity was unpatriotic but also that it actually encouraged the invasion, which would be then perceived as justified punishment for an obstinate disregard of the obvious risks. Yet, at the same time, the invasions predicted and depicted by this genre had a particular side-effect: as Matin notes, such 'acts of aggression ... paradoxically "vaccinate[d]" Britain by stimulating its resistances'.[16] The concept of an immune response after exposure to some attack is obviously borrowed from bacteriology while the identification of the aggressor as foreign and exotic comes directly from tropical medicine.

Furthermore, the issue which sat comfortably in the centre of the triple Venn diagram of invasion literature, bacteriology and tropical medicine, was that of personal responsibility. Robert Koch[17] and other scientists proved conclusively that infections, both domestic and exotic, are not diseases of 'social misery'[18] or barbarity but are caused by germs: tangible infectious agents such as viruses, bacteria and parasites. Still, their discoveries – although widely accepted by medical authorities – barely dented the overwhelming popular conviction that diseases were punishments for negligence or some kinds of transgressive behaviours. Lack of hygiene, improperly ventilated dwellings, overindulgence of any kind, engaging in risky or immoral behaviours, broadly defined savagery – all of these were considered preventable causes of disease, which in effect put the entire blame for the infection on the sick. While on the one hand, such beliefs made the condemnation of certain groups of society easier, they also allowed for creating a very distinct line dividing 'us' – the civilised, the clean, and the healthy – from 'them' – the savage, the filthy, and the sick. In line with such views, those unlucky enough to be placed on the wrong side of this line of demarcation were believed to be easily recognised and branded as the infected – and dealt with accordingly. Bacteriology identified the Other as domestic: those who are socially and financially underprivileged and misrepresented, those in urgent need of moral education, and, finally, those possessing redeemable potential if only they would accept the lessons given by their betters. On the other end of the spectrum of the infected are the colonised nations. Geographically and ethnically distant from the heart of the Empire, they present a different problem: the threat of spreading their infection. Therefore, even if efforts at civilising them are taken up, the most important objective of the medical authorities and their supporters is to isolate and control them and keep them from crossing, or even blurring, the borders between 'us' and 'them'.

16 Matin, '"We Aren't German Slaves Here, Thank God"', 260.

17 Steve M. Blevins and Michael S. Bronze, 'Robert Koch and the "Golden Age" of Microbiology', *International Journal of Infectious Diseases* 14 (2010): 750.

18 Robert Koch, 'The Aetiology of Tuberculosis', np, viewed 16 June 2018, http://www.academia.dk/MedHist/Biblioteket/koch_Aetiology-of-Tuberculosis_1882.php.

Within this context I place infection literature: a sub-genre of invasion literature which as its invading agents, instead of foreign attackers, employs pathogens, combining imperial propaganda with scientific notions of virulence and immunity. Through its combination of notions borrowed from bacteriology, tropical medicine and invasion narratives, infection literature is characterised by a number of essential elements. Since it is indebted to medical science, it utilises the idea that invasion is not necessarily correlated with the number of the invaders. Here, the invasion is characterised by its quality, not quantity: a single invading agent is able to wreak havoc tantamount to an epidemic precisely because they possess the quality borrowed from bacteriology, which is virulence. Moreover, because they are transmitted in a fashion reminiscent of pathogens, these invaders usually rely on carriers or vectors to travel to their destination. Those carriers tend to be presented either as hapless victims of circumstances, which force them to facilitate the travels of their unwelcome guests, or unscrupulous smugglers intentionally putting the Empire at risk. Finally, a medical authority or a scientist must be a prominent character in the narrative of infection. In Doyle's detective fiction, these roles are fulfilled by both Sherlock Holmes and Dr Watson. While the latter is explicitly characterised as a man of medicine and war veteran, Holmes's professional background is less evident; we know, however, that he possesses profound knowledge of chemistry and practical knowledge of anatomy and botany.[19] Yet the way in which he is presented brings to mind a medical professional. Holmes styles himself as a consulting detective but his clients very much resemble those of Watson's: they come with particular problems, expect diagnosis and solutions – which Sherlock, the chemist of London, is most of the time able to offer.

More crucially, because Sherlock Holmes and Dr Watson fulfil the functions of medical authorities in infection literature, their views on what is to be considered pathological are influenced by the state of the medical knowledge of the late nineteenth century. Thus, the stories of infection in the Holmes canon are consistent with Doyle's assumptions regarding the causes of diseases. It is also worth noting that Doyle himself can also be located in the centre of the bacteriology-tropical medicine-invasion literature Venn diagram. He studied medicine during the golden age of microbiology and was an avid admirer of Robert Koch's bacteriological work.[20] He was also a sturdy imperialist.

19 Doyle, *The Sign of the Four*, 13.

20 Laura Otis, *Membranes: Metaphors of Invasion in Nineteenth-Century Literature, Science, and Politics* (Baltimore and London: The Johns Hopkins University Press, 2000), 110.

As Laura Otis notes, 'believing that the Boer War "was a righteous war and well worth sacrifices", he attempted to enlist'.[21] Although Doyle was rejected on the grounds of age – he was over forty at the time – he still went to South Africa in the capacity of a doctor. But, Otis remarks, '[t]he chief enemy Doyle faced in South Africa was not the irate Dutch farmers but local disease'.[22] In this way he experienced first-hand the challenges and risks faced by tropical physicians, and these experiences to a certain extent shaped his later works, such as a Holmes story 'The Dying Detective'[23] published over a decade after Doyle's return from Africa.

It is of course an act of intentional fallacy to assume that a work of literature is to be reduced to the expression of views, opinions and experiences of its author. Still, when it comes to fiction writing, the authors' background is their most convenient repository of inspiration. The storyteller weaves such stories which speak his or her truth, but they are credible only if they ring true to the readers, too. Drawing on their personal lives is perhaps the most natural way of fiction writers to ensure that their stories are believable.

The Sherlock Holmes stories are texts of culture open to any kind of interpretation, even such without regard for Doyle's biography. Nonetheless, because I read Doyle's work as representative of infection literature – which is in itself a reductive classification – within this framework of interpretation, the state of medical knowledge, political affiliations and literary preferences of the author and the public of the late Victorian period must be taken into consideration. The following sections present my interpretation of Doyle's novel *The Sign of the Four* which identifies the staple elements of infection literature such as the pathogenic characters, the carrier, the medical authority and the ideological biases expressed explicitly or only suggested by the narrative.

3 The Voiceless and the Rewarded

To fit the definition of an invading force in infection literature, the characters presented as infective agents must be easily identifiable. Laura Otis points out that in this respect one of the identifying markers is the size, in either a literal or figurative sense.[24] In my reading of Arthur Conan Doyle's *The Sign of the*

21 Otis, *Membranes*, 92.

22 Ibid.

23 Arthur Conan Doyle, 'The Adventure of the Dying Detective', in: *His Last Bow: Some Reminiscences of Sherlock Holmes* (London: Collins Classics, 2016).

24 Otis, *Membranes*, 96.

Four there are three characters which I interpret as 'pathogenic': the escaped convict Jonathan Small, who fulfils the function of the carrier; the poisoned-dart shooting cannibal Tonga, who may be read as the embodiment of an exotic, virulent germ; and, the collective character of the Baker Street irregulars – Holmes's unofficial force. All of them, through either physical appearance or nominal identification, have some connection with 'smallness'.

Composing his novel, Doyle employed a technique which I would call distorted mirroring: many characters in the story have their narrative twins; these, however, are not their exact reflections but rather their distorted, exaggerated versions. Those characters who are supposed to be identified as 'us' or non-Other, are presented in a conventional way. However, those who are embodying the vices against which Doyle warns his audience are distorted to the point of ridicule. For instance, the novel opens with a scene in which Sherlock Holmes injects himself with a solution of cocaine; the drug-taking is repeated, or reflected, later, when the reader is introduced to Thaddeus Sholto: an obvious addict constantly 'hooked on the hookah'.[25] But while Holmes is almost robotic in his precision and moderation, the fidgety Sholto puffs with abandon, presenting a laughable yet sad picture of uncontrollable drug dependence.

The example which combines mirroring technique with the themes of invasion and the dreadfulness of the urban Other is the scene of the visit of Holmes's 'unofficial force' at 221B Baker Street:

> As he spoke, there came a swift pattering of naked feet upon the stairs, a clatter of high voices, and in rushed a dozen dirty and ragged little street-Arabs. There was some show of discipline among them, despite their tumultuous entry, for they instantly drew up in line and stood facing us with expectant faces. One of their number, taller and older than the others, stood forward with an air of lounging superiority which was very funny in such a disreputable little scarecrow.
>
> "Got your message, sir", said he, "and brought 'em on sharp. Three bob and a tanner for tickets".
>
> "Here you are", said Holmes, producing some silver. "In future they can report to you, Wiggins, and you to me. I cannot have the house invaded in this way".
>
> …
>
> "Yes, guv'nor", said Wiggins.[26]

25 Joseph McLaughlin, *Writing the Urban Jungle: Reading Empire in London from Doyle to Eliot* (Charlottesville and London: University Press of Virginia, 2000), 59.

26 Doyle, *The Sign of the Four*, 161.

At first this dirty dozen may be read as a distorted reflection of official force; with some show of discipline undermined by the disreputable appearance of the 'Baker Street irregulars'. It is interesting to note that even in their nickname, their incongruity is emphasised. They are 'irregular' in the military sense, but they are also 'contrary to rules and customs', irregular at Baker Street because their right place is outside of proper or fashionable districts of the city; they are at home in the slums. The fact that they dare cross the border between the streets to where they belong and the civilised world of the city centre is tantamount to invasion, as Holmes points out. But the street-Arabs present a home invasion on a low, controllable scale much less dangerous than that presented by the unexplored threats of the exotic East. Once we learn of the villains of the story, we realise the perverse distortion of the chronology of the storyline. It is not the street-Arabs that are a distorted reflection of the official force; it is the two villains who are the distorted reflection of the street-Arabs.

In her reading of this scene, Laura Otis remarks that

> Holmes can track down Small and his tiny cohort only because he forms his own collaboration with "small" people.... Holmes can detect and defeat the "small" because he knows them intimately and can enlist them for his own purposes. Like Small, he despises his little associates, but he respects their power to move freely because of their relative invisibility.[27]

Unlike Otis, I would not go as far as referring to Holmes's reaction to his unofficial force as tantamount to disdain. He seems more amused than condescending at their invasion, and the fact that his little associates are able to blend in the crowd and provide him with useful intelligence clearly impresses him. The street-Arabs may be semantically related to the exotic Other but they are everything but; homegrown and common, they serve to show the propagandist message supported by Doyle: that there is still hope to redeem and discipline the domestic Other in their ways, as long as it is done by the corrective hand of the authority. Their usefulness and discipline locate them above the stereotypical undeserving poor; and for exhibiting such potential for improvement they are rewarded with a power given only to the worthy: a voice. But this reward shows the insidious power play inscribed in the narrative in which the street-Arabs are conditioned and trained like pets: the voice is limited to their leader Wiggins, and to expressions of servitude. Only once both these conditions are met, are they paid for their work.

---

27 Otis, *Membranes*, 96.

The other small disreputable barefoot character, Tonga, is not given the same reward precisely because he goes against the virtues of usefulness and discipline. But, of course, he is not in the same class as the Baker Street irregulars. He is an aberration, the civilised world irregular; to give him a voice is to consider him human.[28] In infection literature, a genre governed by simplicity of its message, there is no room for such generosity. The first time the idea of a cannibal roaming the streets of London is introduced into the plot is when Holmes and Watson examine the room in which the body of Bartholomew Sholto – Thaddeus's twin brother – is found.[29] One of the traces attracts their attention:

> [Holmes] held down the lamp to the floor, and as he did so I saw for the second time that night a startled, surprised look come over his face. For myself, as I followed his gaze, my skin was cold under my clothes. The floor was covered thickly with the prints of a naked foot – clear, well defined, perfectly formed, but scarce half the size of those of an ordinary man[.]
> "Holmes", I said, in a whisper, "a child has done this horrid thing".[30]

The first expression of Holmes's shock to which Watson alludes, is the discovery of Bartholomew Sholto's body whose face is petrified into a terrifying *risus sardonicus* – a reaction to the poisonous alkaloid present in the dart stuck to the side of his head. But while it is understandable that such a sight might shake even the ever-composed Holmes, this second instance seems rather peculiar. Apparently, the idea that the crime might have been committed by a child does not fit Holmes's image of a possible perpetrator. As it is shown in the previous quote, to Holmes the patter of naked feet relates to good news on the one hand and assertion of his authority on the other. He describes the unexpected visit of the street-Arabs as an invasion, but he does it in jest, realising that it does not pose any risk either to his well-being or his power. While he

---

28 In a similar vein, Yomna Saber interprets the voicelessness of the African American protagonist Velma, from Toni Cade Bambara's *The Salt Eaters*, as relating to the loss or lack of agency. Velma, however, is not completely mute in the narrative, as her internal monologue, a crucial part of her story, is available to the reader directly. Tonga is never permitted any unmediated voice. Yomna Saber, 'Toni Cade Bambara's *The Salt Eaters*: Hearing the Silent Voice of Pain', in this volume.

29 The Sholto brothers are of course another instance of distorted mirroring: while Thaddeus is in perpetual motion, fidgeting and twitching restlessly, the dead Bartholomew is in eternal peace.

30 Doyle, *The Sign of the Four*, 141.

is not naive enough not to realise that his unofficial force might employ illegal means to find their way around the metropolis, he does not assume anything more serious than trespassing or petty theft. However, if one of those was to kill an English gentleman with a foreign dart, it would have gone against not just his expectations but the general notion that the urban poor possess the potential to be improved and their wayward ways corrected. The ideological composition of the novel allows for another solution, one that introduces the foreign element, conventionally associated with the dangerous and the illicit, and one that saves the naivety of the social improvement project.

Thus, almost immediately Holmes's apprehension disappears, replaced by his trademark cold logic: '"I was staggered for a moment", he said, "but the thing is quite natural. My memory failed me, or I should have been able to foretell it"'.[31] Since the elements of the puzzle do not seem to fit, he disregards them and turns his attention elsewhere: '"Diminutive footmarks, toes never fettered by boots, naked feet, stone-headed wooden mace, great agility, small poisoned darts. What do you make of all this?" "A savage!"'[32] Although the street-Arabs are introduced as a mock version of the official force, they in fact serve as a counterbalance to the distorted vision of a child, the cannibal Tonga. However, the line that divides the homegrown children from the exotic pseudo child is very thin: physically they are interchangeable, with their small feet and great agility. Only once the murderer is equipped with exotic attributes of poisoned darts and wooden mace, does he become the savage. In this sense, the shock that Holmes expresses at the sight of the small child-like footprints at the crime scene can be read as the shock of realisation that what distinguishes his controlled and useful unofficial force from the uncontrollable savage enemy is just the accessories, items which can switch hands with disturbing ease.

These two images of bare feet present two visions of invasion: one threatening and sinister because it is foreign and unknown and one harmless and almost playful because it is familiar and domestic. Moreover, the level of controllability presented by these two types of savages is diametrically different. Tonga is utterly out of and beyond control, his native instincts break out unexpectedly, without any regulating agents. The Baker Street irregulars, even if they appear wild, possess inherent discipline and need for order, resembling more of a disorderly army than uncontrollable horde. It seems so because the street-Arabs, although as unwelcome in imperial London as Tonga, symbolise the pathogens living in a state of balance with their environment. Inevitably, London is 'a great cesspool into which all the loungers and idlers of the Empire

31 Ibid.

32 Doyle, *The Sign of the Four*, 162.

are irresistibly drained';[33] human scum in all forms come uninvited but they somehow do not disrupt the precious balance. The street-Arabs – whether they were assimilated a long time before or emerged as the result of this environment – have become the integral part of the cityscape to such an extent that the urban organism accepts them as parts of 'self'. The virulence of Tonga, on the other hand, lies in his multilevel strangeness: he is foreign, incongruous, dangerous, and thus he will always be recognised as such – and rejected.

The cannibal of the Andaman Islands never once utters a single word in the course of the narrative; that he can actually speak is only asserted by his companion, Jonathan Small, but we are never allowed to verify it. And while he never speaks, others speak about him, for him, and on his behalf. The multitude of voices related to Tonga: Watson's, Holmes's, Small's, police officers' and even the passage in a gazetteer related to the natives of his homeland do not create a diverse and multidimensional view of him. In fact, all of them reiterate the same message, perhaps most comprehensively expressed by the anonymous author of the entrance in the gazetteer:

> The aborigines of the Andaman Islands may perhaps claim the distinction of being the smallest race upon this earth .... The average height is rather below four feet, although many full-grown adults may be found who are very much smaller than this. They are a fierce, morose and intractable people, though capable of forming most devoted friendships when their confidence has once been gained. ... They are naturally hideous, having large, misshapen heads, small, fierce eyes and distorted features. Their feet and hands, however, are remarkably small. So intractable and fierce they are, that all the efforts of the British officials have failed to win them over in any degree. They have always been a terror to shipwrecked crews, braining the survivors with their stoneheaded clubs or shooting them with their poisoned arrows. These massacres are invariably concluded by a cannibal feast.[34]

Commenting on this particular fragment, Susan Cannon Harris notes,

> Tonga is, it should be pointed out, *Doyle's* idea of an Andaman Islander, which is wide of the mark even for a nineteenth-century British imperialist. As the tireless horde of Sherlockian scribblers are fond of pointing

33 Doyle, *A Study in Scarlet*, 4.

34 Doyle, *The Sign of the Four*, 162–163.

> out, *The Sign of Four* in general betrays what seems to be either massive ignorance of or complete disregard for accuracy as regards Indian culture.[35]

Tonga is not a reflection of a real-life representative of the Andamans, he is a reflection of a foreign danger, the more vilified and over the top, the better. The description from the gazetteer, the 'the very latest authority',[36] is of course Doyle's invention and it betrays the same ideological bias as the rest of his narratives. This makes sense within the convention of detective story as well as invasion/infection literature. Doyle himself explains the instances of crude characterisation in *The Sign of the Four* through the remark made by one of the minor characters:

> It is a romance! ... An injured lady, half a million in treasure, a black cannibal and a wooden-legged ruffian. They take the place of the conventional dragon or wicked earl.[37]

Seeking psychological depth and dimension in characters from a romance is perhaps an exercise in futility. Neither the two knights in shining armours nor the two villains are depicted with solicitous care regarding their personality and internal motivation. In classifying his work as romance, Doyle also signals that he follows the literary convention according to which the good characters are immediately recognised and are strongly contrasted with the equally identifiable evil ones. In romance, as well as in detective fiction or invasion literature, characters fulfil specific functions dictated by such conventions. Sherlock and Watson are the guardians of the Empire while Tonga and Small are the evil invaders and all they are allowed to do in the confines of these genres is to serve their ideological purposes.

4 The Vocal

It is interesting how the most problematic character of the novel is given a platform to explain and justify his actions. In my reading, Jonathan Small's account of his life serves two purposes: it gives him the opportunity to appeal to the reader, if not for forgiveness, then for understanding of his actions, but on

35 Susan Cannon Harris, 'Pathological Possibilities: Contagion and Empire in Doyle's Sherlock Holmes Stories', *Victorian Literature and Culture*, 31.2 (2003): 464.

36 Doyle, *The Sign of the Four*, 162.

37 Doyle, *The Sign of the Four*, 165.

the other hand, it emphatically demonstrates the dangers of the exotic, not only on epidemiological but also on personal level. In the character of Small Doyle shows how vital discipline and control are in the process of maintaining the proper Western backbone. The story of Small is the story of descent, from the humble but proper English beginnings to the state of utter and unredeemable depravation. The story is the more perverse because Small weaves it himself, engaging in narrative self-creation and attempting to whitewash his dark past, thus echoing the practices of proponents and apologists of the imperial project. His example is exceptional, as it combines the experiences and expectations related to the two other pathogenic characters: homegrown but spoilt by his foreign experiences, small in name and humanity, unscrupulous in smuggling a dangerous individual into his homeland, he is nonetheless capable of extracting readers' understanding, if not pity, and suggesting the possibility of redemption.

Through Jonathan Small Doyle challenges his own assumptions of who must be doomed and who can be redeemed. Tonga is undoubtedly a dangerous, undesirable introduction to the tissue of London and thus he must not just be captured, contained and kept mute, but annihilated – which is the case in the end. The Baker Street irregulars are presented positively as useful and manageable but, most importantly, as domestic, an integral part of the cityscape. Small, on the other hand, is somewhere in the middle, his status is unequivocal, his verdict suspended. Perhaps this is why he is allowed to tell his own story and thus allow the readers to decide where to place him themselves.

An impartial reading of his tale is nonetheless rather difficult. Even his proper Worcestershire beginnings show that he is not just mean by name. When he flees England at the age of eighteen, Small leaves behind more than his family of 'steady, chapel-going folk'.[38] As he explains:

> I got into a mess over a girl, and could only get out of it again by taking the Queen's shilling and joining the 3rd Buffs, which was just starting for India.[39]

Thus from the very beginning of his adult life, his fate is shadowed by the need to escape and the subsequent punishment of such choice. It starts with escaping some unspecified responsibility and ends with him being the escaped convict. He never becomes the soldier he sets out to be for a short swim in the Ganges costs him a leg, an example of cosmic karma dealt by a passing crocodile. This

---

38 Doyle, *The Sign of the Four*, 187.

39 Ibid.

incident also marks the moment in which Small becomes a lesser person; in this case – literally. After five months spent in hospital, he emerges, in his own words, 'a useless cripple',[40] with a wooden leg and no future, and his descent begins.

He survives the Indian Mutiny which breaks out when he tends a plantation in Muttra, and finds himself in the city of Agra, 'swarming with fanatics and fierce devil-worshippers of all sorts'.[41] His narrative is peppered with casual offensive remarks towards the Indians, such as this one, as he emphatically tries to distance himself from any association with them. This turns out to be impossible as his destiny is to be inextricably entwined with precisely such people – so much, in fact, that he is soon regarded one of them. In Agra, he joins a volunteer army fighting the rebels where he commands two Punjabis: Mahomet Singh and Abdullah Khan. As the convention dictates, being the fierce representatives of the dangerous Other, they almost immediately turn against their white supervisor during one of their night watches. At this point Small is given an offer he cannot refuse:

> You must either be with us now, or you must be silenced for ever. The thing is too great a one for us to hesitate. Either you are heart and soul with us on your oath on the cross of the Christians, or your body this night shall be thrown into the ditch, and we shall pass over to our brothers in the rebel army. There is no middle way. Which is it to be – death or life?[42]

The thing too great to hesitate that Khan mentions is the great Agra treasure which they intend to steal, first killing the merchant who carries it, and then split between them. Their rationale in 'inviting' Small in partaking of the spoils is that 'the Sikh knows the Englishman, and the Englishman knows the Sikh'.[43] Small identifies himself and is still identified as a Westerner at this point, but he is deficient in his physical appearance and national character to such an extent that Khan does not hesitate to draw parallels between them. And indeed, a few paragraphs later Small confirms their equalisation and his moral descent directly connected with it:

> In Worcestershire the life of a man seems a great and a sacred thing; but it is very different when there is fire and blood all round you, and you have

40 Ibid.

41 Doyle, *The Sign of the Four*, 189.

42 Doyle, *The Sign of the Four*, 190–191.

43 Doyle, *The Sign of the Four*, 191.

> been used to meeting death at every turn. Whether Achmet the merchant lived or died was a thing as light as air to me, but at the talk about the treasure my heart turned to it….[44]

Yet again, however, the universe turns against him. He is not allowed to enjoy the plunder for together with his companions he is condemned to death – although his sentence is later changed to servitude for life – for having murdered the merchant. As a prisoner, Small is transferred to Madras, and then to the Andamans, where he divides his time into planting yams, helping the surgeon stationed in the isles to dispense drugs and devising ways of possible escape, all the while the stolen treasure is safely hidden in Agra. He decides to entice two English officers – Captain Morstan and Major Sholto – with information about the treasure in exchange for facilitating his escape. This plan is ultimately unsuccessful: he is betrayed and robbed by Sholto – for nobody, not even a British major, is safe from the demoralising effect of the exotic. In the end, he escapes the Andaman Islands with the help of his new acquaintance, little Tonga, but not before showcasing the distance of his fall from Western ideals. To get to a boat prepared for him by Tonga, Small must overcome one final obstacle – the guard at the wharf. The manner in which he does it shows how close he has come to the savagery of Tonga:

> [A] queer thought came into my head, and showed me where I could lay my hand on a weapon. I sat down in the darkness and unstrapped my wooden leg. With three long hops I was on him. He put his carbine to his shoulder, but I struck him full, and knocked the whole front of his skull in.[45]

It is crucial to note how this experience completes Small's smallness: at the end of his tale he is nothing more than the cannibal with a wooden mace described by the racist gazetteer. In many respects, he is even worse than his companion. Tonga as a conventional exotic villain is given the conscience of a child or even of an animal, and is assumed to have no mental capacity to know any better. As far as infection literature goes, Tonga's function is limited to that of an infectious agent devoid of free will or voice. Small, on the other hand, is portrayed as a wilful carrier, corrupted to the core by his colonial past and unscrupulous in endangering the heart of the Empire for his personal gain. The fact that despite

44 Doyle, *The Sign of the Four*, 192.

45 Doyle, *The Sign of the Four*, 201.

his Western background and intelligence, he allowed himself to stoop so low – and as a result of such a base motive, greed – proves the extent of his corruption. Yet, because, unlike Tonga, he has the privilege of being able to state his own case, Small's narrative allows for a certain level of interpretive ambiguity. He is both his own accuser and advocate which lets the readers decide whether he possesses the potential to be redeemed or not.

5 Conclusion

As a conventional detective story of the late Victorian period, *The Sign of the Four* utilises narrative and mental shortcuts to arrive at a message that as long as the Empire is protected by its guardian, the consulting chemist Sherlock Holmes, the precious balance between 'us' and the Other will forever be kept in check. As a romance alluded to by Doyle himself, the novel becomes a tale of the good, proper Western values fighting with the evil, exotic unwelcome invaders. Finally, if read as a story of infection, *The Sign of the Four* exhibits the propagandist messages vocalised also by invasion literature, bacteriology and tropical medicine at the end of the nineteenth century: that the domestic Other can be disciplined and trained to become useful; that the foreign is the source of danger and disease which must be contained and controlled; and finally that the exotic possesses a powerful corruptive capacity which only those with the strongest of characters can resist. In all three of its generic incarnations, the novel presents the stereotypes and assumptions which reflect the political, medical and literary *status quo* of the time, giving prominence to a specific viewpoint while disregarding or excluding others. In a sense, then, infection literature is a distorting mirror of the late Victorian era world. It limits its reflection, reducing it to the unrepresentative caricature of those people and such problems that the Establishment wished to draw attention to at the time.

Bibliography

Blevins, Steve M. and Michael S. Bronze. 'Robert Koch and the "Golden Age" of Microbiology'. *International Journal of Infectious Diseases* 14 (2010): 744–751.

Doyle, Arthur Conan. *The Adventures and Memoirs of Sherlock Holmes.* Ware: Wordsworth, 1996.

Doyle, Arthur Conan. *The Hound of the Baskervilles.* London: Penguin Books, 2009.

Doyle, Arthur Conan. *Memories and Adventures.* Ware: Wordsworth, 2007.

Doyle, Arthur Conan. *A Study in Scarlet* and *The Sign of the Four*. Ware: Wordsworth, 2004.

Doyle, Arthur Conan. *The Return of Sherlock Holmes*. Oxford: Oxford University Press, 1994.

Green, Richard Lancelyn. Introduction to *The Return of Sherlock Holmes* by Arthur Conan Doyle, xi–xxxv. Oxford: Oxford University Press, 1994.

Harris, Susan Cannon. 'Pathological Possibilities: Contagion and Empire in Doyle's Sherlock Holmes Stories'. *Victorian Literature and Culture*, 31.2 (2003): 447–466.

Kerley, Paul and Claire Bates. 'The Archers: What Effect Has the Rob and Helen Story Had?'. *BBC News Magazine*. 5 April 2016. Viewed 16 June 2018. http://www.bbc.com/news/magazine-35961057.

Koch, Robert. 'The Aetiology of Tuberculosis'. Viewed 16 June 2018. http://www.academia.dk/MedHist/Biblioteket/koch_Aetiology-of-Tuberculosis_1882.php.

Matin, A. Michael. '"We Aren't German Slaves Here, Thank God": Conrad's Transposed Nationalism and British Literature of Espionage and Invasion'. *Journal of Modern Literature* 21.2 (1997–98): 251–280.

McLaughlin, Joseph. *Writing the Urban Jungle: Reading Empire in London from Doyle to Eliot*. Charlottesville and London: University Press of Virginia, 2000.

Otis, Laura. *Membranes: Metaphors of Invasion in Nineteenth-Century Literature, Science, and Politics*. Baltimore and London: The Johns Hopkins University Press, 2000.

Roberts, Yvonne. 'The Real-World Bonus of The Archers Abuse Drama'. *The Guardian*. 4 September 2016. Viewed 16 June 2018. https://www.theguardian.com/commentisfree/2016/sep/03/archers-shines-light-on-rarely-discussed-issues-domestic-abuse.

Siddique, Haroon and Kevin Rawlinson. 'The Archers: Call to Help Domestic Abuse Victims as Titchener Trial Starts'. *The Guardian*. 4 September 2016. Viewed 16 June 2018. https://www.theguardian.com/tv-and-radio/2016/sep/04/the-archers-call-to-help-domestic-abuse-victims-as-titchener-trial-starts.

Stendhal. *The Red and the Black: A Chronicle of the Nineteenth Century*. Translated by Slater, Catherine. Oxford: Oxford University Press, 1998.

Trueman, Paul. 'The Helen Titchener (nee Archer) Rescue Fund'. *JustGiving*. Viewed 16 June 2018. https://www.justgiving.com/fundraising/helentitchener.

Name Index

Subject Index